www.wadsworth.com

wadsworth.com is the World Wide Web site for Wadsworth and is your direct source to dozens of online resources.

At wadsworth.com you can find out about supplements, demonstration software, and student resources. You can also send email to many of our authors and preview new publications and exciting new technologies.

www.wadsworth.com
Changing the way the world learns®

Groups
Theory and Practice

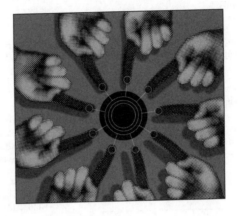

Shawn Meghan Burn

California Polytechnic State University—
San Luis Obispo

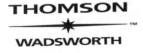
THOMSON
WADSWORTH

Australia • Canada • Mexico • Singapore • Spain
United Kingdom • United States

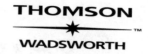

Publisher: Vicki Knight
Sponsoring Editor: Marianne Taflinger
Assistant Editor: Jennifer Wilkinson
Editorial Assistant: Nicole Root
Marketing Manager: Lori Grebe
Marketing Assistant: Laurel Anderson
Project Manager, Editorial Production: Kimberly Adams
Print/Media Buyer: Doreen Suruki
Permissions Editor: Beth Zuber

Production Service and Compositor: Carlisle
    Communications, Ltd.
Copy Editor: Margaret C. Tropp
Cover Designer: Cheryl Carrington
Cover Image: Private Collection/The Bridgeman Art
    Library. *Floating Forms* (1985) by Davidson.
Cover Printer: Webcom
Printer: Webcom

Printed in Canada
1 2 3 4 5 6 7 06 05 04 03 02

For more information about our products, contact us at:
Thomson Learning Academic Resource Center
1-800-423-0563

For permission to use material from this text, contact us by:
Phone: 1-800-730-2214   **Fax:** 1-800-730-2215
Web: http://www.thomsonrights.com

Library of Congress Control Number: 2003100506

ISBN 0-534-52671-3

Wadsworth/Thomson Learning
10 Davis Drive
Belmont, CA 94002-3098
USA

Asia
Thomson Learning
5 Shenton Way #01-01
UIC Building
Singapore 068808

Australia
Nelson Thomson Learning
102 Dodds Street
South Melbourne, Victoria 3205
Australia

Canada
Nelson Thomson Learning
1120 Birchmount Road
Toronto, Ontario M1K 5G4
Canada

Europe/Middle East/Africa
Thomson Learning
High Holborn House
50/51 Bedford Row
London WC1R 4LR
United Kingdom

Latin America
Thomson Learning
Seneca, 53
Colonia Polanco
11560 Mexico D.F.
Mexico

Spain
Paraninfo Thomson Learning
Calle/Magallanes, 25
28015 Madrid, Spain

Brief Table of Contents

Table of Contents

Preface

The study of groups has the potential to be both intellectually stimulating and immensely practical. With that in mind, I have two general goals for this text. One goal is to teach the reader about the scholarly thinking and research in the field of group dynamics. A second goal of the book is to embody group dynamicist Kurt Lewin's philosophy: "No theory without practice, no practice without theory."

The majority of the chapters focus on standard topics in group dynamics such as the functions and features of groups, group structure (norms and roles, status and power, communication), group development, leadership, conflict, group decision making, and productivity; there are also chapters on diversity and teams. In an effort to provide a thorough understanding of the discipline, classic thinking and research on these topics as well as current research and trends, are presented. The book is heavily researched and referenced. After reading the book, the reader will be familiar with basic group processes and essential concepts, theories, and theorists. This, however, is not enough to fulfill the promise of group dynamics, a promise that requires we use our scholarly knowledge to enhance group skills and effectiveness.

With this book, I hope to make good on that promise by providing a mix of theory and research and the practical group skills that logically follow from these. The basic idea is, "Here are the findings from the scholarly study of group dynamics, and here are practical uses of those ideas for improving group effectiveness." I have tried to write a book that will please those instructors with a basic approach to group dynamics and those with an applied focus, and a book that will teach and please readers regardless. Many academic programs require a group dynamics course to prepare students for careers that heavily involve group work. Many people want to better their group skills and increase group effectiveness. This book should serve such programs and individuals well. But I believe it will also serve those who remain unconvinced that the scholarly study of group dynamics should include an applied focus for the learning of group dynamics theory and that research is enhanced when it easy to apply to personal experiences and when people can see its practical use.

Key Content Features

- There is an emphasis on both classic and modern theory and research on group dynamics.

- There is an emphasis on group effectiveness. Recommendations for improving group practice and individual group skills appear after each conceptual presentation.

- There is an emphasis on diversity. In addition to a chapter on diversity in groups, topics are discussed in terms of available research on gender, ethnicity, and culture.

- The book includes many pedagogical features such as a running glossary, study questions, detailed chapter summaries, built-in opportunities to apply the information just read (the *APPLY IT!* activities sprinkled throughout the chapters), and self and group assessment instruments.

- Three student-led group activities, requiring little or no preparation on the part of the instructor, are provided at the end of each chapter (the instructor's manual provides additional instructor-led activities). Activities take a variety of forms, including case study analysis, data collection and analysis, group observations, group discussions, role plays, and simulations.

Key Pedagogical Features

- The book is written in a readable, friendly style, with lots of examples.

- Major terms appear in bold in the text and appear in a running glossary in the margins.

- Bulleted chapter summaries match chapter headings and are divided into separate concept and skills summaries.

- Study questions are provided at the end of chapters.

- The *APPLY IT!* feature reinforces chapter concepts by inviting readers to apply what they have just read to their current or past group experiences. These activities may also be used as essay assignments or for group discussions.

Book Overview

Chapter 1, An Introduction to Group Dynamics, introduces the reader to the field of group dynamics with an emphasis on the characteristics and functions of groups and a brief history of the field. Concepts central to the book appear in this first chapter. These include groups as sources of identity (social identity theory), group structure, the importance of group goals, the social comparative function of groups, and the tension between task and socioemotional goals.

Group dynamics is based on research; **Chapter 2, Research Methods in Group Dynamics,** emphasizes how research on groups is conducted. The major features of the experimental method, meta-analysis, correlational methods, observational methods, surveys and questionnaires, and case studies are all discussed. Internal, external, and construct validity are covered, and ethical considerations in the conduct of group dynamics research are explained.

Group member behavior is strongly influenced by the group's norms and by the member's position or role in the group. **Chapter 3, Norms and Roles in Groups,** explains the importance to groups of norms and roles and how they can be used to promote group effectiveness. This chapter discusses why groups develop norms and roles and why group members conform to them. Culture, gender, and conformity are also discussed. The chapter distinguishes between norms and conformity that contribute to group productivity and member development, and those that are counterproductive to the group and its members. The potential benefits of dissent and how members can change a group's norms or challenge a group majority are explored. Common types of group roles are identified. The importance of clarity regarding norms and roles, especially in regard to the socialization of new members and dealing with problem group members, is emphasized.

Chapter 4, Status and Power Dynamics in Groups, examines groups through the group structure lens of status and power. Of special concern in this chapter are how groups assign status to their members, how group members gain power, how status and power differences affect group functioning, and the effects of status differences on relations between groups. Status hierarchies and their development in groups are major topics. Readers learn how status is earned in groups and how it is often assigned based on status markers and on specific and diffuse status characteristics. The relationship between gender, ethnicity, and status in small groups is discussed. The effect of status differences on group members and their relationships is emphasized. Power is another important topic in this chapter, and coverage is given to the bases of power, the relationship between status and power, influence tactics, and culture, gender, and power. Recommendations for the appropriate assignment of status and the use of power are provided.

A defining feature of groups is that members of groups interact; **Chapter 5, Communication in Groups,** considers the topic of group communication. Topics in this chapter include verbal and nonverbal communication, the importance of congruent messages, cross-cultural communication, gossip and rumor, and electronic communication. After reading the chapter, students will recognize the role of communication structure in promoting group effectiveness. They will also know how to promote a supportive rather than defensive group communication climate. They will understand how to increase verbal and nonverbal effectiveness and how to stand up for themselves in a group without hurting other members. They will have learned about intercultural communication and the challenges of communicating with group members from other cultures and how this may be done more effectively.

Chapter 6, Group Development, is about group development and cohesiveness. The chapter reviews standard sequential stage theories of group development, such as the Tuckman model and Wheelan's integrative model, as well as newer models specific to particular types of groups (such as the Worchel and Gersick models). Group development in therapy groups and models of dyadic group development are included. Suggestions for facilitating group development and cohesiveness are provided throughout the chapter. Group socialization and how groups are affected by membership change are also examined in this chapter.

Scholars of group dynamics agree that conflict has the potential to be constructive or destructive to a group; this is the main theme of **Chapter 7, Understanding and Managing Conflict.** The difference between destructive conflict (conflict spiraling, perceptual distortion, and a competitive goal structure) and constructive conflict (a cooperative goal structure and constructive controversy) are emphasized. Common features of conflict resolution strategies and how to implement them are presented, and negotiation and mediation are discussed. The chapter also reviews individual, cultural, and gender differences in conflict resolution styles. Distinctions are made among interpersonal, intragroup, and intergroup conflict, and the dynamics and resolution of each type of conflict are discussed.

Not all groups are comprised of similar members; **Chapter 8, Member Diversity and Group Dynamics,** considers the important topic of diversity in groups. The similarity attraction paradigm and the social categorization approach are used to explain our discomfort with diversity. The value-in-diversity hypothesis is used to emphasize the potential advantages of member heterogeneity, such as enhanced problem solving and creativity. The intercultural approach to member diversity is also covered in this chapter, including additive multiculturalism and multicultural group skills. Throughout the chapter, guidelines are provided to overcome common group process challenges in heterogeneous groups so as to maximize their potential.

Kurt Lewin once said that "most groups fail to function with the fullest possible efficiency, all will agree. What the major causes of inefficiency are and what can be done to remedy them, however, are not so simply recognized" (Lewin, 1947, p. 14). This is the topic of **Chapter 9, Group Productivity.** Readers first learn that actual productivity is frequently lower than potential productivity because of motivational and coordination losses. The chapter emphasizes the role of group goal setting in preventing motivational losses and how to reduce social loafing according to the collective effort model. Gender, culture, and social loafing are also discussed. Readers learn about tacit and explicit coordination in groups and how group coordination can be improved to reduce coordination losses. A final topic of the chapter concerns group meetings and how to make them productive.

Chapter 10, Leadership, examines traditional and contemporary trait, behavioral, and contingency theories of leadership and the recommendations that follow from each for improving leadership practice. Leadership, gender, and culture are another major topic. Gender and ethnic differences in leadership style and effectiveness and explanations for the lower numbers of women and minorities in leadership roles are reviewed. Findings from the cross-cultural study of leadership and suggestions for improving leadership practice based on diversity research are provided.

Chapter 11, Group Decision Making, describes the situations that lead groups to make poor decisions and the conditions under which group decisions are superior to decisions made individually. Readers learn about some common group decision-making constraints and about groups as collective information processors. Groupthink and group polarization are other major topics in this chapter. Leader decision styles and the influence of culture and gender on group decision making are also discussed. Throughout the chapter, suggestions are provided to help groups make quality decisions efficiently and to build the group rather than dividing it during the decision-making process.

Teams are the primary unit of performance for an increasing number of organizations; **Chapter 12, Teams,** examines the topic of teamwork. A team is not just any workgroup, and the chapter begins by identifying the features of teams and different ways of classifying teams. Teams are bounded social units operating in organizational contexts, and the chapter explains the importance of organizational supports such as team incentives and team recognition. Team effectiveness is a central focus of the chapter. Readers learn about the relationship between cohesion and team performance and the importance of having a team composed of members with the right combination of taskwork and teamwork skills. They also learn about the importance of team-related attitudes, team leadership, and team training in improving team effectiveness. Finally, the chapter includes a discussion of difficult team members and suggestions for dealing with them.

Instructor's Manual

An instructor's manual with learning objectives, chapter outlines, group activities, test items, and ideas for lectures and discussions for each chapter is available from the publisher. The group activities provide step-by-step instructions and materials for teacher-directed activities. The activities are designed to underscore chapter concepts, demonstrate the features of effective groups, and build individual group skills.

Acknowledgments

Although writing a book is in many ways a solitary experience, it is also true that it is something that cannot be done well alone. I am grateful to all the brilliant scholars and researchers whose work informed this book and from whom I learned so much, including Don Forsyth, my undergraduate group dynamics teacher and mentor. And a special thanks to our reviewer/focus group participant, Nancy Zare, of Springfield Community College. I would also like to thank the following people whose comments about what they wanted in a group dynamics text guided me daily.

Survey Respondents:

Roger Smitter, North Central College
Dennis Waller, Northwest Nazarene University
John Heapes, Harrisburg Area Community College
Diane Stevens, University of North Carolina, Chapel Hill
Glynis Holm Strause, Coastal Bend College
Gwen Wittenbaum, Michigan State University
Dennis Gouran, Pennsylvania State University
Lawrence A. Hosman, University of Southern Mississippi
Linda Giesbrecht-Bettoli, Tennessee Technological University
Darwyn Linder, Arizona State University
Elizabeth Yost Hammer, Belmont University
Steve Bradshaw, Bryan College
LaVerne K. Jordan, Olivet Nazarene University
Steve Kramer, Mount Union College
Jonathan Segal, Trinity College
Sue Sehgal, Georgia State University
Peter Jorgensen, Western Illinois University
Rick Houser, University of Massachusetts, Boston
Jonathan Millen, Rider University
Curt Van Geisen, St. Charles City Community College
Richard J. Gaynor, Virginia Western Community College
Salomon Rettig, Hunter College
Lesa Stern, Southern Illinois University Edwardsville
Robert Rugel, George Mason
M. A. Denison, University of Houston–Victoria
Jean E. Perry, Glendale College
J. R. Kelly, Purdue University
Susan Kosche Vallem, Wartburg College
Arlie V. Daniel, East Central University
Nancy Karlin, University of Northern Colorado
Kathy Pounders, University of Colorado, Denver
Rajoy Venzke, Concordia University
Sam Fung, Austin Peay State University
Craig Lundberg, Cornell University
Dorothy Doolittle, Christopher Newport University
Jere Littlejohn, Mississippi State University
Jennifer Johnson, University of Central Arkansas

Barbara Laughlin Adler, Concordia College
William Benoit, University of Missouri
Andrew Guinn, St. Joseph's College
John Showalter, Erskine College
Jim Fernandes, Gallaudet University
Jamie J. Boudreau, Governors State University
Edward Mabry, University of Wisconsin, Milwaukee
R. Mosvick, Macalester College
Michael J. Hostetler, St. John's University
Deborah Burris, Pfeiffer University
Jeana Abromeit, Alverno College
Laurinda Porter, St. Cloud University
Kathleen Propp, Northern Illinois University
Philip Harwood, University of Dayton
Margaret French, Pitt Community College
Roberta Davilla, University of Northern Iowa
Gail Palmer, Oakland Community College
Ed Raymaker, Maine Maritime Academy
Royce Singleton, Jr., Holy Cross
Peter Keller, Mansfield University
Lawrence R. Frey, Loyola University Chicago
Arthur Ferrari, Connecticut College
William E. Lavell, University of Wisconsin–Whitewater
Mariam Suarez, Wichita State University
Marcia Dixson, Indiana–Purdue Fort Wayne
Steve Coffman, Montana State University–Billings

Reviewers:

Robert Mills, DePaul University
Beverly Palmer, California State University, Dominguez Hills
Lynn C. Howell, Queens College
Chalmer Labig, Oklahoma State University
Robin Lockhart, Midwestern State University
Camille Bunting, Texas A&M University
Linda Giesbrecht-Bettoli, Tennessee Technical University
Samuel Fung, Austin Peay State University
Robert Conyne, University of Cincinatti
John Chapin, Pennsylvania State University
Susan Carol Losh, Florida State University
Jayne Proesel, Webster University

My editor at Wadsworth Marianne Taflinger, was a pleasure to work with, as was the production and editorial staff that assisted in turning a manuscript into a book. My faculty group (the Psychology and Child Development faculty at Cal Poly San Luis Obispo), my family group (my husband, stepchildren, and son), and my group dynamics students all taught me a lot about real-world groups and made me practice what I preach. Thanks also to those students who gave me permission to share their group experiences for this book and to Lourdes Greenberg, Joan McCarthy, Patricia Fernandez, Kim VanDiver, and Cheryl Moore, who assisted with clerical tasks. My brilliant, talented, awesome son Kane, one of the brightest lights in my life, deserves credit for listening to me blather on about group dynamics and how it applies to his high school experience. Last, I would like to thank my husband, the gifted clinical social worker Gene Courter, who supports my work in every way and so patiently waits to walk with me and our chocolate Labrador, Floberz. We are a great triad indeed.

About the Author

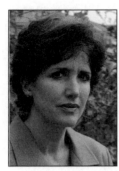

Shawn Burn is Professor of Psychology and Child Development Department at California Polytechnic State University San Luis Obispo. A former department chairperson, she now focuses on student advising and teaching group dynamics, social psychology, research methods, and cross-cultural women's studies courses. She has a B.S. in psychology from Virginia Commonwealth University and her M.A. and Ph.D. are in applied social psychology from Claremont Graduate University. Other books she has authored are *The Social Psychology of Gender* (McGraw-Hill, 1996) and *Women in Cross-Cultural Perspective: A Global Approach* (McGraw-Hill, 2000). She has published articles on a variety of topics such as intergroup conflict, heterosexism, and the use of social norms to promote environmentally responsible behavior. Current group dynamics related research includes a study on social identity deindividuation effects theory in regards to the eruption of crowd violence. She also serves as a group dynamics consultant and program evaluator. She is married with a teenage son and three stepchildren, and enjoys hiking, movies, reading, and writing.

Chapter 1

An Introduction to Group Dynamics

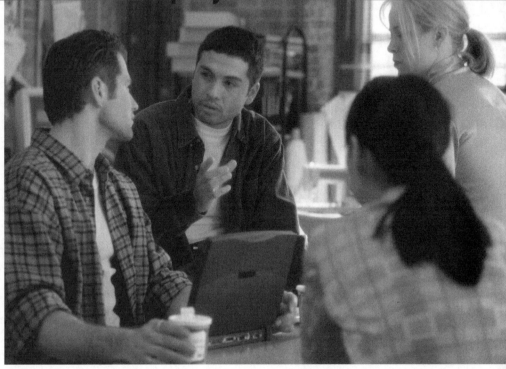

© Jose Luis Pelaez, Inc./CORBIS

Group dynamics

The scientific study of group processes with the goal of understanding and improving groups.

This is a book on **group dynamics,** the scientific study of group processes. After reading this book, you will have a scholarly understanding of groups and how to use that knowledge to improve them.

The Potential of Groups

Regardless of the path your life takes, it is a virtual certainty that much of your work and personal life will be spent as a group member. Human groups can be the source of many great things, personal, professional, and societal. Groups of friends and family have good times and support each other during bad times. Social workers team up with a group of psychologists, physicians, and representatives from social service organizations to serve clients. Counselors and therapists lead therapy groups. Members of support groups find encouragement and information from fellow members. Athletes coordinate team plays to win games. Employees in medical fields, business, education, and social service synchronize with coworkers to deliver services and products. Juries decide guilt and innocence. Students work together on group projects. Citizen groups organize to foster change or to help less fortunate community members. When groups work well, they are sources of meaning, fun, personal growth, societal change, and productivity.

Apprehensions About Groups

Despite the great potential of groups, many people are apprehensive about them and feel they lack important group skills. When you consider that we are born into groups, live in family groups, are educated in classroom groups, work in groups, and often worship and recreate in groups, it seems surprising that so many people feel insecure about their group skills. However, people often resist groups because of a bad experience which may include:

- Being puzzled or distracted by a difficult or different group member
- Unresolved and poorly managed conflicts that pollute the group with mistrust and suspicion
- Having trouble getting work done
- Members' hesitancy to question a poor group decision or challenge group traditions
- Building cohesion by being cruel to a "different" group member or by making enemies of other groups
- Members' lack of cohesion that prevents the group from working efficiently and effectively
- Norms that support violent or disruptive acts
- Conflicts within or between groups that interfere with productivity
- Poorly run meetings and ineffective group leaders
- Members who don't do their share of the group work, dominate the group process, or won't participate

Although these experiences comprise only a small percentage of our group experiences, they are memorable because we often wish we knew how to handle them better.

Most people express some insecurity about their group skills, and a desire to improve them. For instance, **Box 1-1** gives a sampling of some of the group situations my students have trouble with and some of the group skills they would like to develop. Typically, students of group dynamics want to know how to manage group conflict, how to deal with status and power differences, how to deal with diversity, how to communicate in a group context, and how to make groups pro-

BOX 1-1 / A SAMPLING OF STUDENTS' FEELINGS ABOUT GROUPS

"I have trouble when the group has decided to go in a direction that's different from mine. I will retreat and feel stupid and unwanted, even rejected. I need to learn how to take the 'back seat' more. I need to learn how not to be the 'group mom.' I need to detach and allow group members more freedom and space. I need to be more assertive and stand up to authority."

"I have trouble when people do not give input or when people are not willing to compromise. I get frustrated; yet I still try to work with them. Sometimes I get angry; other times I give up. I would like to be able to motivate such nonparticipants."

"I would like to increase my leadership skills, and instead of 'gossiping' about problem people behind their backs, I'd like to confront them."

"I want to be better able to state my beliefs in groups I am new to. I'd like to try to become less stubborn in confrontations, and I'd like to be able to better communicate what I'm feeling to the important people in my life."

"I would like to develop skills that would allow me to communicate my views more effectively in a group. I've often noticed, even when I present a sound idea, that the *presentation* of the idea seems to be as important as the idea itself in its acceptance."

"I have trouble when groups can't reach a consensus in decisions. It's very difficult when half the group is stubborn and won't negotiate."

"I have the most trouble attending a group for the first time, especially if I don't know anyone. I feel extremely nervous and self-conscious. I would like to be more secure in work groups. I would like to be able to walk into an existing group and feel competent to interact and be involved."

"I would like to work on doing things faster in a group. Many groups I've been in procrastinate."

"I would like to become better at disagreeing with group consensus instead of being persuaded because the whole group thinks something is right. I would like to encourage others to be equal participants and stand up to those who dominate the group."

"I would like to develop more trust for group members. I would like to change my skepticism of the ability of group members. I would like to become more open-minded to others' thoughts and be able to work as a group to resolve conflicts and overcome obstacles."

ductive. Fortunately, there is a lot of research on these topics, research reported in this book. Group dynamics and people's group behavior are actually quite predictable, although understandably complex. However, improving group skills requires more than a scholarly understanding of group dynamics. It also requires a special kind of consciousness, a "mindfulness" about groups and our behavior in

Apply It! ••• **Considering Your Group Strengths and Weaknesses**

List the groups that you are a member of. With these in mind, describe your strengths and weaknesses in groups. Which group skills would you like to strengthen? Consider such things as:

1. Whether you are satisfied with your level of participation (Do you over- or underparticipate?)
2. How often you take a leadership role and your leadership style
3. How you deal with difficult group members and situations
4. How you handle conflict in a group and between groups
5. How other members would describe your group behavior

them, an ability to see group dynamics in action in the groups we are a part of, and a willingness to act according to this knowledge. It is up to you to work at applying the suggestions and tools given in this book for improving group functioning. You already know that groups have the power to influence your behavior and affect your life; what you may not know is how much power you have to influence the groups that you are a part of.

Why Groups?

Of course, groups are not all bad. If they were, it is unlikely they would be so common. And common they are. People in every society belong to small primary groups that involve face-to-face interaction (Baumeister & Leary, 1995). As Irving Yalom (1995), the famous group therapist, said, "There is convincing data from the study of primitive human cultures and nonhuman primates that humans have always lived in groups that have been characterized by intense and persistent relationships among members" (p. 17).

Groups Are Sources of Meaning and Belonging

As well as having the potential to provide some of our more frustrating, boring, and noxious experiences, groups are potentially powerful sources of belonging. Many of us have had extraordinary experiences as members of a friendship group or sports team, for example. Indeed, the idea that we have a need to belong and that groups meet this need is an old one in psychology. Chances are that you have studied Maslow's hierarchy of needs. Remember that Maslow (1970, 1971) suggested that the needs for belongingness and for recognition and respect from others (esteem) must be met before we reach the ultimate goal of self-actualization, the realization of our own unique, positive potential. Of course, these are needs met by our involvement with other people.

Baumeister and Leary (1995) propose that the need to belong has two main features. First, people need frequent personal contacts and interactions. Second, people need to perceive an interpersonal bond or relationship that is marked by stability, affective concern, and continuation into the foreseeable future. People look to groups to satisfy these needs. Baumeister and Leary gathered a variety of empirical evidence in support of their hypotheses. For instance, they cite research demonstrating that the deprivation of belongingness causes emotional distress, and that it negatively affects physical and mental health. As shown in a later chapter, the need to belong is one of the major motivations underlying conformity.

Groups Are Sources of Identity

Social identity

That part of a person's self-concept that comes from knowledge of membership in a social group, together with the value and emotional significance of that membership.

What groups are important sources of meaning and identity for you? The groups we belong to are important parts of who we are and how we define ourselves. Pride in our groups contributes to self-esteem, a type of self-esteem called "collective self-esteem" (Crocker & Luhtanen, 1990). This idea comes from social identity theory. Tajfel (1981) described **social identity** as that part of an individual's self-concept that derives from knowledge of membership in a social group, together with the value and emotional significance of that membership. It has long been recognized that our group memberships contribute in a major way to our sense of who we are and of our place in the world (Brown, 1988). Throughout the book, you will learn how this affects a number of different group dynamics, such as conformity, and how it affects relations between groups (intergroup relations).

Groups Are Sources of Information

Groups also provide us with information about the world, and about ourselves. The environments in which we operate are largely created by humans. We get food from a grocery store, which we buy with money obtained from working within a human-created economy, and we get our education and careers by following rules and guidelines developed by people. Negotiating this terrain is hardly obvious, and to survive and have our needs met, we need information from groups. What should we do? What should we think? Our groups help us to decide.

Social comparison theory

A theory emphasizing that people evaluate their own abilities and opinions by comparing themselves to others.

We also use groups to get information about ourselves—in particular, to decide whether we are any good. We do this by seeking feedback from others, by ceaselessly comparing ourselves to others and to standards set by our group. This is the essence of **social comparison theory** (Festinger, 1954). According to social comparison theory, people evaluate their own abilities and opinions by comparing themselves to others. Research indicates that people are especially likely to do this when they are uncertain (Suls & Fletcher, 1983) and that they are more likely to compare themselves to people who are similar to them in relevant ways (Goethals & Darley, 1977; Miller, 1982).

If you are like most people, you compare yourself to your siblings, the people you went to high school with, individuals who have the same job title or degrees that you have, or other relevant groups. Did you do well on a paper or an exam? The first thing my students want to know to decide this is how everyone else did. Indeed, in one study (Klein, 1997), students judging artwork were given false feedback as to the number they got correct and how their scores stacked up to their peers'. Later, when asked about their skill at the task, their assessments were based not on their absolute scores but on the extent to which they did better than their peers.

Social comparison processes are also very important in the workplace. When judging what is "fair," we compare our treatment to the treatment of others. Employees' satisfaction with pay raises and promotions frequently depends on how the raises and promotions compare to the raises and promotions of others with similar backgrounds (Goodman, 1977). These others may be within the same organization or outside of it. These concerns about fairness can have a significant effect on a workgroup. When social comparison leads to the perception of inequity, members may reduce their productivity in protest and may spend a significant amount of time discussing inequities and lobbying for more pay.

Social comparison can have profound effects on self-esteem. Are you attractive? Are you smart? Your answer may depend on who you compare yourself to. To boost their self-esteem, some people engage in **downward social comparison,** comparing themselves to others who are worse than they are on a trait, skill, or ability (Aspinwall & Taylor, 1993; Wheeler & Kunitate, 1992). Could this be why people watch soap operas and daytime talk shows? Do these shows make them feel better because their lives and families look relatively healthy in comparison?

Sometimes, though, a friend, family member, spouse, or coworker is very successful, and **upward social comparison**—the comparison of ourselves to people who are better than us on a particular trait or ability—is unavoidable. According to Tesser's (1988) **self-evaluation maintenance theory,** when another person outperforms us on a behavior that is relevant to our self-definition, the better their performance and the closer our relationship, the greater is the threat to our self-esteem and the more likely we are to experience **social comparison jealousy. Box 1-2** is intended to help you explore the consequences of social comparison jealousy in two-person groups (dyads).

Of course, upward social comparison does not always lead to social comparison jealousy; sometimes we can be very happy about the success of those close to us. For instance, it seems that we can be happy for successful others if they are older or further along in their life plan than we are. In that event, their success is less threatening to our egos, for in time we expect to reach that level of success as well. We also do not experience social compari-

Downward social comparison

The comparison of ourselves to others who are worse than we are on a trait, skill, or ability.

Upward social comparison

The comparison of ourselves to people who are better than we are on a particular trait or ability.

Self-evaluation maintenance theory

A variant of social comparison theory that says when close others do better than we do on things that are important to us, we may experience social comparison jealousy.

Social comparison jealousy

Feelings of jealousy that occur when someone close to us outperforms us on an ego-relevant task.

BOX 1-2 / SOCIAL COMPARISON PROCESSES IN THE DYADIC RELATIONSHIP

Social comparison jealousy provides many challenges to relationships. Social psychologists have long noted that we like those who are similar to us. Relationships with similar others are often successful because similar others are easier to communicate and be with because we have more in common with them. However, in a relationship with a similar other, it is likely that at some point one person will outperform the other on a task that they both value, and social comparison jealousy may result. Those who feel jealous may feel guilty that they cannot be happy for the successful other. They may then distance themselves to avoid these feelings and to avoid the reminder that they are less successful. Those who are successful may feel guilty because they know their success makes the other feel bad. Furthermore, they may feel that they cannot show how happy they are about their own success for fear that it will make the less successful other feel even worse. They too may distance from the less successful other to avoid these feelings.

Some relationships do not survive this dynamic. If the relationship is an important one, it is probably worth talking to the other person about what's going on. The more successful person usually provides the less successful person with reassurance that although this person may have succeeded more in this domain at this time, the other person is just as successful when other things are taken into account. Those who are successful also generally share insecurities or humility, emphasizing that they do not think they are better than the less successful one. They also typically express the desire to continue the relationship. In these ways, one person's success does not have to mean the end of the relationship.

---

son jealousy when others outperform us on a behavior that is *not* relevant to our self-definition. According to Tesser (1988), under these conditions, the better their performance and the closer our relationship, the more we can be proud of them and bask in their success. Sometimes this is called **basking in reflected glory.**

Basking in reflected glory

How we can be proud and happy for a significant other who performs well on a task that is not important to us.

The role of social comparison processes in group dynamics is extremely important. As one of my students once said, "People are often competitive and comparative in groups." In later chapters you will learn how these processes affect conformity, intergroup relations, and reactions to status and reward differences. For instance, people decide whether their group is being treated fairly by comparing it to other groups.

Apply It! ••• **Your Experience With Social Comparison**

Describe a situation in which you have engaged in upward social comparison. Who did you compare yourself to, with what result? Similarly, analyze a situation in which you engaged in downward social comparison. Have you ever experienced social comparison jealousy or "basked in reflected glory"?

Groups Help Us to Accomplish Things

People seek groups to satisfy their needs for meaning, belonging, and information about the world and themselves. People also need groups to get things done, and groups can be the agents of enhanced productivity. It often takes a group to deliver a product or service, or to reach a goal. Much of this book focuses on how to make groups more productive.

Groups Are Change Agents

Groups can be the purveyors of personal change and growth. Yalom (1995) says that groups can help individuals to change by instilling hope (if others can change, so can I), reminding us that everyone has problems, providing alternative methods to solve our problems, and giving us needed feedback about our own behavior and how to improve it. For example, millions of alcohol-addicted people have stopped drinking by participating in Alcoholics Anonymous, a support group for alcoholics. A commonly used method for producing therapeutic change is group therapy, in which a trained psychotherapist leads a group of up to twelve people.

Groups are also significant when it comes to our political and economic interests. Individually, our voices are quiet, but when combined with many others, they are likely to be heard. For instance, globally, the actions of grassroots women's political groups have contributed significantly to progress towards women's equality. Civil rights legislation in the United States might not have happened without organized political action groups. Were it not for unions and labor movements, many of us would work many more hours, for less pay, and under harsher conditions.

Groups Help Us to Survive

Groups also contribute to our survival. Humans have long formed and lived in groups. Some theorists suggest that living in groups increased humans' chances of survival and that the tendency to form groups is biologically encoded (Buss, 1990, 1991). As Barchas (1986, p. 212) said, "over the course of evolution, the small group became the basic survival strategy developed by the human species." The idea is that groups contribute to human survival because groups can share food, provide mates, help care for offspring, hunt large animals, and defend against predators (Baumeister & Leary, 1995). Baumeister and Leary propose that evolutionary selection resulted in a set of internal mechanisms that guide humans into social groups and lasting relationships. For instance, children who desire to stay with a family group are more likely to receive care, food, and protection. Because children with these tendencies were more likely to survive and reproduce, this quality became more common in the gene pool. There is little question that humans are inclined to form groups. However, although we may be born with this tendency, good group skills are often learned through experience and effort.

What Is a Group?

The next task is to get clearer on just what is meant by a "group"—after all, not every collection of people is a group. As groups are referred to throughout the book, you will notice that these are not random collections of folks. A group, in the group dynamics' sense, has some special qualities that distinguish it from a "bunch of people."

Members of Groups Interact

A number of definitions emphasize the idea of interaction and interdependence among group members. For instance, Shaw (1981, p. 454) said: "A group is defined as two or more persons who are interacting with one another in such a manner that each person influences and is influenced by each other person." Likewise, Homans (1950, p. 1) said: "We mean by a group a number of persons who communicate with one another often over a span of time, and who are few enough so that each person is able to communicate with all the others, not secondhand, through other people, but face-to-face." Of course, Homans was writing before teleconferencing and computer chat rooms existed.

Groupness

The extent to which an aggregate functions as a group. Smaller groups with a high level of interaction and a past and future are higher in groupness.

McGrath (1984) suggests that the more interaction between members, the more of a group they are, and the more **groupness** they possess. Three criteria—size, interdependence, and temporal pattern—determine groupness, because each one is positively related to interaction among members. What McGrath says is that social aggregates (collections of people) are "groupier" when groups are small, are able to interact on a variety of issues, have a past in common, and envision a future together.

When the situation or group size is such that one-on-one interaction among members is not possible, the potential for true "groupness" is lost. For instance, physical distance and large collections of people both make interaction unlikely. All the employees at a large organization do not constitute a group in the group dynamic sense because members from one unit rarely come into contact with members from other units and are unable to interact with every other member. It is unlikely that your larger classes function as true groups. If you live in a dorm, it is unlikely that the whole dorm operates as a group, although it is likely that your floor of the dorm does, especially if interaction is fostered by activities created by the resident advisers. If you are a nurse in a large hospital, your unit or the nurses who work the same shift may comprise a group, but there are probably too many nurses in the entire hospital to function at a high level of groupness.

An essential part of interaction is communication, and many problems in groups are problems of communication. Chapter 5 is devoted to the topic of group communication. Another part of group interaction concerns the coordination of the group such that goals may be reached. Chapter 9 focuses on group productivity.

Groups Have Structure

Group structure
The group's norms and roles, patterns of prestige and authority, and communication network.

It is almost impossible to describe what happens in groups without using terms that indicate the "place" of members with respect to one another (Cartwright & Zander, 1968). This is why some definitions of groups focus on **group structure**—the fact that groups have rules or norms that govern the group, members have different roles, patterns of power and authority are relatively stable, and there is an established communication network. When a group acquires some stability in the arrangement of relationships among members, it is structured (Cartwright & Zander, 1968). To understand group structure, consider that you are probably central in one group but marginal in another. You know everything that's going on in one group, but in another you are "out of the loop" and have to depend on gossip. In one group, it is acceptable for you to dress informally; in another, it is not. In one group, you talk a lot, and the group takes up many of your ideas; in another group, you are quiet, and when you do make suggestions, they are ignored.

Norms
Group rules or expectations that specify appropriate behavior for group members.

According to Levine and Moreland (1995), three critical aspects of structure are norms, roles, and status systems. **Norms** are group rules or expectations that specify appropriate behavior for group members. Groups may have norms that tell us how to dress, what topics are acceptable for discussion and which are off-limits, who we are allowed to talk to and how, who we can sit with, whether touching is allowed, how decisions are to be made, and so on. Typically, those who conform to the group's norms are rewarded and those who do not are punished with some form of social disapproval, and sometimes with expulsion from the group. **Roles** are positions that people occupy within the group, each with different expectations for behavior. Different behaviors are expected of a student and a professor, an employee and a manager, a doctor and a nurse, for example. **Status systems** reflect the distribution of power and prestige among members. Not all members are equally valued, and it is usually the case that the ideas and suggestions of some members carry more weight than ideas and suggestions from other members. In many groups, some individuals have the power to issue direct orders and other members do not. Cartwright and Zander (1968) emphasize that an important part of a group's structure is its **communication structure**—the communication channels in the group and who communicates with whom. For instance, one member may be in a central position, connected to everyone else through a relatively small number of communication links, whereas another may be removed by many links from other group members.

Roles
Positions that people occupy within the group, each with different expectations for behavior.

Status systems
The distribution of power and prestige among members.

Communication structure
The communication channels in the group and who communicates with whom.

The group dynamics that arise out of group structure are powerful influences on group behavior and are seen in family groups, friendship groups, and work groups. Norms and roles are the topic of Chapter 3, status and power systems are discussed in Chapter 4, and communication structures are explored in Chapter 5.

Groups Have Goals

Goals

The mission, purpose, or objectives that guide the group's actions and allow the group to plan and coordinate members' efforts.

Still other definitions emphasize that groups exist for a purpose and are used to accomplish **goals.** The idea is that people join groups to achieve goals they are unable to achieve by themselves. Goals guide the actions of group members. Goals let the members know where the group is going and whether it is getting there. Goals allow members to plan and coordinate their efforts. McGrath (1984) discussed four basic task goals of groups: *generating* (ideas and plans), *choosing* (how to solve a problem and where to get answers), *negotiating* (to resolve conflicts of interest and conflicts of viewpoint), and *executing* (performances, tasks, and contests and battles with other groups).

Bales (1950, 1953) made a very important observation about group goals. He noted that people's actions in a group are geared toward the accomplishment of the group's goals but that a basic tension exists between the group's goal of task accomplishment and the goal of meeting group members' socioemotional needs. As members engage in instrumental activities (tasks that get the job done and accomplish goals), conflicts, sensitivities, and dissatisfactions invariably arise. These are dealt with through socioemotional behaviors (expressive, emotional behaviors), in which members show concern for the feelings of others, make jokes, soothe hurt feelings, and otherwise do things to maintain the integrity of the group so that it can return to the task at hand. People are both irritating and irritable, and this leads to inevitable bumps in groups' functioning. Managing this delicate balance between group members' feelings and getting the job done is one of the focuses of this book. Goals are also important to group output and are discussed further in Chapter 9 on group productivity and Chapter 12 on teams.

Members Identify Themselves as a Group

There is an old saying that "If it looks like a duck, and quacks like a duck, it is a duck." Likewise, if it looks like a group and acts like a group, and the members consider it a group, then it is a group. Brown (1988, pp. 2–3) stated that "a group exists when two or more people define themselves as members of it and when its existence is recognized by at least one other." As you read earlier, groups are often psychologically significant to us in the sense that our identification with them is an important source of meaning and belonging. Social identity theory highlights the idea that an aggregate becomes a group when its members share a social identity. Turner (1982, p. 15) emphasized this point when he said that a group exists "when two or more individuals . . . perceive themselves to be members of the same social category."

Groups Have Two or More Members

There is some disagreement about how many people it takes to make a group. Some say it takes two or more people, and others say it takes three or more. For

Dyads
A two-person group.

Group
Two or more interacting, interdependent people.

instance, Shaw (1981, p. 8) defines a group as "two or more persons who are interacting in such a manner that each person influences and is influenced by each other person." In contrast, Levine and Moreland (1995) argue that **dyads** (two-person aggregates) should be treated separately from groups because they are different in some significant ways. For example, they are destroyed by the loss of one member. Dyadic relationships frequently affect the larger group that the individuals are a part of. For instance, a conflict between two employees may affect the cohesion of the workgroup. A romance between two friends may change the dynamics of a friendship group. Also, dyads do possess the central features of groups, such as interaction, interdependence, shared identity, and structure. Therefore the focus of this book is primarily on groups with three or more members, the definition favored here is that a **group** is two or more interacting, interdependent people.

A related issue surrounds the distinction between interpersonal and group processes. Some group theorists believe that interpersonal processes (the dynamics of relationships between individuals) are separate from group processes and, as such, should not be included in the study of groups. The idea is that groups are unified systems with dynamics that go beyond the relationships between the individual members. Brown (1988) distinguishes interpersonal from group behavior by saying that when people act interpersonally, they act according to their distinctive personal characteristics, whereas group behavior entails acting based on group memberships. In group situations, diverse individuals act in remarkably uniform ways (Brown, 1988).

Although it is true that interpersonal processes and group processes are not the same, there is also little question that one of the things that makes groups so complex are the multiple interpersonal dynamics that overlay and affect group processes. As the well-known group researcher Robert Freed Bales (1988) noted, a complete understanding of a group requires an understanding of its members, their relationships to one another, the overall dynamic tendencies of the total group, and the impact of broader organizational culture on the inner workings of the group. Intragroup processes—the interactions that take place among members, including communication, coordination, and conflict, as well as reactions to leadership and to one another—all affect group outcomes.

Even intrapersonal dynamics (within the individual) are relevant to the study of group dynamics. The famous group psychotherapist Irving Yalom (1995) emphasized the subtle dynamic interplay between the group member and the group environment, noting that over time group members frequently enact their own characteristic maladaptive interpersonal behaviors in the group. In the therapy group, the examination of this "baggage" from past groups is a rich source of material for exploration and growth. But in many groups, bringing issues from past group experiences can lead to biased reactions to events in the group and to other group members, greatly influencing the group process and taking up a lot of group time. For these reasons, a more comprehensive understanding of groups involves considering the interplay of intrapersonal, interpersonal (between individuals), and group dynamics.

Apply It! ••• **What Is Your "Group Baggage"?**

What types of group situations and group members do you have trouble with? How might these be related to your past group experiences, including those with your family group? Can you think of any critical group experiences that have colored your later experiences in groups? How can understanding these make you a better group member? Do you agree or disagree with the notion that we carry our past "group baggage" into new group experiences?

A Brief History of the Study of Group Dynamics

The Late Nineteenth Century and Gustave LeBon

The scholarly study of groups originates in the late 1800s and has roots primarily in psychology and sociology.

Gustave LeBon was one of the first to study groups. Trained as a medical doctor but more interested in writing on scientific topics for the masses, he was fascinated by mob behavior such as that which occurred during the French Revolution. In the late nineteenth century, he wrote about crowd psychology in a book titled *The Crowd* (1895/1968). LeBon suggested that crowds come to act as "one mind," called the **"collective mind,"** which overrides the mind of the individual. LeBon (1895, 1968 p. 12) said "by the mere fact that he forms part of an organized crowd, a man descends several rungs in the ladder of civilization. Isolated, he may be a cultivated individual; in a crowd, he is a barbarian." Furthermore, he viewed the process by which a collection of individuals becomes a crowd with a collective mind as being like a disease that starts with one or two people and then spreads throughout the group. He called this the process of contagion. For example, if one person coughs in a movie theater or during a lecture, suddenly many people start coughing. LeBon said of contagion, "it must be classed among those phenomena of a hypnotic order. In a group every sentiment and act is contagious, and contagious to such a degree that an individual readily sacrifices his personal interest to the collective interest" (p. 10).

Modern group theorists have challenged and greatly refined LeBon's ideas. However, LeBon deserves credit for being one of the first to draw attention to the fact that groups can lead individuals to behave more destructively than they would as isolated individuals.

Collective mind
LeBon's name for his idea that crowds come to act as "one mind" that overrides the minds of individuals.

The Early Psychological Perspective

The newly developing field of psychology, with its emphasis on scientific methods, was not entirely comfortable with LeBon's dogmatic and largely unscientific presentation of the "group mind." His work was clearly influenced by his political views (which were contemptuous of the working class that led the French Revolution), and his work was more of an essay than a scientific study. An 1898

Social facilitation

How the presence of others increases performance on well-learned tasks.

study by Norman Triplett on a group phenomenon now known as **social facilitation** demonstrated that groups could be studied using scientific methods, but this work was little noticed. Triplett studied cyclists and children, and found that the presence of others increases performance. Indeed, despite Triplett's studies, some influential psychologists of the early twentieth century continued to argue that the group concept was unscientific. For instance, F. H. Allport (1924) argued that groups aren't "real" because they cannot be seen, felt, heard, or smelled as something distinctively different from the individuals who are their members (Steiner, 1986). After all, he noted, no one ever tripped over a group, so how can they be real? For those of us who have witnessed group violence, been excluded from a group, undergone an us–them conflict, or experienced a sense of we-ness as a group member, the notion that groups are not real is almost nonsensical. However, it is important to realize that in an effort to gain credibility as a science, the newly developing field of psychology was distinctly interested in those concepts that were objectively measurable and observable.

Meanwhile, studies on social facilitation continued through the early part of the 20th century, and the 1920s saw the first glimmers of the group as a therapeutic agent. Burrow (1924) suggested that because emotional disorders result from unresolved problems that originate in group contexts (the family), treatment should occur in a group context that illuminates the patients' way of relating to others. But Burrow's argument was not well received, and group therapy lay dormant until World War II, when posttraumatic stress syndrome and a shortage of therapists led to its adoption. Today there is a large research literature on the study of groups as therapeutic change agents.

In 1936, social psychologist Muzafer Sherif began the scientific study of social norms and conformity, a topic that remains central in the modern study of groups. In a now classic study, Sherif (1936) showed how in ambiguous (unclear) situations, individuals rely on groups for information. The study also traced the development and persistence of norms within a group. Sherif also made important contributions to group dynamics through his work on intergroup conflict (conflict between groups). We return to Sherif's studies in later chapters on group influence and intergroup conflict.

The long-standing tradition of studying group dynamics in the workplace also began in the 1930s. For instance, in a series of studies now known as the Hawthorne studies (because they were conducted at the Hawthorne Electric Plant), Elton Mayo (1933) demonstrated that workgroup relations influenced productivity. Mayo was studying the effects of lighting on performance but found that lighting had less effect on productivity than did workgroup norms.

Kurt Lewin and the Research Center for Group Dynamics

The 1940s saw what many believe to be the founding of modern group dynamics, with a focus on the scientific study of groups. Kurt Lewin, one of the most influential figures in modern group dynamics, attempted to persuade the psychological community not only that groups were worth studying, but that they could be studied scientifically. Lewin saw groups as more than the sum of their parts. As he once said (1947/1997, p. 303), "there is no more magic behind the fact that groups have properties of their own, which are different from the properties of their subgroups or their individual members, than behind the fact that molecules have properties which are different from the properties of the atoms or ions of which they are composed."

Field theory

Theories suggesting that the behavior of group members is due to an interactive field of influences, including personal, interpersonal, group, and situation.

Lewin's (1946/1997a) **field theory** of human behavior suggests that the behavior of group members is a function of both their personal qualities and the environment (environment is defined broadly to include other group members). Lewin elegantly captured this idea in the formula $B = f(P,E)$. If you take a moment to reflect on one of your recent group experiences and your behavior in the group, you will see the beauty and complexity of this seemingly simple idea that behavior (B) is a function (f) of both the person (P) and the environment (E).

Lewin (1951/1997) emphasized that to understand the group, one must understand the group's position in the "social field"—that is, how it is a result of many coexisting social entities, including other groups, subgroups, members, barriers, channels of communication, and so on. Lewin called this a "field theory" of human behavior and used the term *lifespace* to represent the combination of the person and his or her psychological environment. His idea was that each person is surrounded by a "life space," a dynamic field of forces within which his or her needs and purposes interact with the influences of the environment. Social behavior can be schematized in terms of the tension and interplay of these forces and of the individual's tendency to maintain equilibrium among them, or to restore equilibrium when it has been disturbed.

Lewin (1947) noted that too often "social action at any level is based to a high degree on opinion and tradition rather than on rational understanding about possible alternatives or on clear foresight about what the effects of different social actions would be" (p. 7). He argued that "the study of group life should reach beyond the level of description; the conditions of group life and the forces which bring about change or which resist change should be investigated" (p.9). He used the term *dynamics* to refer to these forces.

Lewin was optimistic that such group dynamics could be studied scientifically and founded the Research Center for Group Dynamics (RCGD) in 1945. The mission of the RCGD was to advance the scientific knowledge of group processes through theory building and group experiments, and to foster the application of scientific knowledge to the solving of social problems (Deutsch, 1992). As Gordon Allport noted in 1948, Lewin's methods have a pioneer characteristic because he was one of the first scientists to successfully adapt experimentation to the complex problems of group life (Allport, 1948/1997).

A good example is a 1939 study by Lewin, Lippit, and White that systematically studied the effects of leadership style on productivity and aggressiveness. The researchers assigned 10- and 11-year-old boys to one of three after-school groups composed of five boys each. One group had an autocratic leader who gave orders and criticized. A second group had a democratic leader who provided in-struction and guidance but invited the boys' input into decisions. A third group had a laissez-faire leader who took a more "hands-off" approach, participating little in the group. The researchers observed the groups, recording the amount of time they spent working as well as the levels of aggression displayed. The re-searchers found that the children in the authoritarian-led groups worked more, but only when the leader watched them; the democratically led groups contin-ued working even after the leader's absence; and the laissez-faire groups worked the least. The children in the authoritarian group were more hostile, picking on group members more and engaging in destructive behavior. At this point in your education, you have probably heard of many studies using this type of format to study human behavior, and the Lewin, Lippit, and White study may not seem like a big deal. However, it is important because it was one of the first studies to use this now standard research design to investigate people.

Those who worked with Lewin at RCGD remember him as an intellectu-ally stimulating and personally supportive colleague and mentor. Indeed, one of Lewin's contributions to the study of groups was the inspiration he provided to a number of young researchers. These researchers went on to generate a variety of theories and research on the topic of groups, including research on group co-hesiveness (Festinger, Schacter, & Back, 1950); cooperation (Deutsch, 1949a, 1949b); group decision making (Guetzkow & Gyr, 1954); leadership (Lippit & White, 1958); and power (French & Raven, 1959). In many ways, their work formed the backbone of the field of group dynamics.

Another of Lewin's greatest contributions to group dynamics was his idea that theoretical and applied psychology are not mutually exclusive, and indeed should go hand in hand. This idea is essential to modern group dynamics, for it is only through rigorous scientific work, including that done with real-world groups, that we can develop the theories and practices to improve groups. As Lewin (1948) said, "research that produces nothing but books will not suffice" (p. 203). However, he was also aware that too often applied research lacked rigor and a theoretical basis. He emphasized the bidirectional relationship between theory and practice:

> Many psychologists working today in an applied field are keenly aware of the need for close cooperation between theoretical and ap-plied psychology. This can be accomplished in psychology as it has been in physics, if the theorist does not look toward applied problems with highbrow aversion or with fear of social problems, and if the ap-plied psychologist realizes that *there is nothing so practical as a good theory.* (Lewin, 1951a, p. 169)

Unfortunately, the study of groups by psychologists took a detour of sorts when Lewin, the champion of studying groups in all their complexity, died unexpectedly in 1947 at the age of 57. His students, such as Leon Festinger of cognitive dissonance fame, did their part to encourage the growth of social psychology as a scientific discipline. However, the way they went about it detracted from Lewin's vision of theory and practice as symbiotic. In an effort to gain academic and scientific credibility, social psychologists focused on hypotheses that could be tested using the experimental model because this method is similar to the methods used by the hard sciences. Jones (1985, in the *Handbook of Social Psychology*) calls this the "Rodney Dangerfield era" in social psychology when social psychology was trying to gain respect.

The result was that despite Lewin's intention for group dynamics to involve a mix of research methods, the social-psychological study of groups became dominated by the study of the small group in the laboratory setting (a controlled research setting as opposed to a real-world or "field" setting). These groups were composed of strangers (usually undergraduates) brought together by researchers under controlled conditions. To maximize control and enhance the ability to establish causality, the researchers would systematically vary some factor while holding all other aspects of the environment constant. In this way, they could, with some degree of certainty, make cause–effect assertions.

During the 1960s and 1970s, group research in psychology focused mostly on conformity and "group polarization" (Tindale & Anderson, 1998). Group polarization is the idea that group discussions solidify and strengthen people's initial inclinations as others provide them with additional reasons to think what they do and as they try to support the dominant group position. As a result, groups make more extreme decisions than would individual members.

Topics such as helping behavior, social facilitation, and group aggression were also explored using clever experiments, and it became more common to study how the group affects the behavior of individuals than it was to study the dynamics of the groups themselves. For instance, Darley and Latane (1968) conducted laboratory studies on altruism (helping behavior) in groups of strangers. They expected that as the number of people present in an emergency increased, helping would decrease. The idea is that in group situations, responsibility is shared, and the more people present, the less responsible each one feels (this is called *diffusion of responsibility*). Also, in ambiguous situations, as emergency situations often are, people will take their cue as to what to do from the group that is present. Ironically, everyone is looking to everyone else for a cue, but no one does anything because no one else is doing anything (this is called *pluralistic ignorance*).

To test their hypothesis, Latane and Darley staged emergencies while systematically varying the number of bystanders present and then measuring how long it took research participants to get help. They took care to make sure that the experimental conditions were identical for all participants and that the only thing that varied was the number of people present, which the researchers controlled. Because they had controlled everything, they could assert with confidence that the amount of helping was a direct result of the number of people present. If the participants were treated identically except for the number of people present, then differences between them had to be due to the number of people present.

Although productive in the sense that many basic group principles were scientifically established, laboratory experiments were limited in a number of ways. In particular, they could not begin to mimic the complex environments in which groups operate, nor the ebb and flow of groups over time. For instance, we know a lot more about how groups of strangers respond to crisis than we do about the dynamics of helping in groups where members know one another. Critics such as McGuire (1973) expressed concerns that the manipulational laboratory experiment (where one causal factor is systematically varied while everything else is held constant) merely demonstrates obvious truths rather than dealing with more complex or contradictory features of human behavior. The original promise of psychology for the study of groups was temporarily lost.

The Early Sociological Perspective

Sociologists were also beginning to consider groups at the end of the nineteenth century. The sociological perspective contrasted with the psychological perspective of Allport and others, for whom groups did not really exist as entities distinct from the individuals that comprised them. Indeed, sociologists such as Emile Durkheim (1895) emphasized that a group "is not identical to the sum of its parts, it is something else with different properties than those presented by the parts of which it is composed. . . . It cannot be understood by a piecemeal examination of its parts" (pp. 126, 128). As Charles Horton Cooley (1909/1998, p. 184), one of the founders of modern sociology, said,

> We must learn to see mankind [sic] in psychical wholes, rather than in artificial separation. We must see and feel the communal life of family and local groups as immediate facts, not as combinations of something else. And perhaps we shall do this best by recalling our own experience and extending it through sympathetic observation. What, in our life, is the family and the fellowship; what do we know of the we-feeling?

Cooley's point was that that we cannot think of individuals entirely apart from their social groups, and conversely, we cannot think of social groups without also thinking of the individuals that comprise them. In Cooley's work we also find some of the first writings on topics that remain central in the modern study of groups: group communication and conflict, social comparison processes, the situating of groups in larger social contexts, and the role of groups in the development of our identities.

Another early and important sociologist, George Herbert Mead (1934), also asserted that a full understanding of groups and their individual members requires that we observe complex group activity. The idea is akin to saying that you cannot understand a cake by looking at its ingredients in isolation from one another. A cake is more than the sum of its parts, in the sense that the ingredients must interact to produce it. The ingredients apart do not look, taste, or smell like a cake. Likewise, interacting individuals produce something distinctive in the form of group.

Sociologists continued to make important contributions to group study. In the 1940s, Jacob Moreno (1953) developed a technique called sociometry to measure the relationships between workers. Moreno asked group members a series of questions, such as who they liked and did not like. He then constructed a sociogram, a visual display of member relationships. He used this information to diagnose group problems and resolve them. Today, software is available to process sociometric data, and you can use sociograms to measure group members' respect and liking for one another as well as group communication patterns.

Robert Freed Bales, IPA, and SYMLOG

In the 1950s, sociologists looked at small groups as miniature social systems. The work of Robert Freed Bales continues to be influential; you have already seen his name earlier in the chapter in regard to the task and socioemotional goals of groups. Bales began his research on small groups in 1943 with a field study of Alcoholics Anonymous meetings (A. P. Hare, 1996a). It was at this time that he began developing a system of categorizing group processes, later known as Interaction Process Analysis (IPA). For instance, he examined how friendly group members were to one another, the dynamics of dominance in the group, and the balance of task-oriented and socioemotional behaviors and related these factors to group effectiveness.

Like Lewin's theory, Bales' was a field theory that emphasized an interactive field of influences including personal, interpersonal, group, and situation. He hoped that the observation and categorization of group behaviors using his system would reveal how groups deal with "universal systems problems." For instance, typical systems problems include how to adapt to the immediate situation, how to accomplish the group's goal, how to hold the group together, and how to satisfy member needs (Mills, 1967). Using IPA, Bales made a number of "discoveries." These included the common role differentiation between "task" leaders and "social" leaders, patterns of group problem solving, and the developmental phases that occur over a series of meetings (A. P. Hare, 1996a). In the 1970s, Bales introduced a more detailed and structured observational measure known as SYMLOG (System of Multiple Level Observation of Groups). You will read more about IPA and SYMLOG in Chapter 2.

Today's Group Dynamics

Several writers (Bargal, Gold, & Lewin, 1992; Levine & Moreland, 1990; Steiner, 1986) have noted that theory-driven research on groups has declined. In recent years, it has also become more common to study real-world or "natural" groups and the influence of group dynamics on organizational and social problems such as gang violence or youth tobacco use. The experimental laboratory study that once dominated the study of small groups has given way to more applied research methods such as surveys and observational techniques (Levine & Moreland, 1990). As Levine and Moreland point out, this is mostly a good thing in that practical information may be obtained along with the development of theories that can account for complex behavior in natural groups. This approach reflects group study as envisioned by Lewin, an "action research" model in which research simultaneously solves problems and generates new knowledge. Lewin's former student Deutsch (1992) characterized it as a "tough-minded" but "tender-hearted" approach.

Today neither psychology nor sociology dominates the study of groups. Instead, research on real groups in all their complexity is now conducted in a variety of disciplines. For instance, organizational psychologists conduct research on teams and workgroup productivity, communication researchers examine small group communication, social workers and clinical and counseling psychologists explore the dynamics of therapeutic change groups, and sociologists examine status dynamics in groups.

Concept Review

Why Groups?

- People in every society belong to groups, and there is evidence that humans have always lived in groups.
- Groups satisfy a number of human needs. Groups are sources of belonging and provide us with meaningful social identities. According to social comparison theory, groups also provide us with needed information about ourselves, information that can affect our self-esteem. Groups also help us to accomplish things, including goals of personal change and growth. Groups also contribute to our survival.

Definitions and Features of Groups

- A group is defined as two or more interacting people.
- Members of groups interact and influence one another.
- Groups have structure in that norms and roles govern them, they usually have relatively stable patterns of power and authority, and some group members have greater power and prestige than others.
- Groups have goals that guide the actions of the group by helping them to plan and coordinate their efforts. Because people are so sensitive, there are

often tensions between the group's goal of task accomplishment and the goal of meeting members' socioemotional needs.

- Some group definitions emphasize that group members share a group identity and say that a group exists when two or more people define themselves as a group.
- Interpersonal and group processes are not the same but they do affect one another. The multiple interpersonal dynamics that overlay and affect group processes mean that a more comprehensive understanding of groups involves considering the interplay of intrapersonal, interpersonal, and group dynamics.

History of Group Dynamics

- The scholarly study of groups originated in the late 1800s and has its roots in psychology and sociology.
- Gustave LeBon (1895) was one of the first to study the behavior of groups when he studied crowd behavior. Around the same time, a study by Norman Triplett (1898) on what was later called social facilitation found that the presence of others increases performance, although some psychologists at the time questioned the idea that groups could be studied scientifically.
- The 1920s and 1930s saw some of the first studies on group norms, groups in the workplace, and groups as therapeutic change agents.
- The 1940s ushered in what many believe to be the founding of modern group dynamics, stimulated by the work of psychologist Kurt Lewin. Lewin advanced the notions that through rigorous scientific work we can develop theories and practices to improve groups, and that theory and practice should go hand in hand.
- In the 1950s, sociologists made important contributions to the study of groups by looking at groups as miniature social systems. Sociologist Robert Freed Bales developed a system for categorizing group processes now known as Interaction Process Analysis. His theories emphasized how groups respond to individuals and situations. In the 1970s, Bales developed a detailed system for understanding a group known as SYMLOG.
- After Lewin's death in 1947, the study of groups by psychologists focused on the use of laboratory experiments to study how groups affected individuals' behavior. Although these studies established many basic group principles, they limited the study of groups to phenomena that could be studied in a laboratory setting.
- Today, research on groups is conducted by a variety of disciplines that use a number of different research methods. Much of this research focuses on real-world (natural) groups.

Study Questions

1. In what way are groups potentially powerful sources of belonging?
2. How are groups sources of identity?
3. What does it mean to say that groups are sources of information?
4. How do groups contribute to human survival?
5. How can groups can be "agents of change"?
6. What are the key features of groups described in the chapter?
7. What is groupness? What factors influence it?
8. According to Bales (1950, 1953), what basic tension exists in groups?
9. Who was Gustave LeBon, and what contribution did he make to the study of groups?
10. In the late nineteenth and early twentieth centuries, what did the new field of psychology have to say about groups?
11. What was the sociological perspective on groups in the late nineteenth and early twentieth centuries?
12. Who was Kurt Lewin, and what was his approach to the study of groups?
13. What contributions did Robert Bales make to the study of groups?
14. Describe the study of group dynamics following Lewin's death.

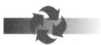

Group Activities

Activity 1: Make Your Class a Group

With your group, review the features of groups discussed in the chapter and evaluate your class as a group. To what extent is your class a group in the group dynamics sense? What would have to happen for your class to become more "groupy"?

Activity 2: Collect Data: How Uncomfortable Are People in Groups?

This chapter suggests that many people are apprehensive about groups and feel that they lack important group skills. In this activity, you will collect some data to try to find out how comfortable people feel in group situations.

   With your group, go out and ask people the following questions (each member should write the answer options on an index card to show to interviewees). Ask the interviewee to write answers on a slip of paper (while you look the other way) and then place it into an envelope. Combine all members' data and summarize your findings.

1. Would you say that in general you are very comfortable, comfortable, somewhat comfortable, somewhat uncomfortable, or very uncomfortable in group situations?

2. In general, how confident are you in your group skills? Would you say that you are very confident, confident, somewhat confident, somewhat unconfident, unconfident, or very unconfident?

3. In which of the following group skills would you most like to grow and develop—conflict resolution, leadership, making a group more productive, or dealing with difficult group members?

Activity 3: Identify Your Class's Group Goals

According to this chapter, groups have goals that let members know where the group is going and whether they are making progress. With your group, make a list of goals for your group dynamics class that you all agree on. Share your goals with the class.

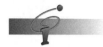

InfoTrac College Edition Search Terms

To do research for your papers and assignments, use InfoTrac that's provided free with new copies of this book. Go to http://infotrac.thomsonlearning.com and enter the following search terms:

- Functions of Groups
- Social Comparison
- Self-help Groups
- Social Identity Theory

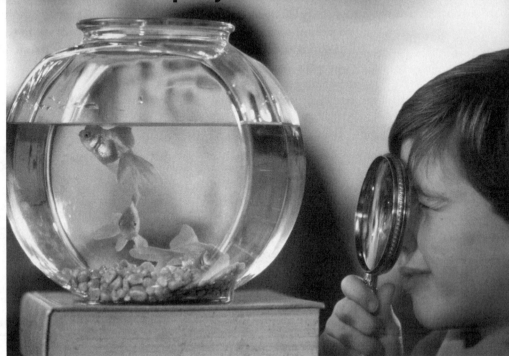

© Tom & Dee Ann McCarthy/CORBIS

Variety is evident in who studies groups (organizational psychologists, clinical psychologists, sociologists, social workers, and others) and in the types of groups and group processes studied. However, the field of group dynamics is unified in its agreement that research can help us understand groups and provide us with information useful for group improvement. Research involves the use of objective, precise, and verifiable methods to gain knowledge and test ideas about the causes of and influences on human behavior. Chapter 1 explained that the study of group dynamics is largely research based and that the field developed after social scientists such as Kurt Lewin and Robert Bales demonstrated that groups could be studied scientifically. In this chapter, you will learn in more detail about how group dynamics research is conducted.

Many students expect research methods to be boring or intimidating; thoughts of taking a nap or running away are not uncommon. However, if you think about it, the idea behind research methods is an intriguing one. How do we know whether our hunches about human behavior and groups are correct? How do we design studies so that we are confident about the nature of the world, including groups? Also, bear in mind that research methods have a great deal to offer us in terms of broadening our knowledge and testing interventions. Because virtually all organizations do some research, you have an advantage if you have a decent understanding of research methods. Familiarity with research methods is also important in terms of being a good consumer of research findings. You do not want to change an attitude, belief, behavior, or organizational practice based on faulty research findings.

The Experimental Method

Experimental method

A research method designed to test cause–effect relationships by systematically manipulating hypothesized causal variables while holding all other variables constant.

Many different research methods are available. The **experimental method** is designed to test proposed cause–effect relationships between variables. In an experiment, the researcher carefully varies the variable expected to cause some change in another variable (the effect) while holding everything else steady (constant). That way, if the effect variable changes, the researcher can conclude there is a cause–effect relationship between the two variables.

The Ad Hoc Group Laboratory Experiment

Ad hoc groups

An artificial group created solely for the purpose of studying it in a controlled laboratory setting.

Experimental confederate

A researcher's accomplice who is part of the independent variable manipulation or experimental situation.

Much of group dynamics research has been done on **ad hoc groups**—artificial groups concocted solely for the purpose of studying them in a controlled laboratory setting for a period of one to two hours (McGrath, 1993, 1997). Consider this classic study conducted by Stanley Schacter (1951) on how groups respond to "deviates"—individuals who do not go along with the group's majority. Schacter randomly assigned college students to groups and planted one of his accomplices in each group. The groups were asked to decide the fate of a juvenile delinquent named Johnny Rocco. In some of the groups, the researcher's accomplice (called an **experimental confederate**) was instructed by the researcher to always go along with the group (this confederate was called the "mode"). In some of the groups, he was instructed to always go against the group (the "deviate"), and in yet others, he was told to begin by disagreeing with the group's majority, but over time to change to going along with them (the "slider"). After the group discussions, Schacter asked the participants a number of questions to see how groups responded to members based on their level of conformity to the majority. Just as your instincts may have told you, the deviate was not well liked, was eventually all but ignored by the group, and was assigned the least desirable of the group's tasks. The other two confederates fared well along these lines; they were rewarded with acceptance and liking for their conformity to the group's majority. Historically, this type of research paradigm—the laboratory experiment conducted with ad hoc or artificial groups (groups of strangers brought together for purposes of the study)—has been one of the most popular research designs in group dynamics.

Independent and Dependent Variables

Recall that the experiment is a method used to test cause–effect predictions or hypotheses. The experimenter systematically manipulates (changes around) a manageable number of causal variables, while holding all other influences on behavior constant. Other variables are then measured to see whether they are affected. The **independent variable (IV)** is the name of the manipulated variable. The IV is expected to cause changes in the **dependent variable (DV).** In Schacter's (1951) study, the IV was the level of conformity as represented by the three types of experimental confederates. The dependent variable is the name of the measured variable (the effect or behavior expected to be influenced by the IV). Schacter's experiment had several dependent variables, including liking for the experimental confederate and the tasks assigned to the confederate by the group.

Independent variable (IV)

In an experiment, the hypothesized causal variable, systematically varied (manipulated) by the researcher.

Dependent variable (DV)

In an experiment, the measured "effect" variable, expected to change depending on the level of the independent variable.

In the Lewin, Lippit, and White (1939) leader experiment described in Chapter 1, the experimenters systematically varied the type of leader (autocratic, democratic, or laissez-faire), which was thus the independent variable. The dependent variables included the number of aggressive actions observed and liking for the leader (obtained from interviews with the research participants). The idea behind the experiment is that if there is a cause–effect relationship between the IV and the DV, then groups that differ on the IV will differ on the DV. For instance, Lewin and his colleagues found that liking for the leader changed depending on the type of leader being rated (the boys did not like the autocratic leaders and preferred the democratic ones).

Random Assignment and Control

Two central features of the experiment are random assignment and control over the experimental situation. Remember that the purpose of the experiment is to demonstrate that there is or is not a cause–effect relationship between the variables. If you do not find a difference between the IV groups on the DV, you want to be confident that in fact the IV has no effect on the DV. If you find that the IV groups do differ on the DV, you want to be able to say that the IV caused these differences. To draw this conclusion, you must be able to say that the groups are virtually identical except for the independent variable. If they are not, how do you know that these other differences are not the true causes of the difference between the groups on the DV?

Making sure that the groups are the same except for the IV is done in two ways. One way is to make sure that the groups are treated identically except for the independent variable. This is called **experimental control.** For instance, researchers typically make sure that instructions to participants are delivered in the same way and that experimenters are the same across IV conditions. The second way is to guarantee that the groups are equal in terms of the kinds of people in them. This is done by **random assignment** of participants to the different IV conditions. Both of these techniques reduce **experimental confounds,** extraneous factors in the study that "confound" (confuse) our ability to draw clear conclusions about our findings.

With random assignment, participants have an equal chance of ending up in any of the IV groups. Random assignment is like a promise that IV groups are equivalent on any participant variables (such as age, education, or experience) that may affect the DV. Think of it this way: If you wanted to divide a large group into two equally talented teams to play basketball, you could toss a coin for each individual—tails they go on one team, heads they go on the other. Height, athleticism, age, and basketball playing experience and talent would be evenly distributed between the two groups. Random assignment rules out the possibility that changes in the dependent variable were due to preexisting group differences and were not caused by the independent variable.

For instance, many studies have been conducted on brainstorming, a technique for generating ideas in which group members are encouraged to speak freely without criticizing their own or others' ideas. Random assignment is important to the validity of these studies. Osborn (1957) claimed that the productivity of problem-solving groups would be enhanced if members were encouraged to first say whatever came to mind and to later evaluate the ideas generated. If you are like many people, you might assume that group brainstorming is effective for producing more and higher-quality ideas. However, laboratory research does not support this hypothesis. Indeed, an equal number of individuals working alone are about twice as productive as a brainstorming group (Mullen, Johnson, & Salas, 1991).

In brainstorming studies, participants are often randomly assigned to one of two independent variable groups. One IV group brainstorms with others on a task, such as generating ideas on how to increase tourism in the United States. Participants in the other IV group brainstorm alone, and their results are combined with those of other group members. Random assignment is important in these types of studies. We want to be sure that there is an equal number of creative people in all IV groups. We want to know that recreation majors who have taken a class on tourism are not all in one IV group. Random assignment ensures that these and other qualities that could affect the dependent variable are evenly distributed across the IV groups. Then, if differences between the IV groups are found in the number of quality ideas generated, the researchers can safely con-

Experimental control

A key experimental feature that requires that everything in the setting stay the same except for the independent variable.

Random assignment

A key experimental feature in which research participants have an equal chance of ending up in any of the IV groups.

Experimental confounds

Extraneous factors in a study that confuse our ability to draw clear conclusions about our findings.

Apply It! ••• Identifying Key Experimental Features

Social loafing is the name given to people's tendency not to work as hard or to "slack" on collective (group) tasks. Latane, Williams, and Harkins conducted one classic experimental study of social loafing in 1979. College student participants cheered and clapped alone and in groups of two, four, or six persons (each person performed in each condition). They were told to clap or cheer as loudly as possible at specific times, so that the researchers could "determine how much noise people make in social settings." Although larger groups made more noise, the amount of noise generated by each participant dropped as group size increased. What is the independent variable in this study? What is the dependent variable? Why is random assignment important here?

clude that the differences are due to the IV and not to other ways in which the groups differ. For instance, we would not want someone to look at our study and say, "All the recreation majors were in the IV group in which participants worked alone. How do I know that this factor is not responsible for the better performance of this group?" Random assignment takes care of that possibility.

Internal Validity and External Validity

Internal validity

The ability to conclude from the study results that there is or is not a cause–effect relationship between the variables.

Experiments are usually high in **internal validity**—the ability to conclude from the study results that a cause–effect relationship does or does not exist. A research design is internally valid if it rules out alternative explanations for a relationship, or lack of one, between the variables. Random assignment to manipulated independent variable conditions, along with the control of the experimental situation, enhances internal validity. In short, if you compare groups that are virtually identical except for the independent variable, and these groups differ on the dependent variable, you can be reasonably sure that changes in the dependent variable were caused by the manipulation of the independent variable. Paradoxically, though, the very features of the laboratory experiment that contribute to internal validity also contribute to some of the shortcomings of the method.

Group dynamics researchers sometimes use artificial (ad hoc) groups because when researchers study real groups, they have no control over how the groups' histories might affect the variables under study. Studying new groups, with no history, keeps things neater because the researcher does not have to worry about how past history may influence current group behavior or interact with the independent variable. Short-term studies of ad hoc groups are also less expensive in terms of researcher time and resources. Although short-term laboratory studies of artificial groups have made significant contributions to the understanding of groups, this type of research paradigm has its critics. One such critic is McGrath (1990) who said:

Much of the empirical foundation of group theory derives from study of a limited range of types of ad hoc groups under controlled experimental conditions. Most of that work involves very small groups (two to four members) with constant membership arbitrarily assigned by an experimenter that exist only for a limited time without past or future as a group, isolated rather than embedded in any larger social units (organizations, communities). These groups are studied while performing single and relatively simple tasks arbitrarily assigned to them by the experimenter. . . . Such limiting features of the groups on which empirical evidence has been gathered systematically constrain the scope of the theories built on that evidence. (pp. 148–149)

McGrath (1990) emphasizes that real-world groups are complex social systems that engage in multiple, interdependent functions and concurrent projects while partially nested within, and loosely coupled to, surrounding systems. Groups, he says, are "multifunctioned"; they contribute to the systems in which they are embedded (such as organizations), their members, and themselves. Studies of ad hoc groups are limited in their ability to shed light on these more complex group dynamics because they are short-term and because they strip away contextual factors for the sake of experimental control (McGrath, 1997). For instance, using the short-term group study, it is difficult to study group development, termination, member socialization, and how various kinds of changes affect groups (McGrath, 1993). Furthermore, research findings from short-term temporary groups may not apply to longer-term groups. McGrath (1993) gives the example of the repeated finding of short-term research that computer-mediated groups produce lower-quality and lower-quantity work, but longer-term studies do not find this to be the case.

External validity

The extent to which a study's findings can be applied or generalized to other people and settings.

External validity is the extent to which your study's findings can be applied or generalized to other people and settings. Some critics of the experimental method note that laboratory settings may be so unlike the real world that the results from experimental research may not be applicable outside of the laboratory setting. Human participants, unlike atoms or rats, know they are being studied, and this knowledge may motivate them to impress, assist, or confound the experimenter (Steiner, 1986). The term **mundane realism** is sometimes used to refer to the extent to which an experiment is similar to real-life situations (Aronson, Wilson, & Akert, 1999). Generally, researchers work to make their experiments as realistic as possible. For instance, in group simulation research, a number of persons are brought together and, after a lengthy "get acquainted" session, are asked to work on a task, discuss an issue, or play a game. Independent variables such as the size of the group or the nature of the task are manipulated, after which the experimenter becomes as inconspicuous as possible (Steiner, 1986). However, the ad hoc group is by definition an ar-

Mundane realism

The extent to which an experiment is similar to real-life situations.

tificial group and, depending on the group phenomena being studied, may pose a problem for external validity.

Another external validity concern stems from the fact that sometimes the way a concept is represented in an experiment is unlike the way it is represented in real life. For instance, in some studies, an independent variable is manipulated and group productivity is measured in terms of how many uses an artificial group can generate for a brick. Can results from studies using these types of measures of productivity be applied to real group productivity in general? Detractors of the method might answer "No" or at least "We don't know for sure." Supporters of experimental research would say "Yes, even if the situation is artificial, you can still have **psychological realism** if relevant psychological and group processes are triggered" (Aronson, Wilson, & Akert, 1999). Who is right? We only know the answer after hypotheses that have been tested using the ad hoc group experimental method are repeated, or replicated, outside of the laboratory with real groups in real settings.

Psychological realism
The extent to which an experiment triggers relevant psychological and group processes.

Another external validity concern arises from the people that are most often studied by ad hoc experimental group researchers. Most of this research involves Euroamerican (white) college student participants and may or may not be applicable to people who are not white, American, and college aged. Until the 1980s, it was also typical for most experimental studies to be conducted with primarily male participants. Of course, this is not a problem if group processes operate the same in all people and are not influenced by gender and culture, but it is unlikely that this is the case for all group processes. The truth is that we cannot know how gender and culture affect group processes without conducting research with diverse samples of participants across cultures. Fortunately, there is a growing research literature on the role of gender and culture in group behavior, but because this is a relatively new area of study, there is still a lot we do not know.

Field Experiments

Field experiments
Experiments conducted in real-world settings.

The Lewin, Lippitt, and White (1939) study mentioned earlier is what is known as a field experiment. **Field experiments** are experiments conducted in real-world settings. They involve manipulation of an IV, random assignment to IV groups, and measurement of a dependent variable, but are not conducted in a laboratory setting. In principle, field experiments should enhance both internal and external validity. After all, if there is random assignment to IV conditions such that the groups are essentially equivalent except for the IV, then we should be able to say with some certainty whether changes in the DV are the result of the IV. And the fact that the experiment is in a real-world setting rather than an artificial laboratory one should boost external validity.

The reality, though, is that field experiments are seldom conducted in group dynamics. The reason is that it is exceptionally rare to have the power in a real-world setting to randomly assign people to independent variable groups.

Those who control the settings in which real groups operate, such as administrators and managers, are interested in getting the work of their organizations done. They are much less interested in furthering a scientific understanding of groups by letting a researcher systematically monkey around with factors such as group size, task, composition, leadership, or decision-making strategy. Furthermore, controlling the situation so that the groups remain equivalent except for the IV is also challenging. For instance, something unintended by the researchers, such as a drastic membership change, can happen to one of the IV groups but not the other. It then becomes difficult to say how this event influenced differences between the groups on the dependent variables.

Typically, there is a trade-off between internal and external validity because the control that gives us internal validity frequently reduces the similarity of the experimental situation to real-world situations. Conversely, when we study real groups over time, their sheer complexity makes it difficult to make causal claims with any certainty. A quick glance at the lengthy references of this book will tell you that this problem has not stopped group dynamics research. Instead, those studying group dynamics try to make up for the shortcomings of one method by studying the same phenomena with different methods. The idea is that we can get a more complete picture if we apply a variety of techniques and if we repeat studies with different people in different settings.

Meta-Analysis

It is risky to draw conclusions based on one study because there is always some chance that the results were obtained by chance and are not reliable. This is why you will generally find multiple research studies on any group topic. In order to reach conclusions about a phenomenon, it is necessary to compare and contrast the research findings (Johnson & Eagly, 2000). Those who study group dynamics often review past research to determine what we already know about group function and group process and to formulate plans of action to address critical problems in groups (Mullen & Driskell, 1998). After dozens of studies on a topic, it is time to see what the overall pattern of results tells us.

The Narrative Review

Narrative review
A method for examining the research literature on a topic by counting the number of studies that support a particular hypothesis.

Before the mid-1980s, these reviews typically involved examining the research literature on a particular topic, counting the number of studies that supported a particular hypothesis and the number that did not. Sometimes called the voting method of review, this approach is also called a **narrative review.** Narrative reviews had a number of problems. Independent narrative reviews of the same literature often reached differing conclusions; the reviewers examined a limited sample of studies and failed to consider how differences in study results might have led to differing research findings (Johnson & Eagly, 2000). For instance, one narrative review of the relationship between group cohesiveness and group performance concluded that research does not support a relationship, whereas another asserted with equal confidence that cohesion promotes productivity (Mullen & Copper, 1994).

The Quantitative, Statistical Review

Meta-analyses

A quantitative, statistical integration of the research literature done to arrive at an overall estimate of the size of the differences between groups.

In the past fifteen years, researchers have increasingly favored quantitative, statistical integrations of the research literature, called **meta-analyses.** In most chapters of this book, you will read about at least one meta-analysis. Meta-analyses involve the use of statistical techniques to combine information from many studies to arrive at an overall estimate of the size of the differences between groups (see Johnson & Eagly, 2000, for a detailed discussion). Whereas narrative reviews are qualitative syntheses, meta-analyses are quantitative. Unlike the narrative review, meta-analysis tells us more than how many studies found a statistically significant difference between IV groups. Meta-analysis tells us whether there is a difference between groups on some variable and gives us an estimate of the

Effect size

In meta-analysis, a statistic that indicates across studies how strong the research finding is.

effect size—how large the difference is or, to put it another way, how strong the finding is. This is important because researchers have traditionally reported only whether a difference between the IV groups is greater than that expected by chance (statistically significant), but even small differences between the groups can be statistically significant if variability within the groups is low. Even when a finding is generally accepted in group dynamics, it is useful to confirm it and to know how strong an effect the independent variable has on the dependent variable. For instance, Mullen, Salas, and Driskell's (1989) meta-analysis confirmed the belief among group dynamists that one of the strongest determinants of who emerges as the leader in an initially leaderless group is the group member with the highest rate of participation.

Statistical power

The ability to detect a difference between groups; when low, we may fail to detect a relationship between the variables even when one exists.

Meta-analysis also increases **statistical power**—the ability to detect a difference between groups. It is more difficult to obtain a significant effect when differences or effects are small, especially if you do not have many people in your study. In other words, small effects and sample sizes reduce statistical power. As a result, a statistical test may fail to detect a difference that is actually there (this is called a Type II or beta error in statistics lingo). Thus, we might falsely conclude there is no difference between the groups when in fact there is. Because meta-analyses combine data from a number of studies, statistical power is boosted. This means that sometimes a meta-analysis will find a difference between groups that was not revealed by the voting method (Lipsey & Wilson, 1993).

Meta-analyses are increasingly relied upon to inform us about the knowledge that has accumulated on various research topics (Johnson & Eagly, 2000). Standards for conducting such meta-analyses are thorough and precise. Great effort is made to collect all available research studies on the topic, including unpublished ones. Meta-analytic researchers carefully consider the independent and dependent variables that characterize the literature, and how they have been measured. They code each study on a number of factors that may affect research findings, such as methods, measures, and people studied.

Commonly, an effect size (d) is computed for each study by subtracting the mean of one group from the mean of the other and dividing this difference by the pooled within-group standard (Lipsey & Wilson, 1993). Cohen (1969) suggests that a d of 0.20 indicates a small effect size, 0.50 a medium effect size, and 0.80 a large effect size. The ds from each study are then averaged to get an idea of the overall size of the effect across studies (add up the ds and divide by the number of ds). A comparison of ds from studies from different time periods, or using different measures, methods, age groups, or contexts, may be also be undertaken in order to see how differences change over time and across situations. For instance, in a meta-analysis of social loafing studies (the tendency for people to slack off in a group), Karau and Williams (1993) found that the effect was larger for males than females and more pronounced as groups increased in size.

Mullen (1989) used meta-analytic techniques to compare group dynamics studies using ad hoc groups and real groups in naturalistic environments. Webster (1994) expected that results from artificial laboratory groups would be stronger because of the degree of control in the laboratory. Others, such as Shaw (1981), expected that independent variables might be more potent in real-world settings, and, therefore, that stronger effects might be seen there. After comparing the effect sizes of studies from four different topic areas in group dynamics (leadership, brainstorming, cohesiveness, and intergroup conflict), Mullen (1989) concluded that the study of artificial groups in the laboratory produces weaker effects than those in the real world.

Correlational Methods

Correlational methods
Nonexperimental methods that tell us whether variables are statistically related but cannot tell us about causality.

Many group topics that are worthy of study cannot be studied experimentally. Researchers do not always have the power to randomly assign participants to different types of group experiences and then measure and compare their behavior. **Correlational methods** are nonexperimental methods that tell us only whether variables are related, not whether one causes the other. In correlational research, the researcher does not manipulate any independent variables. Instead, a number of individuals or groups are measured on two or more variables, and statistics are used to determine if the variables are statistically related. As you'll see, the absence of experimental control and random assignment to independent variable conditions means that correlation is not causation.

The Correlation Coefficient

Pearson *r* (correlation coefficient)
A statistic, ranging from −1 to +1, that indicates how strongly two variables are related to one another.

The statistic that is used to indicate how strongly two variables are related to one another is called the **Pearson *r*, or correlation coefficient.** The correlation coefficient, which may range from −1 to +1, indicates the relative strength of the relationship between the two variables. The stronger the relationship, the more closely a change in one is mirrored by a change in the other, and the easier it is to predict the value of one variable if you know the value of the other. The *strength* of the relationship is indicated by how close the coefficient is to 1: The closer *r* is to 1 in either direction (+ or −), the stronger the relationship is between the two variables.

The positive or negative sign indicates the *direction* of the relationship between the two variables. If two variables are negatively related, it means that as one variable increases, the other tends to decrease. For instance, you might predict a negative correlation between member satisfaction and leader authoritarianism. In other words, the more leaders act like dictators, the less satisfied the members are. If the two variables are positively related, it means that they vary in the same direction; as one goes up, so does the other, and as one goes down, so does the other. Participatory leadership, in which leaders consult subordinates on important decisions that affect their work, is positively correlated with member satisfaction and commitment. This means that, in general, member satisfaction goes up as participatory leadership increases, and goes down as it decreases. However, we would not expect a strong correlation between the two variables because other factors such as pay, coworker relations, and the nature of the work also affect member satisfaction.

The Quasi-Experiment

Quasi-experiment
A correlational method in which real-world groups that differ on a quasi-IV are compared on a dependent variable.

One type of correlational method is called a **quasi-experiment.** At first glance, it looks like an experiment because groups that differ on some hypothesized causal variable are compared on a dependent variable. *Quasi* means "sort of" or "imitation," so a quasi-experiment is essentially an imitation experiment. In the quasi-experiment, real-world groups that differ on some variable such as gender

---

Apply It! ••• The Relationship Between Group Cohesiveness and Performance

How strong a relationship would you expect between group cohesiveness and group performance? Would you expect the two variables to be positively or negatively related? Correlational studies on the relationship between group cohesion (members' liking for one another and commitment to the group) and performance often find a small to moderate (0.30 to 0.50) positive correlation between group cohesion and performance. What does this mean? Why isn't the correlation stronger?

are compared on a dependent variable such as leadership style. The big difference between quasi-experiments and true experiments is that the researcher does not manipulate the IV; that is, participants are not randomly assigned to IV groups. The IV is a quasi-IV, not a real manipulated IV. For instance, Ennett and Bauman (1993) studied the role of peer group structure in adolescent cigarette smoking. In particular, they were interested in whether ninth-grade "clique members," "liaisons," or "isolates" smoked more. Clique members are those adolescents who are part of a small, closely knit collection of friends. Liaisons have at least two links with either clique members or other liaisons but are not clique members. Isolates have few or no links to other adolescent networks; they are not part of a clique and generally do not have friends that are either. Note that an experiment is not possible in this situation because the researchers could not manipulate the independent variable. They could not assign some students to be isolates, some to be clique members, and others to be liaisons. These are real-world groups, and students are what they are.

Correlation Is Not Causation

Researchers are fond of saying that correlation is not causation, meaning that correlational methods are low in internal validity. A correlation can tell us whether variables are related, but it does not tell us much about causality. When two variables are correlated, change in one is tied to change in the other, but there are three possible explanations for this relationship. It could mean that Variable A causes changes in Variable B, or that Variable B causes changes in Variable A. For example, a correlation between group cohesion and performance could mean that increased group cohesion causes increased performance, but it could also mean that when groups perform well, cohesiveness is enhanced. A correlation between two variables can also be spurious (coincidental or due to their joint relationship to some other variable). For instance, good leadership might be responsible for both higher performance and greater group cohesion.

Causality is a problem for the quasi-experiment as well. The lack of random assignment lowers the internal validity of the quasi-experiment. If the quasi-IV groups differ on the DV, we cannot easily rule out the likelihood that other differences between the groups, besides the quasi-IV, are actually responsible for the differences on the DV. For instance, Ennett and Bauman (1993) found that isolates smoked at significantly higher rates than did clique members or liaisons. However, because the study is a correlational one, there are a number of possible ways to interpret the findings. Social isolation may cause cigarette smoking due to stress or boredom (A may cause B). Or cigarette smoking could cause social isolation if peers reject smokers (B may cause A). Alternatively, smoking and social isolation may not cause each other but may both be caused by other factors such as deviant tendencies, loneliness, or depression (Variable C is responsible for the relationship between A and B).

Fortunately, advanced statistical techniques such as regression, path analysis, and structural equation modeling can make it easier to rule out the role of other variables in a correlation. For instance, you can statistically hold the effects of possible confounding variables "constant" so that you can see what the relationship between two variables is with the influence of others taken out. Even so, it is still true that correlation is not the same as causation. That being said, correlational research is useful. For instance, Ennett and Bauman (1993) note that their research findings suggest that the common emphasis of smoking prevention programs on cliques may be misplaced and that the peer group may be an ally in the prevention of smoking. Just keep in mind when reading correlational findings that correlation is not causation, and remember to consider the different possibilities for interpreting the findings.

Observational Techniques

Many years ago, Muzafer Sherif and his colleagues (Sherif, Harvey, White, Hood, & Sherif, 1961) conducted a classic study on conflict between groups (intergroup conflict). They took over a boys' camp in Oklahoma for several weeks and assigned incoming 11-year-old campers to one of two groups. After that, they introduced various factors to increase cohesion within each of the groups and to increase competition and conflict between the groups. Most of the data Sherif and his staff collected were derived from careful observations that he and his staff made of the campers as they went about performing their tasks (Kerr, Aronoff, & Messe, 2000). For instance, here is how Sherif (1966, in Kerr et al., 2000) described the cookout:

> The staff supplied the boys with unprepared food. When they got hungry, one boy started to build a fire, asking for help in getting wood. Another attacked the raw hamburger to make patties. . . . A low-ranking member took a knife and started toward the melon. Some of the others protested. The most highly regarded boy in the group took the knife, saying, "You guys who yell the loudest get yours last." (p. 77)

Observational methods
A set of nonexperimental methods in which observers watch groups to gather information.

Sherif used observational techniques. **Observational methods** are another set of nonexperimental method used by group dynamics researchers. The general idea is that an observer watches a group in order to determine what is really going on. As you are about to see, these methods vary in the degree to which the observer is an active part of the group. They also vary in how structured the observations are—that is, whether what they are looking for is clearly defined ahead of time (structured methods) or the observations are not made according to any prearranged criteria (unstructured methods).

Unstructured Observational Methods

Unstructured observational methods

A type of observational method in which observers provide impressionistic, descriptive accounts of the group.

Participant observation

An observational method in which the researcher becomes a member of the group being studied and keeps thorough field notes.

Observational methods may be unstructured or structured. In **unstructured observational methods,** observers offer impressionistic, descriptive accounts of the group. The researcher carefully observes the group and keeps a detailed diary (*field notes*) of the group's dynamics as s/he sees them.

One type of unstructured observational method is **participant observation.** In participant observation, the researcher becomes a member of the group being studied and keeps thorough field notes. An often-cited example of participant observation is an early study of gangs by sociologist William Whyte (1943). Whyte joined an Italian American gang in Boston and studied its leadership and structure for three and a half years. Another classic example comes from the work of Festinger, Reiken, and Schacter (1956). These researchers joined a "doomsday cult" and pretended they believed that the world was going to end. Their goal was to observe what happened when the group's prediction did not come true (followers convinced themselves that their faith had spared the world).

Participant observation is still used to study groups, often in combination with informal interviews with participants. For instance, Ezekiel (1995) attended meetings of neo-Nazi and Klu Klux Klan groups to get an insider's look at the nature of these groups. Martel (2001) studied Jewish masculinity in a group of Jewish Harley-Davidson riders. Drury (Drury & Reicher, 2000; Drury & Stott, 2001) used participant observation to study crowd behavior at political protests. Bock (2000) was a participant observer in two "single mothers by choice" support groups. Evans (2001) studied the normative structure of a cyberspace chat room as a participant in a "married life" chatroom.

One criticism of participant observation is that by being a participant, the researcher cannot help but alter the group in some way. Another concern is that in many cases, group members are unaware that the participant observer is observing them. Generally, ethical guidelines for research with human participants require that people give their informed consent before we involve them in our research. However, not only is this sometimes impractical when studying real-world groups, but when people know that they are being observed, they may change their behavior. Observers, especially a long-term observer of an ongoing group, should be prepared for the possibility that their observational role will be

Apply It! ••• Your Reaction to a Participant Observation

Imagine that you live in a fraternity or sorority house or with a group of roommates that you like quite well. At the end of the school year, a group member announces that s/he was not a "real" member but was in fact observing and recording the group's behavior all year long for a senior thesis. Would this be ethical? What would your reaction be?

discovered and the group will be angry at the deception. People do not like the idea that someone has been spying on them and feel betrayed and foolish when they find out.

Another problem with unstructured observational methods is that they easily permit the introduction of observer biases. You could go to the mall right now and take "field notes" on a group of teenagers. You could note who talks the most, the members who appear to be on the fringes of the group, and what the group does. Just write down everything you observe. However, if both you and I were to observe the same group, it is likely that we would perceive the group through our own personal lenses. For instance, once the researcher has formulated ideas about the group, s/he may be more likely to notice and interpret things in ways consistent with those ideas.

Unstructured observational methods provide data rich in detail but hard to quantify. They tend to be descriptive methods that give us impressionistic accounts of groups. However, some new statistical programs are useful in summarizing and categorizing unstructured observations.

Structured Observational Methods

Structured (systematic) observational methods

Quantitative observational methods in which group behaviors are observed and recorded with an objective coding system.

Structured (systematic) observational methods are more quantitative—that is, more easily reducible to numbers and statistical analysis. Behaviors that occur in the group are recorded in some systematic fashion. For instance, each time a behavior occurs, it is coded according to a set of categories designed ahead of time. Systematic observation methods were developed in part to solve some of the problems presented by unstructured observational studies (Bakeman, 2000). The idea is to develop a system of observation that is free from the biases and desires of the observers.

To use structured observational methods properly, researchers must meticulously develop their recording systems. Coding systems come from the research questions of interest to the researcher. The observer does not code everything, only those things relevant to the research question. The coding system serves as the "lens" of observational research (Bakeman, 2000). Therefore, it is essential that it be a well-focused lens providing an undistorted view. Another important consideration is that observers be carefully trained to ensure agreement among them about how to classify different group behaviors or events. Agreement across raters on how to code the activities of the group is called **interrater reliability.**

Interrater reliability

The extent to which the ratings of different observers are in agreement; boosted by careful training.

Observations may be made directly, by observers who are present while group members interact, or indirectly (by viewing videotapes). Some researchers observe the group "live," sometimes from behind a one-way mirror in a laboratory setting. Some observers sit quietly in the same room. Although observing and recording simultaneously is tiring, direct observation may allow the observer to better tune in to what is going on in the group (Bottorff, 1994). Many researchers prefer indirect observation. Videotaping the group and coding from the tape provide the advantage of repeated viewing so that the group experience can be more carefully analyzed by an unlimited number of judges (Bottorff, 1994). Indirect observation may also provide less interference with the natural flow of group activities (Cunningham & Olshfski, 1985). However, technical problems and group members' resistance to being videotaped can interfere with the effectiveness of indirect observations (Kacen & Rozovski, 1998).

Interaction Process Analysis (IPA)

Interaction Process Analysis (IPA)

An observational coding system developed by Bales to reliably measure six task and six socioemotional activities in a group

System for the Multiple Level Observation of Groups (SYMLOG)

A multimethod scheme for studying group behavior developed by Bales and intended to measure member personalities, member relationships, the group's dynamics, and how the group is affected by its organizational context.

The fact that observational methods have been used to study groups for more than fifty years has provided us with some important lessons (Kerr et al., 2000). One lesson is that efforts to capture the full spectrum of group activity should include categories of both task and socioemotional behavior because all groups face the problem of control and the problem of bonding (Kerr et al., 2000). IPA and SYMLOG are two widely used structured observation systems that rely heavily on this categorization.

In Chapter 1, you read briefly about **Interaction Process Analysis (IPA)** (Bales, 1950, 1970). IPA is designed to reliably measure task and socioemotional activities in a group. Recall that Bales proposed that these are the two basic activities of groups. Task activities are concerned with directing members to address the tasks with which they are confronted, and socioemotional activities are attempts to create and maintain bonds between members. IPA involves converting these broad categories into clear behavioral definitions that can then be observed and measured reliably.

Trained observers watch a group from behind a one-way mirror and rate behaviors using the twelve categories of the IPA system—six group task behaviors and six socioemotional categories (see **Box 2-1**). Examples of task (instrumental) behaviors include suggestions or questions about how to proceed and answers to factual questions. Socioemotional (expressive) behaviors include complimentary remarks, laughter, and statements of support or hostility. IPA is useful because it records the number of times a particular type of behavior has occurred and allows comparison across categories and group members (Forsyth, 1999). IPA is still used by researchers. For instance, in one study, IPA was used to investigate whether female and male groups of college students differed in their interaction style (Hutson-Comeaux & Kelly, 1996). The researchers found that females engaged in more positive socioemotional behavior and males engaged in more task-oriented behavior.

SYMLOG

Bales's (1988) **System for the Multiple Level Observation of Groups (SYMLOG)** provides one of the most detailed observational schemes for studying group behavior. Bales, the originator of SYMLOG, was a field theorist, and

---

BOX 2-1 / INTERACTION PROCESS ANALYSIS: TWELVE SCORING CATEGORIES

Socioemotional Categories

1. Shows Solidarity: jokes, raises others' status, gives help, rewards
2. Shows Tension Release: laughs, shows satisfaction
3. Shows Agreement: passive acceptance, understands, concurs, complies
4. Shows Disagreement: passive rejection, formality, withholds help
5. Shows Tension: asks for help, withdraws "out of field"
6. Shows Antagonism: deflates others' status, defends or asserts self

Task Categories

1. Gives Suggestion: direction, implying autonomy for others
2. Gives Opinion: evaluation, analysis, expresses feeling, wish
3. Gives Information: orientation, repeats, clarifies, confirms
4. Asks for Information: orientation, repetition, confirmation
5. Asks for Opinion: evaluation, analysis, expression of feeling
6. Asks for Suggestion: direction, possible ways of action

Source: Hare (1996b).

Upward-downward (U-D) dimension

In SYMLOG, whether the behavior of a group member, group, or organization demonstrates values of dominance (U) or submission (D).

Positive-negative (P-N) dimension

In SYMLOG, whether the behavior of a group member, group, or organization is friendly (P) or unfriendly (N).

Forward-backward (F-B) dimension

In SYMLOG, whether the behavior of a group member, group, or organization supports the task orientation of the established authority (F) or opposes the established authority (B).

SYMLOG measures the interactive "field" of influences on the group. SYMLOG uses a number of methods to achieve an understanding of (a) the internal dynamics of individual personalities; (b) the relationships of the particular group members to one another; (c) the overall dynamic tendencies of the total group; and (d) the effects of the broader organizational culture on the inner workings of the group (Bales, 1988). In contrast to IPA, SYMLOG is based on the systematic observation of real groups (rather than ad hoc laboratory groups), and ratings are usually made by group members (rather than observers) who know each other well (Bales, 1988).

One basic idea in SYMLOG theory is that three sets of general value dimensions can be used to characterize individuals, groups, and organizations (Hare, 1996b). The **upward-downward (U-D) dimension** represents whether the behavior of a group member, group, or organization demonstrates values of dominance (U) or submission (D). For instance, is an individual active, dominant, and talkative, or passive, introverted, and quiet? The **positive-negative (P-N) dimension** refers to friendliness (P) or unfriendliness (N). Is the person's behavior friendly and democratic or disagreeable, self-interested, and self-protective? The **forward-backward (F-B) dimension** has to do with values supporting the task orientation of the established authority (F) or values opposing the task orientation of the established authority (B). Authority is defined broadly to include customs, group norms, and rules as well as people in positions of authority. The general question is whether the person favors conservative, established, "correct" ways of doing things, or change and creativity.

SYMLOG instruments usually measure twenty-six different combinations of the three dimensions and how frequently an individual or group exhibits a value or behavior (Hare, 1996b; Polley, Hare, & Stone, 1988). For instance, someone who scores high on the NB (negative-backward) combination values nonconformity and seems cynical, irritable, and uncooperative. A DNB (downward-negative-backward) person acts alienated, quits, and withdraws. A UNB (upward-negative-backward) person is a rugged individualist who "shows off" in the group. A person high on the PF (positive-forward) combination would be agreeable and cooperative, and would be idealistic and helpful to others. A UPF (upward-positive-forward) person appears as a purposeful, democratic leader. A DPF (downward-positive-forward) person is gentle, respectful, and willing to accept responsibility.

It is also common to ask individuals to use the twenty-six categories to answer a number of questions. such as "In general, what kinds of values do you personally wish to show in the group?" "What kinds of values do you tend to reject in the group?" "What kinds of values need to be shown by your team in the future to be effective?" "What kinds of values are currently shown in the culture of your organization?" "What kinds of behaviors does Member X show in the group?" The questions asked depend on the purpose of the consultation or study. Respondents answer each question by indicating for each of the twenty-six descriptive values how often it is represented (rarely, sometimes, or often).

SYMLOG is often used by organizational consultants (Hare & Hare, 1996). Computer technology permits the integration and analysis of data so that individual SYMLOG reports can be provided to each group member and an overall report provided to the group. The intention is to provide information to the group that indicates the changes needed to enhance group performance. For instance, one measure permits individuals to diagnose their own interpersonal effectiveness. Other measures identify the values among the individuals that contribute to or interfere with effective teamwork. Reports include tentative suggestions as to why a group member or the group may be viewed in a particular way and what changes would improve teamwork (Bales, 1988). For example, an individual's report may suggest that his group members' ratings of him indicate that he may underemphasize important team behaviors such as being friendly and cooperative, and overemphasize behaviors that undermine teamwork such as being pessimistic, rebellious, and cynical. The consultant may then suggest awareness and skill building or may recommend moving the individual to a role where teamwork is not required. **Box 2-2** adapts some concepts from SYMLOG to help you consider your group behavior.

HW
D

BOX 2-2 / CONSIDERING YOUR GROUP BEHAVIOR

Choose a group that you are a member of and rate your behavior in the group using the following scale:

Strongly Agree	Agree	Neutral	Disagree	Strongly Disagree
5	4	3	2	1

1. _____ "Uninvolved" is a word that group members would use to describe me.
2. _____ Other group members would say that I have a good sense of humor.
3. _____ Group members would describe me as pessimistic and cynical.
4. _____ "Group oriented" would be used by group members to describe me.
5. _____ Group members might describe me as someone that doesn't care much whether others like me and who "goes it alone."
6. _____ Group members see me as dedicated and faithful to the group.
7. _____ I am viewed by group members as indecisive and hold my thoughts and feelings back from the group.
8. _____ My fellow group members would agree that I foster democratic decision making in the group.
9. _____ Group members would describe me as rebellious and unruly.
10. _____ The words "outgoing," "sociable," and "extroverted" would be used by group members to describe me.
11. _____ Group members perceive me as putting my personal interests ahead of the group.
12. _____ I am viewed by group members as helpful to new members and to established members who need extra support.
13. _____ Group members would describe me as quietly content to do my own thing and let the group do its own thing.
14. _____ "Cooperative," "reasonable," and "constructive" are words group members would use to describe me.

Scoring: Add scores of odd-numbered items (1, 3, 5, 7, 9, 11, 13), and divide by 7. The closer your score is to 5, the more you express values and behaviors that interfere with teamwork. Add scores of even-numbered items (2, 4, 6, 8, 10, 12, 14), and divide by 7. The closer your score is to 5, the more you express values and behaviors that contribute to teamwork.

Reflection: Rate yourself as a member of several different groups—for instance, as a family member, workgroup member, and social group member. Compare and contrast the results. Looking back at your responses, what things were revealed that you are satisfied and proud about? What things were revealed that you would like to work on? How might you do this?

Source: Based on the ideas of Bales (1988).

Researchers also use SYMLOG to study groups and the effectiveness of group training programs. For instance, Lawrence and Wisell (1993) used SYMLOG to measure group and individual effectiveness on the three major SYMLOG dimensions before and after a leadership training program in which managers practiced feedback skills and group process methods in a workshop. The increased use of feedback skills resulted in higher ratings on the SYMLOG values of dominance and friendliness. Another study of managers (Hare, Koenigs, & Hare, 1997) compared managers' ratings of themselves and the values they judged to be effective for a manager. Comparisons were made with coworkers' ratings of the manager and the coworkers' ideal profile for the manager. Managers and coworkers both agreed that model managers should be more dominant and friendly than they were rated to be. However, coworkers thought the managers should be less task oriented while managers thought they should be more task oriented.

Sociometry

Sociometry

A technique for analyzing the pattern of relationships among group members—in particular, hierarchies, friendship networks, and cliques within the group.

Sociometry is a technique for analyzing the pattern of relationships among group members—in particular, hierarchies, friendship networks, and cliques within the group. First described by Jacob Moreno (1934), sociometry can be used in a variety of ways, from studying peer relations in children to studying power relations in organizational settings. Although sociometry as practiced today is largely a quantitative method dominated by the use of complex statistical programs, it was originally intended as a simple way to depict the structure of relations among the members of a group.

Sociogram

In sociometry, a graphic display of group members' ratings of one another.

A **sociogram** is a graphic display of group members' ratings of one another. Typically, each group member uses a five-point scale to rate his/her liking of other group members. For instance, each member of your workgroup assigns one of the following ratings to every other member in the workgroup:

1. "I would like to have this person as one of my very best friends."
2. "I would enjoy working with and doing things with this person."
3. "I do not know whether I would like to spend time with this person since I don't know them very well."
4. "I do not care very much for this person but I would be nice to them if I saw them."
5. "I speak to this person only when absolutely necessary."

(derived from Berg, 1998)

This information can be presented in several different ways. A sociogram can be created with circles representing individual group members and arrows between them labeled with the ratings. Often individuals who are preferred by many group members ("stars") are placed in the center, those who are preferred by few ("isolates") are put on the edges, and members who form cliques are grouped together ("chains"). Sociometric information may also appear in tabular form. For instance, ratings for each individual can be presented in a **sociomatrix** with members' names across the top and down the side. Ratings can be averaged to indicate the **sociometric status** of each group member (the average level of liking by other members).

Sociograms and sociomatrices are starting points for understanding a group, not an endpoint. By revealing the group structure, they provide the researcher with a clear direction as to how best to proceed. For instance, identifying stars can be important for knowing who best to approach to disseminate information, introduce changes to the group, or gain access to the group (Berg, 1998). Sociomatrices and sociograms may also indicate where interpersonal problems are in a group, which individuals need coaching, which relationships need strengthening, and what disputes need resolution (Hoffman, Wilcox, Gomez, & Hollander, 1992). As Hoffman et al. (1992) say, sociometry is especially effective because it builds on data that group members accept, enables members to see themselves as others do without provoking defensiveness, and frames interpersonal problems objectively.

Sociomatrix
In sociometry, a tabular presentation of group members' ratings of one another.

Sociometric status
In sociometry, an average rating of how much a member is liked by other group members.

Surveys and Questionnaires

Surveys/questionnaires
Paper-and-pencil instruments used to measure various aspects of group functioning, dependent variables in experimental studies, and variables in correlational studies.

Surveys and **questionnaires** are frequently used as tools by group dynamics researchers. These paper-and-pencil instruments are used when there is no other way to get the information but to ask people. They can be used to measure various aspects of group functioning, such as the extent to which a group operates as a team, or to measure individuals' group skills such as conflict resolution. They can be used to measure dependent variables in experimental studies and variables in correlational studies, or they may be used simply to provide feedback to a group and its members.

Open-Ended and Closed-Ended Survey Items

Open-ended items
Questionnaire items that permit participants to answer in whatever way they choose, with no preset options to choose from and no rating scales.

Open-ended items permit participants to answer in whatever way they choose; there are no preset options to choose from and no rating scales. For instance, "Please comment on what happened in your group today" is an open-ended item. An advantage of open-ended items is that they frequently produce rich and detailed answers. However, they are also frequently difficult to interpret and to quantify. It is sometimes challenging to figure out what participants meant and to combine different participants' responses to make some definitive statements about how many people fall into different categories. For these reasons, open-ended questions are often used more *qualitatively* (to add depth to the inquiry), and closed-ended questions are used more quantitatively (for the computation of statistics and scores). Open-ended questions are also useful in developing options for closed-ended items when you do not know what the range of responses might be.

Closed-ended items require that participants respond to items using the options provided. For instance, one common closed-ended format uses a Likert scale that ranges from Disagree Strongly (1) to Agree Strongly (5). Participants use the scale to indicate the extent to which they agree with survey items. **Box 2-2** is an example of a questionnaire that uses this format. Other types of rating scales are common as well. The semantic differential format requests that the person taking the questionnaire answer in terms of a series of bipolar adjective scales. For example, you could be asked to rate your leader on a seven-point scale anchored at one end by the adjective *democratic* and at the other by the opposite adjective, *autocratic*. Variations on these themes are also found. You might respond to statements about your group using a scale anchored at one end by *Very True of My Group* and at the other by *Not At All True of My Group*, or to statements about your group behavior on a scale ranging from *Always* to *Never*. Oftentimes, questionnaires are designed so that the different items measure different aspects of the same underlying concept, such as group cohesiveness. In these cases, the person's scores on the different items are combined to provide an overall score.

Both closed-ended and open-ended items have advantages and disadvantages. Closed-ended items are easier for participants because they have to write less, but they interfere with creative responses and lack the personal flavor provided by open-ended items. On the other hand, responses to closed-ended items are easier to code, analyze, and summarize. Responses to open-ended items are often difficult to read, may be interpreted in several different ways, and are difficult and time-consuming to analyze. Despite these problems, though, open-ended questions often provide a depth and insight that closed-ended questions do not. Given the relative advantages and disadvantages of the two types of items, many researchers use both.

Closed-ended items
Questionnaire items that require participants respond to items using the options provided.

Designing a Valid Questionnaire

Regardless of whether open-ended or closed-ended items are used, several things are important to consider. One of these has to do with question wording. Items must be developed carefully to avoid biased, leading, or confusing items. The point is not to ask the question in a way that gives you the answer you'd like to hear, but rather to ask the question in a way that best gets at the truth as the respondent sees it. The items must be as clearly stated as possible so that the different respondents understand items in the same way. Otherwise, it is as if participants are not answering the same questions. In the case of closed-ended questions, it is important that the options provided cover all possible responses so that people are not forced to choose an answer that does not really represent them.

Construct validity

The extent to which a research instrument measures what it is intended to measure.

It is challenging to construct a measure that is high in **construct validity**—that is, one that measures what it is intended to measure. To develop a valid measure, researchers spend a lot of time defining the concept and then trying to capture the concept through questionnaire items. For instance, Henry, Arrow, and Carini (1999) developed a measure of "group identification"—members' identification with an interacting group. To do this, they carefully reviewed past writings on the topic and noted similarities and differences between group identification and related concepts. Then, they developed fifty-six items that appeared to correspond to their theoretical definitions. Next, they collected data five times using five different sets of items with 965 college students so that they could identify the survey items that best measured group identification. Ultimately, they ended up with twelve items that measured three different components of group identification. For instance, participants who strongly identify with their group are expected to agree with items such as "I enjoy interaction with the members of this group," "All members need to contribute to achieve the group's goals," and "I think of this group as part of who I am."

Reliability

An indicator of whether a measure consistently measures what it is intended to measure.

A measure may be subjected to a number of different tests of validity. For example, the test should measure what it appears to measure. This type of validity, called *face validity*, is often measured by showing the instrument to those who are knowledgeable in the field. To assess *convergent validity*, the instrument may be correlated with other instruments that are known to measure similar concepts. Correlating the measure with some behavioral outcome assesses *predictive validity*. In addition, for a measure to be valid, it must consistently measure whatever it is that's being measured. This consistency is referred to as the **reliability** of a measure. Using the instrument more than once with the same people and correlating the scores from the different test administrations typically demonstrate test–retest reliability. If the measure is reliable, then individuals should score roughly the same at different testings. Researchers also correlate items with other items or with the total score and then average the correlations to determine whether the items are all tapping into the same thing.

Social desirability bias

In research, the tendency for people to act in a socially desirable manner or give a socially desirable response instead of a more honest one.

One problem with surveys and questionnaires is the **social desirability bias.** People often do not want to admit to less than socially desirable behaviors or thoughts. They may also want to "help" by giving the answer that they think the organization or the researcher wants. For these reasons, it is generally a good idea to emphasize in the instructions the importance of honesty. Also, if possible, responses should be either anonymous (no personally identifying information) or confidential (identities are known by the researcher but are not revealed). The instructions should specify this information as well.

Apply It! ••• **Your Experience With Surveys and Questionnaires**

What is your experience with surveys and questionnaires? Have you taken surveys with closed-ended items that restricted you to answers that did not accurately describe your response? Have you been asked questions on a survey or by an interviewer that were confusing or unclear? Have you ever answered less than honestly due to the social desirability bias?

Case Studies

You have probably seen or at least heard of popular television shows like *Survivor,* and *Boot Camp,* and *The Real World.* These shows are in many ways what researchers would call case studies of a single group. You could watch these shows and identify leaders, group norms, cliques, and communication networks, among other things. **Case studies** are in-depth profiles of groups. There are case studies of cults, government leaders at international summits, religious communes, and rock bands (Forsyth, 1999). Case study researchers often use a variety of research methods to gather data on a group. For instance, a case study of a coronary care unit conducted by Manias and Street (2001) included participant observation, individual interviews, focus groups, and an examination of journals kept by group members. Historical records such as biographies or newspaper accounts are also used to analyze what happened in a group.

Case studies
In-depth profiles of groups.

Case studies are often conducted with the intention of saying something about a particular type of group. An example is the work of Hackman (1990), who conducted a **collective case study** of 33 different workgroups (collective case studies involve the study of several cases). The goal was to identify the factors leading to effective teamwork. Based on these cases, Hackman (1998) concluded that the majority of work teams are ineffective. They make such mistakes as using a group to do a task better done by a talented individual, and expecting a group to operate as a team when members are not skilled and experienced in teamwork. Hackman (1998) acknowledges that this type of research is unable to definitively identify the causes of team success but notes that experimental research on the impact of varying team designs is not viable in real-world organizations. For instance, managers would not tolerate random assignment of people to teams, and teams to varying independent variable conditions. This is a common criticism of case studies—they may provide us with rich information, but few definitive conclusions. Case studies are a popular method for studying actual group performance but require that researchers have direct access to the facts and circumstances surrounding an actual case of effective or ineffective group performance (Hirokawa, De-Gooyer, & Valde, 2000).

Collective case studies
In-depth studies of several cases with the goal of saying something about a particular type of group.

Apply It! ••• **Do Your Own Group Case Study**

Many movies and television shows focus on a small group. For instance, the movie *A Perfect Storm* is about a crew of fishermen, and MTV's *The Real World* is about a group of roommates, and *That 70s Show* is about a friendship group. Do your own case study of a group on a television show or in a movie. Who are the members of the group? Who is the leader of the group, and how does s/he lead? Who is the most liked person? The least liked? What are the norms of the group? What conflicts were present, and how were they resolved?

Ethics in Group Dynamics Research

When conducting research, group dynamics researchers must take care to protect the rights of the groups and people they study. Harm to groups or their members should never occur as a result of research. In general, this means that privacy must be respected, dignity preserved, and information kept confidential. Researchers follow a number of guidelines to ensure that their work is ethical. These guidelines are detailed in publications such as the American Psychological Association's (1992) *Ethical Principles of Psychologists and Code of Conduct*. If researchers do not conduct research in an ethical manner, their professional reputation is harmed, and they will be unable to publish or present their work.

Informed Consent

Informed consent

A statement signed by research participants prior to participation in a study; it provides enough information that they can make a knowledgeable decision.

Prior to collecting data, most researchers have research participants sign a statement, called an **informed consent,** indicating that they were not coerced into participation and freely gave their consent to participate. These informed consent statements include enough information that potential participants can make a knowledgeable decision about whether they want to participate. For instance, participants are told whether their responses are anonymous or confidential and are informed of any potential risks associated with participation. In most cases, they are given a general description of the study's purpose. They are also told how the findings will be used and who to contact in case of questions or distress. It is also typical to inform them that they may withdraw at any time during the study.

Informed consent is not usually obtained when the study is an observational one conducted outside of an organizational setting. It is generally agreed that if a public behavior is easily observable, and the identities of those observed are concealed when reporting is done, then it's "no harm, no foul." Also, in some cases, the study description in the informed consent is deliberately inaccurate because if participants were told the true purpose or topic of study, they would behave differently. In cases like this, and in others where deception is part of the research design, the informed consent includes information suggesting that deception may be used in the study.

Confidentiality

Confidentiality

The researcher's commitment to protect the identities of those studied.

It is important to protect the identities of research participants to safeguard their dignity and maintain their privacy. In addition, research participants may not be honest in their responses if they believe that these responses can be traced back to them. For these reasons, researchers often promise participants **confidentiality** (the researcher knows participants' individual responses but removes all identifying information before reporting study results) or anonymity (even the researcher does not know which participant said what). Even when informed consent is not used, when reporting results, researchers take care to disguise the identities of those studied.

Debriefing

Debriefing

Sharing the details and results of the study with research participants at the study's conclusion.

When possible, researchers share the results of the study with the research participants. This **debriefing** involves giving participants a fairly detailed description of the study's purpose, explaining any unusual procedures (such as deception) and why they were necessary, and telling them how they contributed to scientific knowledge through their participation.

Ethical Review Boards

Ethical review board

A government or university committee that reviews proposed research to determine whether it is in accordance with standard ethical guidelines.

In most cases, researchers have to get their proposed study approved by an **ethical review board** before they can proceed. Most universities and government agencies require that proposed research be reviewed by a committee of researchers knowledgeable in the ethical guidelines developed by the government or by a discipline's national professional organization. These committees, which go by various names including Ethical Review Boards, Human Subjects Committees, and Institutional Review Boards, scrutinize the methodology and make a decision about whether the proposed study is ethical. They are especially concerned with protecting participants from physical, social, or psychological harm. Before granting approval, the committee may require changes in the informed consent or in the procedures to better protect participants.

Concept Review

Experiments

- Experiments are designed to test cause–effect relationships and involve the systematic manipulation of an **independent variable** and measurement of a **dependent variable.** In group dynamics research, it is common for experiments to be conducted with **ad hoc (artificial) groups** brought together for the purposes of study.

- **Experimental confounds** are extraneous factors that confuse our ability to draw clear conclusions. **Experimental control** and **random assignment** are used so that any changes in the dependent variable can be attributed to the independent variable.
- Although experiments are high in **internal validity** (the ability to conclude a cause–effect relationship from the study results), their artificiality and limited samples mean that they are sometimes low in **external validity** (the extent to which the study results can be generalized to other people and places). **Field experiments** maximize internal and external validity but are uncommon because in real-world settings, researchers rarely have the degree of control required.

Meta-Analysis

- **Meta-analyses** are quantitative, statistical integrations of a research literature. Meta-analyses tell us whether there is a difference between groups on some variable and how large the effect is. Standards for conducting meta-analyses are thorough and precise, and great effort is made to collect all available research studies, including unpublished ones.

Correlational Research

- In **correlational research,** nonmanipulated variables are measured to see whether change in one variable is associated with change in another variable. In some correlational research, a **correlation coefficient** is computed that indicates the relative strength and direction of the relationship between two variables. Another type of correlational research is the **quasi-experiment,** in which real-world groups are compared on a dependent variable. Although correlational methods are useful, they are low in internal validity, and results must be interpreted cautiously.

Observational Research

- **Observational techniques** are another nonexperimental method. Observations may be unstructured or structured, with the former offering more qualitative data and the latter providing more quantitative data.
- In **participant observation,** the researcher becomes a member of the group being studied. Critics of the method note that observer biases are likely with this type of **unstructured observation** and that ethical concerns are serious when group members are unaware that a fellow member is actually a researcher.
- **Structured observational methods** require that group behaviors be observed and recorded according to a set of categories developed before the observations are made. Recording systems must be carefully developed and observers carefully trained so that **interrater reliability** is high.

- **Interaction Process Analysis (IPA)** is an observational system in which trained observers rate a group on six categories of task behavior and six categories of socioemotional behavior.
- **SYMLOG (System for the Multiple Level Observation of Groups)** measures a number of different influences on the group, including members' personalities and the effects of organizational culture. SYMLOG assumes that three sets of value dimensions characterize individuals, groups, and organizations: dominance–submission, friendliness–unfriendliness, and adherence to authority–opposition to authority.

Sociometry

- **Sociometry** is a technique that uses group members' ratings of one another to analyze the pattern of relationships among group members. These relationships may be depicted graphically in a **sociogram** or in a chart called a **sociomatrix.**
- Sociometry can be used to identify who is best to approach to disseminate information or introduce changes to the group. It may also be used to indicate where interpersonal problems lie in the group.

Surveys and Questionnaires

- **Surveys** and **questionnaires** are paper-and-pencil measures used to measure various aspects of group functioning or individuals' group skills.
- **Open-ended items** permit participants to answer in whatever way they choose; **closed-ended items** provide answering options. One especially common closed-ended item rating scale is the Likert scale, in which participants indicate the extent of their agreement with various statements.
- For all types of survey items, it is important to carefully word items and options and to take the time to construct a valid measure of the concept under study. It is also important to take steps to reduce the **social desirability bias**—people's tendency to provide the socially desirable response even when it is inaccurate.

Case Studies

- **Case studies** are in-depth profiles of groups. Case study researchers may use a variety of research methods, such as observation, interviews, and surveys, to gather their data.
- **Collective case studies** involve the study of more than one group and are used to gain information about a particular type of group.
- Although case studies provide rich information, causal conclusions are not possible, and it can be difficult to gain access to all relevant facts and circumstances surrounding a group.

Ethics in Group Dynamics Research

- Group dynamics researchers protect the rights of the groups and people they study by following a number of ethical guidelines.
- Prior to collecting data, researchers may have participants sign a statement, called an **informed consent,** indicating that they were not coerced into participation and freely gave their consent to participate. These informed consent statements include enough information that potential participants can make a knowledgeable decision about whether they want to participate.
- Researchers take care to maintain **confidentiality** by disguising the identities of those studied or having participants respond anonymously.
- When possible, researchers **debrief** participants by sharing the results and details of the study.
- **Ethical review boards** examine proposed research studies to determine whether they are in accordance with standard ethical guidelines. Their job is to protect participants from physical, social, or psychological harm. Before granting approval, the committee may require changes.

Study Questions

1. How do the main features of the laboratory experiment conducted with ad hoc groups enhance internal validity? What criticisms are made of this research paradigm?
2. What is meta-analysis, and why is it favored over the narrative review?
3. When is correlational research used? What is a correlation coefficient, and what does it indicate? What is a quasi-experiment? What does it mean to say "correlation is not causation"?
4. What is the difference between structured and unstructured observational methods? What is the difference between qualitative and quantitative observational methods? Why is interrater reliability important to structured methods?
5. What is participant observation? What are some criticisms of it?
6. What is IPA, and how is it used?
7. What is SYMLOG? How are SYMLOG instruments used to provide feedback on the three value dimensions that characterize individuals, groups, and organizations?
8. What is sociometry, and what are sociograms and sociomatrices used for?
9. What are the advantages and disadvantages of closed-ended and open-ended questionnaire items?
10. What should one consider when constructing questionnaire items?
11. How do researchers evaluate their measures to make sure that they are valid and reliable?
12. What do group dynamics researchers do to ensure that their research is ethical?

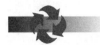

Group Activities

Activity 1: Make a Sociogram

Many television shows are about a group of friends or coworkers. Choose such a show that all group members are familiar with. Make a sociogram in which each TV show member is represented by a circle and arrows from one circle to another represent whether the relationship is positive or negative (use a + or − sign). Place individuals that are preferred by many group members ("stars") in the center, and put those that are preferred by few ("isolates") on the edges.

Activity 2: Design a Measure

Researchers spend many months, if not years, refining their measures. This activity will give you some hands-on experience with part of this process. You (or you and your group) will construct a ten-item measure of a group concept such as leadership ability, conflict resolution skills, or "slacking" (you do not have to choose one of these).

Begin by writing down ideas that you think represent the concept. Next, think about how to turn these ideas into closed-ended items. It may be helpful to review the section of the chapter on closed-ended items, in particular the part on Likert and semantic differential rating scales. Include instructions at the top and, possibly, self-scoring and interpretation at the bottom. Refine your measure by having several people fill it out. Ask them to note whether any of the items were confusing or hard to understand, and whether the response categories exhausted all meaningful answers. Obtain some measure of validity. Make a final version after changes based on the feedback you received. For what purpose(s) could your instrument be used?

Activity 3: Discuss the Ethics

With your group, discuss whether the following research studies are ethical.

1. A researcher wants to study group dynamics in social change groups. To do this, he joins an environmental group trying to stop logging in a remote wilderness area. He attends every meeting, which he secretly tapes, and afterwards makes detailed notes. Although they know he is a group dynamics researcher at the university, they do not know that they are the objects of his study. He plans to publish his findings but will disguise the identity of the group and use pseudonyms for the members.
2. A researcher wants to study group dynamics in groups of adolescents. She has discovered that several groups of teens hang out daily at the mall. She can observe them easily while appearing to be studying at the mall's eateries.

InfoTrac College Edition Search Terms

To do research for your papers and assignments, use InfoTrac that's provided free with new copies of this book. Go to: http://infotrac.thomsonlearning.com and enter the following search terms:

- Small Group Research, Psychology
- Meta-Analysis Groups
- Observational Research
- Sociometry

Chapter 3 Norms and Roles in Groups

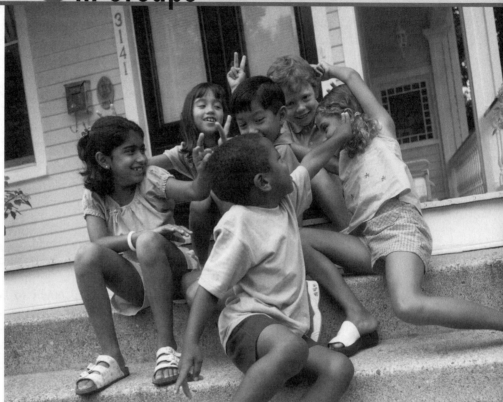

© John Henley/CORBIS

This chapter is on group norms and roles. Group member behavior may be based in part on member personality, but it is also strongly influenced by the group's norms, and by the member's position or role in the group.

As noted in Chapter 1, one important feature of groups is that they are *structured,* and two components of a group's structure are its norms and roles. One of the first things people think of in regard to groups is that groups have rules about what is acceptable in the group and most people experience some pressure to conform to these rules. That we know the power of group norms is illustrated by worries that our children will become part of peer groups with norms that require them to smoke or do illegal drugs. We know that group norms in cults can be so powerful that members will give all their material possessions to the group, marry complete strangers, or commit suicide. We are aware that at times we change our behavior to be accepted, even though internally we don't agree. We fear groups, such as gangs, that have norms supportive of violence. We like leading groups whose members agree on norms conducive to productivity. We love being part of a group whose members share values and develop group norms based on these values. We appreciate groups with norms that require that all members be included and valued and that encourage cooperation among members. When we are new to an established group, we are grateful for clear communication regarding what is expected of group members, and what is expected of us in our new role.

Why do groups develop norms and roles? Why do we conform to them? How can we change a group's norms? What group norms have positive outcomes, and how can we promote these in a group? When do norms lead to destructive group behaviors, and what can we do about this? These are the topics explored in this chapter.

Group Norms

Norms

Shared expectations about how the members of a group ought to behave.

Norms are rules regarding what group members should think and do, what is okay, and what is not okay, according to the group. Norms are the group's standards as to what constitutes normal behavior in the group. They are shared expectations about how the members of a group ought to behave (Levine & Moreland, 1990). Norms may be formal, stated in regulations and handbooks, or verbally and explicitly agreed upon. They may also be informal, never explicitly discussed, but nonetheless important to the group.

Why Groups Have Norms

On the television cartoon show *The Simpsons,* Bart establishes an exclusive club headquartered in a treehouse, complete with a set of detailed rules. Indeed, one of the first orders of business for a new group is often to establish norms. Groups establish norms for a variety of reasons. One prominent reason is that by structuring member behavior, norms enable the group to function more efficiently and smoothly. Festinger, Schacter, and Back (1950) call this source of group norms "group locomotion" because uniformity of group standards helps to "locomote," or propel, the group toward its goal.

People like the predictability and comfort that norms and conformity to them provide. Norms have heuristic value (a *heuristic* is a strategy that reduces the amount of thinking we have to do). After a time, we know the group's norms and comply with them almost unconsciously. Norms also reduce uncertainty in the group by helping us know what to expect of others. Once norms are established or learned by new members, members can simply behave accordingly with relatively little thought and little negotiation. This frees up energy for task performance and reduces member stress.

Norms may also contribute to groupness, because these shared standards may distinguish the group from other groups. The group's norms often represent the group's identity by signifying members' shared values and assumptions. Familiarity with the group's norms is one way to distinguish insiders from outsiders, thereby norms contribute to the group's cohesion.

How Norms Develop in Groups

The initial patterns of behavior in a group often solidify into norms (Feldman, 1984). Over time, most groups develop standardized operating procedures (SOPs)—that is, customary ways of doing things. They begin doing something in a certain way, and that becomes the group's common practice or tradition. For instance, members of a friendship group may arrive at a routine way to celebrate birthdays, and that becomes the group's tradition. Members of a workgroup or roommate group begin handling cleanup chores in a particular way and adopt this as a permanent practice. A student club or community service organization always does the same thing every year for a particular event. Critical events in the group's history may also lead to the development of group norms (Feldman, 1984). For example, groups often develop rules to deal with problem member behaviors.

Institutional norms
Norms that originate in a group's leader or external authorities.

Voluntary norms
Norms negotiated by a group, often to resolve conflict and promote smooth functioning.

Evolutionary norms
Norms originating in a member's response to a situation that is adopted as a norm by the group.

Norms can arise in three ways (Opp, 1982). **Institutional norms** are determined by a group's leader or by external authorities. Maintaining accreditation from a national accrediting body may require that a hospital unit enact norms regarding infection control. A college class may have a norm of taking a break at a particular time, but it is an institutional norm if the professor decided it. The group negotiates **voluntary norms,** often to resolve conflict and contribute to the smooth functioning of the group. For instance, a group of housemates may agree that members must wash their dishes immediately after a meal so that they are available for others to use. After fighting over toys, a group of children agree that if a toy is put down on the ground, other members are free to play with it. A workgroup agrees that meetings will start on time and that latecomers will be responsible for taking meeting minutes. Finally, **evolutionary norms** develop when a member responds to a situation in a particular way and other members adopt that response as well. One time I observed a member of a new student project group immediately denounce the task as stupid (actually, I believe the word "sucks" was used). Other members adopted this attitude as a norm, and this dramatically affected what happened in this group in comparison to other class groups that evolved positive norms.

Members who have experienced norms in other groups that seem appropriate for this group also import norms into the group (Bettenhausen & Murninghan, 1985; Feldman, 1984). From past group experiences, people have scripts that specify proper behavior in various situations (Levine & Moreland, 1990). You will often hear group members say things like "In this other group I was in, we did such-and-such and it worked pretty well." The speed with which norms develop and the amount of negotiation they require depend on the extent to which group members share scripts for situations (Levine & Moreland, 1990).

Members are generally good about conforming to group norms and doing what the group expects of them. Although we may not like to think of ourselves as conformists, the reality is that most of us are, and it usually benefits us to be so. As you will see next, the tendency to be influenced by group norms is a natural one, rooted in our need to belong and our reliance on others for information.

Conformity Due to Informational Pressure

Life and what to make of it is not always self-explanatory, and we rely on information from others to help us make sense of it. In Chapter 1 you read that one function of groups is that they provide us with needed information. Think back to your first day at a new school or job. Did you proceed cautiously, following the lead of others, because you were not sure what to do and assumed they did? Have you gone along with a group's majority because you had not yet formed an opinion and so trusted that they were right? Have you been uncertain what to think about a new policy or new group member and talked with other uncertain group members to arrive at a joint decision about what to think? These are examples of group influence due to **informational pressure.** This occurs when members conform because of a need for information. Not knowing what to think or what to do, a member goes along with the group on the assumption that the group is right. Or when the group is uncertain, members talk and arrive at a group decision about what to think or do.

Informational pressure

The pressure to conform because of uncertainty and a need for information.

Sherif's Classic Study on Informational Pressure

Perhaps the most famous study of informational pressure is Muzafer Sherif's 1936 study showing the development of norms in a group. The Sherif study is important because it demonstrates conformity due to a need for information and shows that conformity due to informational pressure produces real changes in both behavior and belief. The study also shows the formation of norms in a small group.

Sherif took advantage of the *autokinetic effect,* a perceptual illusion in which a pinpoint of light in the dark will appear to move erratically. For instance, sometimes a star in a very dark sky will appear to move, the taillights of a car at night will appear to trail, or as we turn off a television in a dark room the light of the dimming picture will appear to dance ever so briefly. The autokinetic effect is an ambiguous stimulus because it is hard to say with certainty how much movement occurred.

In the Sherif study, participants seated in a totally dark room saw a small dot of light appear fifteen feet in front of them for two seconds. Asked to esti-

Figure 3-1

Sherif's Study of Informational Influence

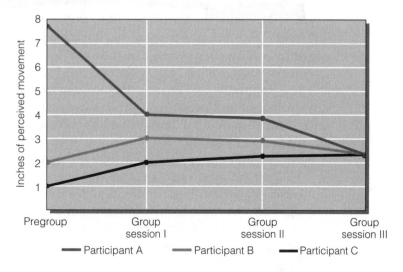

As shown in the graph, participants' estimates of the light's movement were quite different when made independently, but over a three-day period the estimates converged and a group norm was born. The study demonstrates the formation of group norms and how group members arrive at a joint perception when situations are ambiguous.

Apply It! ••• How Groups Form Opinions of New Members and Policies

In what way is a new group member, leader, or policy an ambiguous stimulus? Think of three cases: one in which your group arrived at a group norm regarding what they were to think of a new member, one in which it was a new leader, and one in which a new policy was introduced. Did the process the group went through in each case mimic the one described in the Sherif study? Did the norms persist?

---

mate how much the light had moved, participants gave estimates varying from one to ten inches. Next, they performed the task in three-person groups for three days. The dot was flashed, and people announced their estimates. On day one, the members quickly adjusted their estimates toward the others. By day two, the convergence was even greater, and by day three, the group arrived at an agreement as to how much the light was moving (see Figure 3-1). Later, members were tested away from the group. This time, their estimates reflected the group's norm, rather than their initial estimates. In other words, they came to believe the estimate established by the group.

Informational Pressure in Ambiguous and Stressful Situations

Informational pressure is more likely when a situation is ambiguous and members are uncertain (Baron, Vandello, & Brunsman, 1996; Wooten & Reed, 1998). This makes sense when you think about it: If the situation is clear-cut, there is no need for information, and members will not need to turn to others to decide what to think or do. Crises are especially ambiguous because the group does not usually have established procedures for behaving and may receive conflicting information regarding the severity of the situation and how to handle it. Research in social psychology shows that in a crisis, people will take their cue about how to respond from others (see, for example, Latane & Darley, 1970). For instance, you can imagine that the hijacked plane passengers on September 11, 2001, took their cue from other passengers. On three of the planes, the scared passengers complied with the hijackers. However, on the fourth plane, it appears that a few passengers redefined the situation as one requiring intervention. They shared their view with the others, and the passengers stormed the hijackers. Although the plane crashed, it did not crash into the intended political target in Washington, DC.

In general, it serves us well to look to others for information in ambiguous situations and in crises. However, group members may unwittingly conform to the wrong informational cues, as demonstrated by **pluralistic ignorance.** Pluralistic ignorance describes how bystanders in an emergency fail to act because of faulty assumptions about what is appropriate. Because no one else is doing anything, bystanders assume that nothing should be done, but of course they are all looking to other ignorant bystanders for cues as to what to do. Pluralistic ignorance is a case of informational pressure backfiring; everyone is misled by everyone else's inaction.

Pluralistic ignorance

Occurs when group members mistakenly assume that others know what's going on; a backfiring of informational pressure.

Most studies of pluralistic ignorance involve groups of strangers. However, long-term groups often face uncertain environments and crises when, for instance, they hear there may be company layoffs, cutbacks, or takeovers. In such cases, members will seek information. Unfortunately, group leaders sometimes keep the group in the dark about the details of changes that may affect the group. Often they are just too occupied with managing the change, do not want to alarm members, or do not want to deal with members' emotional reactions. But what leaders should keep in mind is that in an uncertain organizational or group climate, members share what little information they do have and arrive at a group judgment. These judgments, which may be based on inaccurate information, can affect morale and member behavior.

Mass psychogenic illness

The occurrence in a group of people of similar physical symptoms with no apparent physical cause.

One extreme case of informational pressure gone awry is **mass psychogenic illness,** the occurrence in a group of people of similar physical symptoms with no apparent physical cause (Colligan, Pennebaker, & Murphy, 1982). The group "illness" usually begins with a report by one or two group members of vague illness. Other group members then experience similar symptoms triggered by false information or fear. Frequently, group members are under stress and misattribute their physical stress symptoms based on a label provided to them by the social context.

A number of psychologists have studied real-life cases of psychogenic illness (for example, Colligan & Murphy, 1979; Singer, Baum, Baum, & Thew, 1982). In one classic case during World War II, a woman in a small town in Illinois claimed that a stranger had sneaked into her bedroom in the middle of the night and "gassed" her, resulting in partial paralysis and illness. Soon, many residents were making similar charges. An expensive state investigation uncovered no evidence in support of the phantom. Once police announced that they thought it was a case of mass hysteria, there were no more incidents (Johnson, 1945).

Mass psychogenic illness is not merely a relic from the past. In 2001, many Americans were fearful following several bioterrorist incidents involving deadly anthrax bacteria. In one month, at least three different groups falsely thought they had become victims (Roan, 2001). In Maryland, a mentally ill man sprayed a substance in a subway, and several dozen passengers experienced headaches, nausea, and sore throats. In Tennessee, an office worker claimed to have opened a foul-smelling envelope, and soon she and sixteen coworkers complained of dizziness. In Washington State, more than a dozen middle-school students and a teacher claimed they smelled fumes and became faint. In all three cases, health officials could find no evidence of dangerous substances.

Informational Pressure and Improving Group Effectiveness

Since most of the problems that arise in connection with informational pressure can be said to come from *mis*informational pressure, the key is to obtain or supply accurate information and to reduce uncertainty.

1. Avoid pluralistic ignorance. In ambiguous situations, be aware of the tendency for groups to form opinions based on misinformation and misinterpretation of the situation. Do not be too quick to assume what others are thinking or that what appears to be the group's perception is the correct one. Ask questions, seek evidence, and encourage discussion. If your "gut" tells you that the group may be wrong, check it out.

2. If you are in a leadership position, and you want to influence or manage member perceptions, it is best to share information about changes that will affect the group. Do what you can to reduce uncertainty and ambiguity. Otherwise, the group will come up with their own version of reality, a version that may hurt morale and productivity.

3. Members can be mistaken about what is normative in the group and can misinterpret social informational cues. To prevent such mistakes, be open and specific about the sentiments of the group or leaders. For instance, Prentice and

Miller (1996) found that most students overestimated their peers' support for heavy alcohol consumption and that many then conformed to this misperception. Students who participated in discussion sessions in which these misperceptions were corrected drank less alcohol six months later than members of a control group who took part in discussions focusing on personal responsibility.

Conformity Due to Normative Pressure

Group members definitely conform because of a need for information, but they are also likely to conform so that they will be accepted by the group. You probably learned this lesson as a child when peers shunned children who were different from the average. You also know that, to some extent, adult groups are not much different. A neighbor who violates neighborhood norms regarding landscape maintenance may not be invited to neighborhood parties or spoken to at the mailbox. A coworker who arrives late and leaves early may no longer be invited to lunch with the group. A group member who questions the group's normal ways of doing things may be ignored. A family member who violates the family norm that requires marrying a person from the family's religion may be scorned.

Normative pressure

The pressure to conform in order to be socially accepted and avoid rejection.

The pressure to conform in order to be socially accepted and avoid rejection is called **normative pressure.** Chapter 1 emphasized that humans have a basic need to belong. Our motivation for conforming to group norms stems partly from our desire to be accepted and included in the group, and a basic desire to be liked by other group members. One of the worst feelings in the world is to be shunned or avoided by other group members—to have them communicate, in essence that maybe we don't really belong after all. Psychologically, the experience of being an outsider or "deviant" is difficult, and we avoid this experience through conformity to group norms. Obviously, the more important the group is to us, the greater is the motivation to conform and avoid social punishment. As Cartwright and Zander (1968, p. 145) note:

> Rejection of a deviant can be accomplished in various ways. He may be set apart so that no one talks to or listens to him, he may be dropped from activities of the group, or he may be expelled. Obviously, the more attractive the group is to a member, the more he wishes to avoid such extreme sanction. Paradoxically, the greater the cohesiveness of the group is, the more likely the members are to reject the deviant member.

Chapter 2 described a famous study conducted by Stanley Schacter (1951), in which those who disagreed with the group were the least liked group members and were assigned the most undesirable of the group's tasks. At first, the groups spent a lot of time trying to get the deviate to conform. If he did, he was accepted completely; if he did not, he was rejected. According to Levine (1989), a number of studies confirm the general finding that groups reject deviates, especially when the group is cohesive and the deviance seriously interrupts progress toward a group goal.

Research also indicates that the group's tolerance of a member's deviation is based partly on the member's status. Members who have earned a high status in the group through a history of conformity to group norms are allowed to deviate more, with fewer punishments (Giordano, 1983; Hollander, 1960), unless their deviance creates a major obstacle to goal attainment (Levine, 1989). In cases where the deviance interferes with group locomotion, it appears that deviance hurts the evaluation of a high-status member more than it does a lower-status person because we expect less from a low-status member. We have a strong expectation that high-status members will act in the best interests of the group; therefore, a failure to do so is experienced as an especially serious violation.

Asch's Classic Study on Normative Pressure

The fear of social rejection and the uncomfortable feeling of being a "freak" are so strong that it may be hard to go against group norms even when the group is obviously wrong. This was documented in a classic study conducted by Solomon Asch in 1956. Asch was not surprised that conformity was so great in the Sherif autokinetic study; after all, the situation was ambiguous. But what about a crystal-clear situation? Would individuals conform to an obviously wrong majority? To find out, Asch had research participants perform a line-judging task in which they determined which of three lines was similar to a "comparison" line (see Figure 3-2). Participants made their judgments after six experimental confederates (accomplices of the experimenter) had expressed their estimates. For the first two trials, the confederates gave correct judgments. However, on the third trial, the confederates one by one made an obviously wrong choice. In all, the confederates gave a clearly wrong answer on 12 of the 18 trials, and participants conformed to the wrong estimates approximately 37 percent of the time. About 50 percent of the participants conformed 50 percent of the time, and 76 percent conformed at least once. A replication of the study in the 1990s yielded similar results, although participants did not conform quite as much (Larsen, 1990).

Most of Asch's participants did not believe the majority's estimates and conformed only to avoid looking unusual. Alone, they had no uncertainty regarding the task. Unlike Sherif's participants, they did not come to believe the group. As Moscovici (1985, p. 349) noted, it is a matter of "going along with the group, even when the individual realizes that by doing so he turns his back on reality and truth." When Asch (1956) interviewed participants afterward, they reported that it was hard to publicly disagree with the majority—they felt "crazy," "conspicuous," and like a "misfit." Nonetheless, they did resist to some

Figure 3-2

The Line Judgment Task Used in Asch's Study of Normative Influence

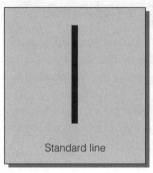 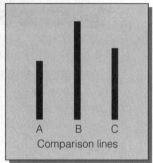

Standard line   A   B   C
                                 Comparison lines

Participants were asked which comparison line, A, B, or C, was the same length as the "standard line." The task was clear-cut. When Asch's participants conformed to a wrong majority about a third of the time, it was taken as evidence of normative pressure—conformity due to a desire to be liked, not right.

extent. Although Asch's participants conformed 37 percent of the time, they did not conform the other 63 percent of the time, and 25 percent refused to conform to any of the majority's wrong answers (Friend, Rafferty, & Bramel, 1990).

Factors Enhancing Normative Pressure: Social Impact Theory

Social impact theory
A theory stating that conformity depends on strength (how important the group of people is to you), immediacy (how close the group is to you in space and time), and number (how many people are in the group).

You do not conform to the norms of every group. According to **social impact theory** (Latane, 1981), conformity depends on three factors: (1) *strength*—how important the group of people is to you; (2) *immediacy*—how close the group is to you in space and time; and (3) *number*—how many people are in the group.

If you do not care about a group or what members think of you (strength), then you will not be motivated by normative pressure. Conversely, when we are highly attracted to a group and identify strongly with it, we are more likely to conform due to normative pressure (Abrams, Wetherell, Cochrane, Hogg, & Turner, 1990; Clark & Maas, 1988; Nowak, Szamrej, & Latane, 1990). This is probably why the tendency to conform is especially great in adolescence when individuals define themselves in terms of their peer groups and so desperately want their approval (Brown, Clasen, & Eicher, 1986; Gavin & Furman, 1989).

In terms of immediacy, the visibility of our behavior also makes a difference: the more public the behavior, the greater the conformity. If the group will not know you did not conform, then of course the negative consequences of deviation are unlikely. Asch (1956) demonstrated this in a variation of his original study when he had participants write their answers on a piece of paper instead of

Apply It! •••	**Normative Pressure and Voting in a Small Group**

Think back to situations in which a group vote was taken and *how* the vote was taken. Explain why voting by a show of hands (or by saying "aye" or "nay"), rather than by anonymous ballot, may influence the results of a group vote. Are you more likely to vote your conscience when an anonymous ballot is used?

saying them aloud. Conformity dropped dramatically (occurring on average 1.5 times out of 18 trials) because the participants no longer had to worry about what others would think if they went against the group.

With regard to number, social impact theory suggests that conformity increases, at least to a point, when the group size is three or more. Research indicates that each additional person in a group increases conformity until the group reaches a size of four or five people, after which adding additional conforming members does not increase the level of conformity. In other words, we are no more likely to conform in an extremely large group than we are in a small group, but we are more likely to conform in a group of five than we are in a group of three. We are also more likely to conform when the group is unanimous. A little later in the chapter, you will learn that the presence of even a single dissenter can encourage others to disagree with the majority.

Tight cultures
Cultures in which norms are clear and reliably imposed and deviance is punished through criticism and rejection.

Culture, Gender, and Normative Pressure

Culture also makes a difference when it comes to normative pressure because some cultures and subcultures have more tolerance for deviation than do others. Triandis (1994) writes that **tight cultures** tolerate much less deviation than **loose cultures.** For instance, Japan is a tight culture, in which norms are clear and reliably imposed and deviance is punished through criticism and rejection. In general, the United States is a loose culture, in which norms are less clear and deviance more tolerated, although some subcultures such as gangs or cults are tight. Triandis suggests that cultural homogeneity (similarity among people in a culture) and isolation from other cultures leads to a tighter culture because there is more agreement about what is correct behavior. Looser cultures tend to have many cultural influences and so may decide that no one norm is "correct."

Loose cultures
Cultures in which norms are less clear and deviance is tolerated.

Culture also makes a difference in conformity to norms because some cultures emphasize the importance of the group and values such as social harmony and cooperation (**collectivistic cultures**), whereas others emphasize the importance of the individual and values such as independence (**individualistic cultures**). People in collectivist cultures, such as many Asian, African, and South American cultures, value conformity for the sake of group harmony and because their fate is seen as interdependent with that of others (Hofstede, 1980; Smith & Bond, 1999). People in individualistic cultures, such as the United States, The

Collectivistic cultures
Cultures that emphasize the importance of the group and community and that value conformity.

Individualistic cultures
Cultures that emphasize the importance of the individual, value independence, and view conformity negatively.

Netherlands, Great Britain, and Canada, value independence of judgment and see conformity negatively (Smith & Bond, 1999). In a meta-analysis of cross-cultural replications of the Asch (1951) line-judging study, Bond and Smith (1996) found that conformity was highest in cultures with higher collectivism scores. Effect sizes were smallest in the North American and Western European studies.

Social stereotypes about the genders might lead us to believe that in comparison to men, women are more conforming because they are more dependent and submissive (Eagly & Wood, 1985). A meta-analysis of 148 studies from 1949 to 1977 found a small effect for gender: 56 percent of the males were less influenceable than the average woman in the studies, but 44 percent of the men were more influenceable (Eagly & Carli, 1981). The effect was largest for studies on group pressure in which the subject is pressured by other group members to change beliefs or behavior. This effect may occur because females are more "communal" and committed to preserving social harmony and good feelings among group members (Eagly & Wood, 1985) or because social norms suggest that men should be independent and not easily influenced (Eagly et al., 1981). Eagly et al. found that men conformed less when they thought group members had access to their opinions than they did when others presumably did not know what their opinion was. This factor did not affect women's conformity.

One interesting finding in regard to gender and influenceability is that the gender of the researcher seems to make a difference in whether gender differences are found. Eagly and Carli (1981) reported that men conducted 79 percent of the studies finding that females were more influenceable and that male researchers tended to find larger differences than did female researchers. Eagly and Carli suggest that perhaps researchers are more likely to design, implement, and report their studies in ways that flatter their own gender.

Maupin and Fisher (1989) found that gender differences in influenceability are affected by the gender-related content of the influencing task and whether female or male superiority on the task is evident. In other words, when we feel competent, we conform less. Eagly and Wood (1982) and Eagly (1983) suggest that women's lower social status in both the home and the workplace may contribute to the perception that women conform more than men. Persons who are lower in power and status are generally expected to yield to the influence of higher-status others. Because individuals have seen more instances of males than females occupying higher-status roles, they have also seen more instances of females being submissive and conforming than males. The studies on gender differences and conformity are now old, and gender roles have changed. Without new research, it is hard to say whether the small gender differences found so many years ago persist.

Normative Pressure and Improving Group Effectiveness

The average person cares what others think, and the average group uses this to ensure conformity to group norms. Normative pressure can be useful in getting members to comply with norms that help the group meet its goals. But it can also encourage conformity to norms that are harmful to the group or its members. For instance, Crandall (1988) studied two sororities with norms supportive of bulimia, an eating disorder characterized by binge eating and self-induced vomiting. Popularity in the sororities was partly a function of conformity to the group's bulimia norms.

Here are some suggestions for using normative pressure to improve group effectiveness.

1. Group pressure can be brought to bear on deviant members whose actions hurt the group, but it is important that the group clearly communicate what norm was violated and why it is important to the group. Immediate feedback, even nonverbal feedback (such as shaking your head to indicate "no"), is better than a later exclusion that the "deviant" may not connect with the relevant norm violation.

2. If conformity is important to the accomplishment of the group's task, you may wish to do things to foster group cohesiveness (see Chapter 6 on group development).

3. To change maladaptive norms or create new norms, enlist the help of high-status group members who agree to discuss, model, and reinforce new norms. Burn (1991) created new recycling norms in neighborhoods by appointing neighborhood "block leaders" (neighbors who already recycled) to talk with their nonrecycling neighbors. Informational communications should also suggest that the new norm is now socially appropriate by including proof that "everyone is doing it" and "experts" recommend it (Burn, 1991; Cialdini, 2001).

4. To really find out what group members think, ask them privately and, ideally, anonymously. This will reduce the influence of normative pressure.

5. Make desired norms clear and specific. Members have to be aware of what attitudes and behaviors will result in approval before they can comply with group norms.

Dissent

Conformity to group norms has its good and bad points. On the one hand, going along with group norms usually contributes to the smooth functioning of the group, and it certainly reduces the amount of thinking we have to do (simply comply with the group rule!). Conformity is also rewarded with social approval and acceptance. On the other hand, though, conformity to outdated norms can reduce group productivity and stifle creativity by preventing change when change is needed. Rigid conformity can also lead to bad decision making when members are reluctant to go against what they think is majority opinion by expressing reservations about the direction the group is headed. There are even times when groups develop norms conducive to unethical or antisocial behavior. In short, there are times when it is appropriate and desirable to challenge group norms—that is, to **dissent**. Furthermore, there is evidence that such dissent improves the quality of group decision making.

Dissent
To challenge group norms.

Minority Influence

Dissenters give others that disagree with the majority the courage to voice their disagreement, but can these minority members influence the majority members to change their minds? Although it is certainly true that groups may apply considerable pressure to members that do not conform, and may even ignore them or force them out of the group, the case should not be overstated. Indeed, years of research suggest that a small chorus of dissenting voices can significantly sway the group. For instance, in one classic study (Moscovici, Lage, & Naffrechoux, 1969), a minority of two people in a six-person group significantly influenced judgments about the color of slides. The blue and blue-green slides were proclaimed by the minority to be green. Most of the majority changed their characterization of the blue-green slides from blue to green, consistent with the minority, and nearly 9 percent of them went along with the minority in judging the blue slides as green. The idea that a minority of group members can influence the majority is called **minority influence.**

Minority influence
The idea that a minority of group members can influence the majority.

Idiosyncrasy Credits

There are several approaches to minority influence. Earlier in the chapter it was suggested that higher-status members are given more leeway in going against the group's norms. For this reason, some experts recommend that if you want to be effective in going against the group, you must first earn the right to do so. This is the basic idea behind Edwin Hollander's (1958, 1960) **theory of idiosyncrasy credits.** To be idiosyncratic is to act according to one's eccentricities, or as a distinctive individual. Hollander suggests that over time, being a good little group member who conforms most of the time earns us the right to be idiosyncratic. In other words, idiosyncrasy credits are essentially conformity "brownie points" that, once earned, may be cashed in later. Also, once you have spent time in the group conforming, you are likely to have earned a higher status in the group. This means that when you challenge a group decision or practice, others are more likely to conform, either because your status enhances your credibility or because they believe there may be negative consequences to them if they do not. Several studies support the idea that the strategy of first conforming and then dissenting is effective (Bray, Johnson, & Chilstrom, 1982; Lortie-Lussier, 1987).

Theory of idiosyncrasy credits
A theory suggesting that to dissent effectively, you must first earn the right by paying conformity dues called idiosyncrasy credits.

Innovation

One advantage of biding your time and waiting before you risk challenging group norms is that once you are established in the group as a well-liked, higher-status member, you can deviate with less risk to your popularity. However, at times it may feel wrong to sit back and let a majority's poor group decision or tradition go by without comment, despite the potential popularity risk. In such

Theory of innovation
A theory suggesting that a strong, persistent minority can effectively sway the majority and cause true change.

cases, can a minority change the mind of the group's majority? According to Serge Moscovici's (1985, 1994) **theory of innovation,** the answer is yes—a strong, persistent minority can effectively sway the majority. The minority will initially be thought to be in error, and will be probably be disliked for disrupting the group's process, but as long as the minority is persistent, consistent, and rational, and not biased, stubborn, or crazy, members will usually rethink their positions (Moscowitz, 1996). Even if the group does not make a direct or immediate movement to the minority position, the group may change the way it thinks about the issue (Nemeth, 1994).

Moscovici's theory is called "innovation" because it is assumed that a group that changes its mind as a result of minority influence has changed because the minority ideas have merit. In other words, when people go along with the majority or a high-status other, they often do so for social approval (normative pressure in action), without really thinking deeply about an issue. Therefore, oftentimes, their conformity is merely external compliance, not internal conversion. In contrast, when they go along with a minority, it is usually because the conflicting viewpoints have provoked them to reexamine the situation and make real changes in their opinions (informational pressure in action). In other words, there is genuine change and conversion. A meta-analysis of nearly 100 studies (Wood, Lundgren, Ouellette, Busceme, & Blackstone, 1994) supports this idea. The minority's introduction of information challenging to the group causes the group to examine the situation more carefully, leading the group to adopt all or part of the minority view. The idea that majorities and minorities both exert influence on the group but in different ways is often called the **dual-process approach to minority influence.**

Dual-process approach to minority influence
The idea that majorities and minorities both exert influence on the group, but in different ways.

The Importance of Minority Positions

Meetings may drag on and decisions may take longer when some members insist on questioning the group. Minority views create stress, anger, and irritation in the group (Nemeth, 1994). But before you get too irritated with minority members or hesitate to express your own minority views, you should keep in mind that minorities can positively influence group performance. In one study, groups with one dissenting confederate came up with more original solutions to difficult business problems than did groups without such a confederate (Van Dyne & Saavedra, 1996). According to one of the leading minority influence researchers, Charlene Nemeth (1994, p. 11), "We find that minority dissent appears to provide practical benefits. Our research shows that exposure to minority dissent stimulates us to take in more information, to think about that information in more divergent ways, to perform better, to think more creatively, and to detect correct solutions that otherwise would have gone undetected." The minority view may be true or only partially true, but either way, it stimulates the detection of correct solutions (Nemeth & Wachtler, 1983).

Dissenters are also important because they give others the courage to go against the group's majority. For instance, when Asch (1955) planted a confederate in the group who agreed with the participant, conformity was reduced by almost 80 percent. Later studies indicated that it does not matter whether the person agrees with the dissenter or even whether the dissenter is a respected group member; the mere presence of a dissenter is enough to break the spell of the majority (Allen & Levine, 1969, 1971). Dissenters model courage and, in doing so, foster independence (Nemeth & Chiles, 1988). Dissenters can change our perception of the situation. When at first it appeared that we should keep dissent to ourselves, now it appears okay to have a different opinion. Dissenters can dispel our perception of an unanimous majority where our disagreement would be useless.

Occasionally, the willingness of one person to speak up can change the whole course of the group's plans as it becomes evident that the majority position was illusory—that everyone agreed because of a false assumption about what everyone else wanted. Sometimes called the **Abilene paradox,** this is especially likely when members are highly motivated to maintain good group relations (Harvey, 1988). Here is a version of the story often used to illustrate. Imagine a Texas family on a 110-degree day. One member suggests that they go to Abilene (a 60-mile drive without air conditioning). He does not really want to go but is trying to be nice. He thinks that the others are bored and probably want to go where more is happening. The next person to speak up also does not want to go but, to be supportive, says "Maybe that would be fun." So, a third person (who also does not want to go) says "Well, yeah, we could do that." The fourth person is thinking to herself "I'd rather drive to hell," but because she has the impression that everyone else wants to go, she says "Okay, let's go." And so they go to Abilene in the sweltering heat. No one has a good time. Upon their return, one person remarks, "That was terrible. I didn't even want to go to Abilene." It quickly becomes apparent that no one wanted to go, and they all realize that if even one person had spoken up they all could have avoided a miserable trip.

Abilene paradox

Occurs when members are so motivated to get along that they all end up agreeing to something no one wants.

The Implications of Deviance for Enhancing Group Effectiveness

You have just learned that dissent can play an important role in a group. Here are some related suggestions for improving group effectiveness.

1. Encourage the expression of minority viewpoints because they may bring to light information that will result in a better group decision.
2. If you are a low-status or new group member and it is apparent that the group tolerates little deviation, the safest strategy for deviating from the group is to first earn high status.
3. If you have not yet earned high status in the group and are a relatively new group member, you can still influence the group if you calmly and persist-

---

BOX 3-1 / YOUR INCLINATIONS TO CONFORM AND DISSENT

Use the following scale to respond to each item: Strongly Agree (7), Agree (6), Agree Somewhat (5), Neither Agree nor Disagree (4), Disagree Somewhat (3), Disagree (2), Strongly Disagree (1)

1. _____ I am generally a confident person.
2. _____ I like to go against trends.
3. _____ I pride myself in being able to take an unpopular stand in the group.
4. _____ I am generally hesitant to go against the majority.
5. _____ I usually go along with the group even if what I want is different from the group.
6. _____ I might think I know what I want or think, but if the group seems to think differently, I will usually change my mind.
7. _____ Sometimes I find myself resisting the group's will, just to be different.
8. _____ I do not like to "rock the boat" by questioning what seems to be the group's majority opinion.
9. _____ I am often unsure what to think or do.
10. _____ I do not care very much whether group members like me or not.

Scoring: Average your scores for items 1, 2, 3, 7, and 10 to get an indication of how easily you go against group norms. The closer your average is to 7, the stronger are your tendencies not to conform. Next, average your scores for items 4, 5, 6, 8, and 9 to get an indication of your tendency to go along with groups. The closer your average is to 7, the greater are your conformist tendencies. Look back at the items and the way you answered them. Are you satisfied with your typical level of conformity? Does your conformity undermine the group's effectiveness? Does your lack of conformity undermine the group's effectiveness?

---

ently present a reasonable argument. However, it is true that this may negatively affect members' liking of you.

4. Avoid the Abilene paradox. Before going along with what seems to you to be a questionable decision, consider the possibility that others (maybe even a majority) may agree with you but are not speaking up. Gently but assertively question the group's position to provide others with the courage to speak their mind.

Norms and Group Performance

So far, you have learned about the development of norms and why group members conform to them. But what types of norms should be promoted in a group, and how can this be done? How should norm violations that interfere with the group's mission be handled?

Teaching Norms to New Members (Socialization)

One reason why it is very stressful to be a new group member is that a new member may have only a general idea regarding what is expected and acceptable in the group. This unfamiliarity with the group's norms makes the newcomer feel like an outsider in the group. Normally, group norms reduce the amount of thinking we have to do, but trying to discern the group's norms requires a lot of effort on the part of new group members.

The learning of group norms is accomplished largely through observation. New group members typically hang back and observe the group to see how the group operates (and to avoid violating any norms). They watch other members and see what behaviors are rewarded and what is punished. They also learn through trial and error. For instance, they receive praise and acceptance after behaving consistently with the group norms. When they do not conform, they receive criticism, correction, or the "cold shoulder" (members avoid eye contact or conversation with deviants and exclude them from social interactions).

Socialization

The process by which new group members learn the norms of the group.

The more time new members spend figuring out the group's norms through observation or trial and error, the more time it takes them to become productive group members. A conscious effort on the part of the group to socialize new members can significantly decrease the time it takes them to learn the ways of the group. Larger groups often formalize many of the group's norms in handbooks, and these formal norms may be reviewed in official orientation sessions. This can be helpful, but many of the group's informal norms may be equally important. For instance, most workgroups have production norms that specify how hard members are to work. Also, many group members find that what leadership says the norms are and what they are in practice are different. It may say in the employee handbook that coming late or leaving early is unacceptable when in fact it is done all the time without penalty. It is important, then, to teach new members about these other norms.

Unfortunately, it is hard to inform new members of group norms when the group itself is largely unaware of many of its norms. As Forsyth (1999) pointed out, groups rarely vote on which norms to adopt. Instead, norms emerge gradually as members align their behaviors to match certain standards. As a consequence, norms are often taken for granted so fully that members do not realize their existence until a norm has been violated. This is why it often makes sense for members to reflect on their own experiences as new group members and to use these as a guide when socializing new members into the group. It can also be a good idea to have relatively new members who can easily recall the experience of being new to the group serve as mentors to new group members. Such members may be most likely to remember the unspoken norms of the group that they learned the hard way. Mentors also give new members someone to go to with questions about the group's norms.

Apply It! ••• How Did You Learn Norms as a New Group Member?

Describe your experiences as a new group member in an established group and the process by which you learned the norms of the group. For instance, consider experiences such as taking on a new job or joining an existing club or other social group. Family experiences such as moving from one parent's home to the other (in case of divorce), foster care experiences, or being a new member of a romantic partner's family group can also be used to illustrate the concepts discussed in the previous section. What might the group have done to help you learn the group's rules more quickly?

Responding to Norm Violations in the Group

Compliance with group norms is often essential to the smooth functioning of the group. Ideally, the group has norms that support the accomplishment of the group's goals. If these norms are not adhered to, group performance suffers. There are several likely outcomes when members do not comply with norms supporting the group's mission. First, once a member violates the norms without consequence, others will often take this as permission to violate the norm also (informational pressure). For instance, at a regular meeting, leaders will wait to start until everyone arrives, and soon almost no one shows up on time to the meetings. Several employees leave early or take long lunches, and others start doing the same. Once a roommate or family member does not do his or her designated chore and others do it instead, the chore system falls apart as members decide "Well, if that member is not complying, why should I?"

A second likely consequence of persistent norm violations is that in groups with an official leader where members feel they have little power over other members, group members may disrespect or become angry with the leader if the leader does not respond to the norm violations. Although group members may be angry at the norm breaker, they seldom assertively confront the violator. Instead, they will try to express their disapproval of norm violations in socially safe ways—for instance, by making sarcastic jokes about the behavior, raising their eyebrows, or giving the deviant the cold shoulder. Meanwhile, they hope that the leader of the group will take care of the problem. In short, group members are often uncomfortable confronting one another and see this as the role of the leader. Therefore, leaders should respond quickly to norm violations lest their leadership be questioned and the violations become more widespread in the group. For instance, in most classrooms, side conversations during a lecture interfere with student learning and concentration. Students may glare at the perpetrators and dislike them for their insensitivity, but generally look to their instructor to shush the offenders. Teachers that fail to do so usually experience three consequences: loss of respect, more side conversations, and reduced student learning.

Sometimes norm violations occur in a group because the norms interfere with the group's productivity or members do not see the point of them. Norms should not be arbitrary or counterproductive; if no one complies, it could be because the norm has no value to the group. Leaders should occasionally scrutinize norms and change those that are outdated or those that stifle diversity or creativity. Members are more likely to behave consistently with a group norm if (1) they had a say in deciding on the norm and (2) they understand and accept the reasons behind it and believe that the group benefits from having the standard (Zander, 1982). Therefore, it makes sense to provide reasons for a group standard. Members may also violate norms out of ignorance. This is especially likely in the case of new members, who may violate norms because they do not know what the norms are. This should be taken into account before getting too angry or frustrated with them.

Norms of Cooperation vs. Norms of Competition

Norms of cooperation
Norms encouraging members to support one another toward the achievement of the group's goals.

Norms of competition
Norms supportive of members' seeking personal goals at the expense of other members.

Groups can have **norms of cooperation** or **norms of competition.** The cooperative group has norms supportive of sharing materials and information, communicating about the task, and supporting one another toward the achievement of the group's goals (Johnson & Johnson, 2000). In the competitive group, members work against each other to achieve a goal that only few can attain (Johnson & Johnson, 2001). In other words, members seek to attain personal goals at the expense of other members, are reluctant to share with other members or provide help and assistance to them, and do not encourage one another to achieve. Commonly, groups with norms of cooperation are more productive than groups with norms of competition between members. Meta-analyses indicate that cooperation in a group has a number of positive benefits in comparison to competitive or individualistic efforts. For instance, members in cooperative groups are more willing to take on difficult tasks and to persist even in challenging situations, generate more ideas, strategies, and solutions, and have positive attitudes toward the tasks and greater motivation to complete them (Johnson & Johnson, 1989).

Competitive group norms (within a group) may be more common in individualistic cultures such as the United States. A number of studies indicate that people from individualist cultures cooperate less than people from collectivist cultures (Cox, Lobel, & McLeod, 1991; Parks & Vu, 1994). Unlike collectivist cultures that emphasize the goals of the group, people in individualistic cultures give a higher priority to their personal goals, even when they conflict with the group goals (Triandis, 1994). This is not to say that people from collectivist cultures are not competitive. Indeed, they are quite competitive in situations where their group is in competition with another group (Triandis, 1994).

If you are still not persuaded that competitive norms are detrimental to group functioning, you may be confusing norms that support competition *between groups* with norms that support competition *within the group*. Competition *between* groups can foster cooperation and productivity within the group (although there are many cases where it can lead to unproductive conflicts between groups; see Chapter 7). Competition *within* a group can boost the productivity of some members (usually the potential winners) but typically reduces the productivity of members who do not believe they have a chance of winning. Competition between group members usually reduces communication, creates tension between group members, and interferes with the cooperation needed to achieve group goals. The effects of putting group members into competition with one another are likely to be negative unless achieving the group's goals does not require coordination and cooperation among members (Levi, 2001).

Although managers and leaders often say "There is no 'I' in 'Team,' " they often structure the group in such a way that cooperation and teamwork are not rewarded. Indeed, norms of competition usually originate in a leadership that creates a reward structure in which members must compete for limited rewards. For instance, imagine a family in which praise, attention, and warmth are rare and children feel that they must compete for parental approval. In this case, siblings become opponents. Often leaders believe that making members compete for limited rewards will motivate group members to work harder, but what they fail to recognize is the damage to the group that is likely to result. All of this is not to say that group members should not be rewarded for work well done. Ideally, however, this should be done without creating a competitive context in which only a few group members will succeed.

For instance, in one American organization, all employees received a 2% raise but were told that they would now compete with coworkers in their own department for additional raises. Each employee would submit an annual report describing what he or she had done to deserve the additional raise. In the next year, many members were less likely to take on group projects, where their contributions would be less noticeable, and when they did, they tried to take as much personal credit as possible for the group's success. Skilled and experienced members were less motivated to help the less skilled and inexperienced. Employees who were not "stars" in the department and therefore unlikely to receive the rewards, became demoralized and embarrassed. Knowing that they would not look as good in comparison to their colleagues, their performance declined.

Productivity Norms

Production norms

Norms specifying how hard to work and how much to produce.

One early finding from group dynamics research is that workgroups often have productivity or **production norms** specifying how hard to work and how much to produce. For instance, in the mid-1920s, a series of experiments known as the Hawthorne studies were conducted at the General Electric Plant in Hawthorne, Illinois (Roethlisberger & Dickson, 1939). In the "bank wiring assembly operation room experiment," one of several Hawthorne studies, the researchers expected a group piecework incentive plan to increase production (faster workers were expected to pressure slower workers to improve production). This is not what happened, though. Instead, the workers decided on what they thought was an acceptable output and applied social pressure to reach and maintain the standard. Those members who exceeded the group's standard were called "rate busters" or "speed kings," and those who underperformed were called "chiselers."

A group's production norms may or may not be congruent with high performance as defined by the work organization or leadership. Some groups may even take pride in doing little work, especially if they dislike or disrespect their manager or the organization's leadership, or feel that the standards set by the leaders are unreasonable. A group is more likely to have norms favoring production when the group's identity is congruent with high production, the group has shared goals related to production, personal goals are tied to group goals of production, and the group likes and values the leadership (Levine, 1989). One classic study (Coch & French, 1948) found that groups that directly participated in determining changes in work practices were more likely to develop norms consistent with high production. This theme will be picked up later in the productivity and leadership chapters.

Productivity Norms and Improving Group Effectiveness

In this part of the chapter, you learned about new member socialization, cooperative versus competitive norms, and how groups typically have production norms. Here are some suggestions for improving group effectiveness that follow from the material presented in this section.

1. Consciously identify important group norms, and clearly communicate these to group members, especially new ones.
2. To help new members learn the group's norms, assign them a mentor, preferably one who remembers the socialization experience and is very familiar with the group's norms.
3. Do not be so rigid about the group's norms that suggestions for improvement or creative ways to approach tasks are not considered.
4. Examine norms to see if they are outdated, arbitrary, or counterproductive, especially in cases of frequent violation. If so, change them.
5. If members violate a norm that is important to the group's effectiveness, act quickly. Otherwise, more violations may occur, and others may violate the norm as well.
6. To increase compliance with norms, ask for member input, and make sure that members understand the purpose of the group's norms.
7. If you are in a leadership role, be aware that members often expect you to deal with norm violations and their trust in your leadership will decline if you fail to do so appropriately.

8. If reaching the group's goal requires communication, sharing of information and resources, and helping one another, then do not make members compete with each other for limited rewards. Instead, reward the group for working cooperatively.

9. Foster high production norms by consulting with the group about production goals and giving rewards based on achievement of these goals.

10. If you are in a leadership position, remember that an antagonistic relationship with members is likely to result in counterproductive norms.

Roles

Roles
The different positions in the group, each with its own set of norms.

Roles are another important component of group structure. Every group has different jobs or positions, or roles. Levine and Moreland (1990) note that a few roles are found in most groups. One of the most common roles is that of leader; a leader tends to emerge even in an initially leaderless group. Another common role is that of newcomer; newcomers are expected to be anxious, passive, dependent, and conforming and are accepted more if they conform to these expectations. Moreland and Levine suggest that a scapegoat role is also common. Members project their own shortcomings onto the scapegoat and blame this person for problems in the group.

Like norms, roles may be formal or informal. Formal roles are prescribed and official, able to be seen on an organizational chart, or are standard positions in a particular type of group (such as mother and father in a family group or nurse and doctor in a hospital). Informal roles are unofficially designated roles, such as joker (who entertains the group with foolishness), devil's advocate (who always challenges the majority), or entertainment coordinator (who organizes group outings). The leader may be a formal or informal role, and both may coexist in the same group. Formal leaders are officially designated, with leadership titles of some sort, whereas informal leaders emerge as leaders in the group but are not publicly identified as such. With roles come **role expectations**—sets of norms that specify how people in different group positions should behave. We expect different things from different group members, depending on their role in the group. If members violate these role expectations, there are usually consequences. For instance, we can say that an employee who is fired for not doing his or her job is terminated for violating role expectations.

Role expectations
What we expect of members based on their role in the group.

Roles are powerful influences on member behavior. Often, we perceive members' behavior to be a reflection of personality, when in fact they are behaving in accordance with their role. This is why a member can appear to change when his or her role changes. For instance, coworkers are often surprised when one of them is promoted into management and then behaves no differently than the managers who preceded him or her. In one famous study demonstrating the power of roles, students at Stanford University were randomly assigned to be either prisoners or guards at a mock prison (the study is often called the Stanford County Prison Study). Participants became so taken over by their roles that the study had to be prematurely concluded as some of the guards became progressively more abusive and the prisoners passive and depressed (Zimbardo, Banks, Haney, & Jaffe, 1973).

Why Groups Have Roles

Roles usually imply a division of labor—who in the group does what. A division of responsibilities (roles) arises whenever a group exists for some time with group activities to perform (Cartwright & Zander, 1968). As groups go about getting a job done, they often find that it makes sense to specialize the tasks of its members and to come up with a structure that helps organize the work through the regularity of assignments and responsibilities. **Role differentiation,** the development of distinct roles in the group, occurs quickly as group members organize to take on different assignments in the group.

Role differentiation

The development of distinct roles in the group that occurs as group members take on different assignments.

Bales (1950) suggested that roles also arise because individuals desire a stable social environment. The argument is that we like the structure that roles in the group provide. Roles reduce uncertainty. For instance, we know what to expect of others based on their role in the group. Roles tell us what to do and who we are in the group in relation to others. Because member roles exist in relation to other member roles, we can predict how other members will behave toward us and we know how to behave toward them. Also, by telling us what we are expected to do, roles provide safety from negative sanctions; if we do what is expected of us according to our role, we can be reasonably sure that we will not have problems in the group. This is why **role ambiguity** is so stressful. Role ambiguity occurs when there is confusion about what our role is in the group or a lack of clarity about what is expected of us in our role. **Role conflict** occurs when the various demands of our role conflict (*intrarole conflict*) or when the demands of several roles we occupy simultaneously conflict with one another (*interrole conflict*). Research indicates that role conflict and role ambiguity create stress and loss of productivity (Abramis, 1994; Antonioni, 1996; Jackson & Schuler, 1985). Conversely, clearly defined roles increase member satisfaction and performance (Barley & Bechky, 1994).

Role ambiguity

Confusion about what our role is in the group or what is expected of us in our role.

Role conflict

When the various demands of our role conflict (intrarole conflict) or when the demands of several roles we occupy conflict with one another (interrole conflict).

Socioemotional & Task Roles

Socioemotional roles

Roles centered on satisfying the emotional needs of group members by encouraging others, mediating conflicts, and providing warmth and praise.

Bales (1950) also suggested that group roles tend to be of two types, socioemotional or task. **Socioemotional roles** are centered on satisfying the emotional needs of group members. These roles involve encouraging others, mediating conflicts, and providing warmth and praise. For instance, *harmonizers* mediate group conflicts, *encouragers* praise and encourage others, and *expediters* make suggestions to promote group process and make sure everyone is included (Benne &

Apply It! ••• **Do You Tend to Assume a Task or a Socioemotional Role?**
Do you tend to occupy a task or a socioemotional role in groups? How do you respond to extremely task-oriented group members? How do you respond to extremely socioemotionally oriented group members? Why do we need a balance of task and socioemotional roles in groups?

Task roles

Roles focused on getting the job done, including providing information, focusing the discussion on tasks, and assigning work.

Sheats, 1948). **Task roles** are focused on getting the job done; they include providing information, focusing the discussion on tasks, and assigning work. Task roles include *initiator-contributors*, who recommend solutions; *information-seekers*, who try to obtain needed facts; and *recorders*, who take notes and keep records (Benne & Sheats, 1948). Bales' (1955) research suggested most people gravitate toward either a task or a socioemotional group role and that, given the roles' competing demands, it is relatively rare for the same individual to occupy both types of roles in the group.

Gender, Ethnicity, and Roles

Upon learning of the task–socioemotional distinction, many people want to know whether female group members tend to assume more socioemotional roles and males more instrumental (task) ones. They assume, given common gender stereotypes, that this would be true. In fact, some studies do find that in mixed-gender groups, males are more inclined to assume task roles and females socioemotional ones (Wood, 1987). However, other studies indicate that it depends less on gender and more on whether the person feels competent at the task. Regardless of gender, those who feel competent are more likely to assume task roles, whereas those who feel they lack competence tend to assume socioemotional roles (Wood & Karten, 1986). When women and men feel equally competent, the roles they assume and how they act are quite similar (Dovidio, Ellyson, Keating, Heltman, & Brown, 1988).

Because our behavior in a group is often determined by the expectations of our role, people in the same role often behave remarkably the same. However, stereotypes may affect the group's role assignments. We often have a picture in our minds of the type of person that is appropriate for a role (a prototype), and that mental picture often includes gender, age, and ethnicity. We choose members for different roles based partly on how they fit our role prototypes. These beliefs about what type of person is appropriate for what role come partly from the type of person we have seen occupy that role in the past. For instance, all societies are gender-role segregated, viewing most roles as ideally occupied by one or the other gender. Almost every job listed by the U.S. Department of Labor is dominated either by females or by males. As a result, we are more inclined to assign some roles (such as leader) to male members and other roles (such as secretary or recorder) to female members. In the chapters on status, diversity, and leadership, you will learn more about the processes by which demographic characteristics such as gender, age, and ethnicity influence role assignment and member participation in groups.

Roles and Improving Group Effectiveness

When it comes to roles and group effectiveness, the main key is clarity and consistency regarding role expectations.

1. Reduce role ambiguity by clarifying role expectations, especially for new group members. In task groups, job descriptions may be helpful.
2. The tendency for roles to evolve in a group without discussion means that members can have different assumptions about whose job it is do what. Reduce misunderstandings and confusion by discussing role expectations.
3. To reduce intrarole conflict, avoid giving members role assignments with competing demands.
4. Do not develop such rigid role expectations and descriptions that the group cannot respond to change. Otherwise, when new tasks or demands on the group develop, members will be reluctant to respond to them, thus interfering with the group's adaptation to new circumstances.
5. Be careful to assign roles based on qualifications rather than on demographic variables such as gender, age, or ethnicity.

Concept Review

Group Norms

- **Norms** are the group's standards and shared expectations, both formal and informal, about how group members ought to behave.
- Norms contribute to group locomotion, provide predictability and comfort, and contribute to groupness.
- **Institutional norms** are determined by a group's leader or by external authorities. **Voluntary norms** are negotiated to contribute to smooth functioning. **Evolutionary norms** develop when a member responds to a situation in a particular way and other members adopt that response as well. Members also import norms into the group from other groups.

Why We Are Influenced by Group Norms

- We often conform because of **informational pressure.** Not knowing what to think or what to do, we go along with the group on the assumption that the group is right.

- The most famous study of informational pressure is Sherif's 1936 study showing the development of norms in a group using a perceptual illusion called the autokinetic effect. Over the course of three days, groups arrived at a group norm regarding the amount of movement of a light in a dark room.
- Informational pressure is more likely when a situation is ambiguous and members are uncertain. Unfortunately, members may unwittingly conform to the wrong informational cues, as demonstrated by **pluralistic ignorance.** One extreme case of informational pressure gone awry is **mass psychogenic illness,** the occurrence in a group of people of similar physical symptoms with no apparent physical cause.
- The pressure to conform in order to be socially accepted and avoid rejection is called **normative pressure.**
- In Asch's 1956 classic study on normative pressure, participants determined which of three lines was similar to a "comparison" line after six experimental confederates made clearly wrong estimates. Participants conformed to the wrong estimates approximately 37 percent of the time although they had no uncertainty regarding the task.
- According to **social impact theory,** conformity depends on strength (how important the group of people is to you), immediacy (how close the group is to you in space and time), and number (how many people are in the group). We are also more likely to conform when the group is unanimous.
- **Loose cultures** tolerate much more deviation than **tight cultures.** Cultural homogeneity and isolation from other cultures lead to a tighter culture because there is more agreement about what is correct behavior. Looser cultures tend to have many cultural influences.
- People in **collectivistic cultures** value conformity for the sake of group harmony and because their fate is seen as interdependent with that of others. People in **individualistic cultures** value independence of judgment and see conformity negatively. Conformity tends to be higher in cultures with higher collectivism scores.
- Research finds only small gender differences in conformity.

Dissent

- **Dissent,** or challenging group norms, is sometimes appropriate and desirable. Research suggests that a small chorus of dissenting voices can significantly sway the group. This idea is called **minority influence.**
- Hollander's **theory of idiosyncrasy credits** suggests that you must earn the right to dissent by first conforming to earn high status. Moscovici's **theory of innovation** suggests that a strong, persistent minority can change the way the majority thinks about an issue, even if high status has not yet been earned. Research supports both theories.

- Minority dissent stimulates the group to take in more information, to think about that information in more divergent ways, to perform better, to think more creatively, and to detect more solutions that are correct. Dissenters also give others the courage to go against the group's majority. The willingness to dissent may also prevent the **Abilene paradox,** a situation in which members of a cohesive group falsely believe that each of the others wants to pursue a course of action that in fact none of them prefers.

Norms and Group Performance

- The more quickly a new member learns the group's norms, the more quickly he or she can become a full and contributing member of that group.
- Group norms are learned through observation and trial and error. The time it takes to learn norms is decreased when the group makes an effort to **socialize** new members.
- Compliance with group norms is important to group functioning. When members do not comply with norms supporting the group mission, others will often take this as permission to violate the norm (informational pressure). Also, group members may disrespect or become angry with the leader if the leader does not respond.
- Some norm violations occur because the norms interfere with the group's productivity or members do not see their purpose. Members are more likely to behave consistently with group norms when they have participated in their creation, understand and accept the reasons for the norms, and believe that the group benefits from the norms.
- **Norms of cooperation** encourage sharing of materials and information, task communication, and support of one another toward achievement of the group's goals. **Norms of competition** pit members against one another to achieve a goal that only few can attain. Although competition *between* groups can foster productivity, competition *within* a group usually reduces communication, creates tension between group members, and interferes with the cooperation needed to achieve group goals.
- Groups often have **production norms** specifying how hard to work and how much to produce. Norms favoring production are more likely when the group's identity is congruent with high production, the group has shared goals related to production, personal goals are tied to group goals of production, and the group likes and values the leadership.

Roles

- **Roles** are sets of norms that specify how people in different group positions should behave. These roles may be formal or informal. There are different norms for members depending on their role in the group (**role expectations**) and consequences if these are violated.

- **Role differentiation,** the development of distinct roles in the group, occurs quickly as group members organize to take on different assignments in the group.
- **Role ambiguity** occurs when there is confusion about what our role is in the group or a lack of clarity about what is expected of us in our role. **Role conflict** occurs when the various demands of our role conflict (intrarole conflict) or when the demands of several roles we occupy simultaneously conflict with one another (interrole conflict). Role conflict and role ambiguity are stressful and reduce productivity.

Socioemotional and Task Roles

- Bales suggested that group roles tend to be of two types. **Socioemotional roles** are centered on satisfying the emotional needs of group members. **Task roles** are focused on getting the job done. Most people gravitate toward either a task or a socioemotional group role.

Gender, Ethnicity, and Roles

- Some studies find that in mixed-gender groups, males are more inclined to assume task roles and females to take on socioemotional roles. Other studies indicate that regardless of gender, those who feel competent are more likely to assume task roles while those who feel they lack competence tend to assume socioemotional roles.
- Stereotypes may affect the group's role assignments. We choose members for different roles based partly on how they fit our role prototypes. These beliefs about what type of person is appropriate for what role come partly from the type of person we have seen occupy the role in the past.

Skill Review

Prevent Pluralistic Ignorance

- To avoid pluralistic ignorance, ask questions, seek evidence, and encourage discussion before assuming you know what the group thinks or that it is right.
- If you are in a leadership position, share information to reduce uncertainty and ambiguity so that the group does not act according to faulty assumptions.

Prevent and Deal With Norm Violations

- Consciously identify important group norms, and clearly communicate these to members, especially new ones.

- To help new members learn the group's norms, assign them a mentor.
- Increase norm compliance by getting member input and making sure that members understand the norms' purpose.
- To increase conformity due to normative pressure, increase cohesion and meet members' belongingness and identity needs.
- Be aware that members expect leaders to deal with norm violations promptly and appropriately.
- To prevent additional violations, act quickly when norms are violated.
- Use normative and informational pressure on deviant members. Clearly communicate what norm was violated and why it is important to the group.

Change Maladaptive Norms

- Do not be so rigid about the group's norms that suggestions for improvement or creative ways to approach tasks are not considered.
- Evaluate norms and change outdated, arbitrary, or counterproductive norms.
- To change maladaptive norms or create new norms, enlist the help of high-status group members who agree to discuss, model, and reinforce new norms.
- Suggest that a new norm is appropriate by providing evidence that "everyone is doing it" and "experts" recommend it.

Encourage Appropriate Dissent

- Encourage the expression of minority viewpoints because such viewpoints may bring to light information that will result in a better group decision or the changing of outmoded group practices.
- Avoid the Abilene paradox. Speak up before going along with what seems to you to be a questionable decision, because others may feel the same way.

Encourage Norms of Cooperation

- Do not make group members compete with one another for limited rewards.
- Reward the group for working cooperatively.

Foster High Production Norms

- Consult with the group about production goals, and give rewards based on the achievement of these goals.
- If you are in a leadership position, remember that an antagonistic relationship with members is likely to result in counterproductive norms.

Improve Productivity by Proper Role Assignments

- Find out member strengths, experience, and skills before assigning roles, and assign roles based on qualifications rather than on demographic variables such as gender, age, or ethnicity.

Reduce Role Ambiguity and Role Conflict

- Clarify and discuss role expectations to reduce role ambiguity.
- To reduce intrarole conflict, avoid giving members role assignments with competing demands.
- Do not develop such rigid role expectations and descriptions that the group cannot respond to change.

Study Questions

1. What are norms? Why do groups have norms? How do norms in groups develop?

2. What is informational pressure, and how did Sherif's famous study with the autokinetic effect demonstrate it?

3. When is conformity due to informational pressure most likely? How are pluralistic ignorance and mass psychogenic illness examples of *mis*informational pressure? How can knowledge about informational pressure be used to improve group effectiveness?

4. What is normative pressure, and how was it illustrated Asch's classic study?

5. According to social impact theory, what three factors affect conformity due to normative pressure? How can knowledge about normative pressure be used to increase group effectiveness?

6. How do gender and culture affect conformity?

7. How do groups benefit from dissent? How do the theory of idiosyncracy credits and the theory of innovation explain how minorities can successfully influence majorities?

8. How do members learn group norms? What can be done to foster this process?

9. How can norms aid in productivity? How can they interfere with productivity? Why are norms of cooperation more conducive to productivity than norms of competitiveness? What should be done if norms are violated? How can new norms be created in the group?

10. What are roles? Why does role differentiation occur?

11. What are role conflict and role ambiguity? Why are they harmful? What can be done to reduce them?

12. What are task and socioemotional roles? Is it true that women are more likely to occupy socioemotional roles and males task roles?

Group Activities

Activity 1: Analyze the Norms of Your Class

Let's say a new student has just joined your classroom. To ease this student's entrance into the class group, you and your group have to provide a handbook about the group's norms. Create two lists of specific class norms for this new student, one of formal norms and one of informal norms. Include common penalties imposed on group members who violate the norms so that the new member knows what will happen if s/he fails to comply with the group's norms. What other norms should your class consider adopting to deal with any problem behaviors or inefficiencies in how the class works?

Activity 2: Case Analysis: Socializing New Group Members

Read the following case, and answer the questions that follow with your group.

It was the first day of my new job at the bank, and I was nervous because I didn't know what would be expected of me. I felt some relief when my superior told me that she would explain how things worked. We went into a conference room, where we went over many rules. Then, after I signed a statement agreeing to abide by them, we went over banking procedures, including the time sheet process. It was at this time that I began to really learn about the group. It turns out that a new manager was coming in and had formulated the new time sheet process. The woman explaining things to me was not happy about it and had no problem letting me know that her coworkers felt the same way. Then it was time to train. The information I received was contradictory, with three different tellers giving three different sets of instructions for the same task. I was given a small spiral notebook that had been passed down from teller to teller to help the new hires. I asked if there was an official "teller handbook" but was told there was not.

The notebook was vague, and it took me a long time to discover what my job was and how to do it. I just had to watch other tellers, do my best, and get corrected if I did something wrong. It was frustrating because I really wanted to do a good job.

1. Explain how role ambiguity is a problem and how it might reduce productivity.
2. If your group was hired as an organizational consulting team, what exactly would you recommend to this organization based on the problems described in this case?
3. Share experiences as members of new groups. How did you learn the norms of the group? What would have made your experience easier?

Activity 3: Learn About Norms and Roles: A Card Game

Each four-person group is given a deck of cards and is given fifteen minutes to choose a card game and clarify the rules to all members. Next, play the game for at least a half hour. When time is called, answer the following questions.

1. What formal norms guided the group's behavior? What informal norms guided the group's behavior? Identify any institutional norms, voluntary norms, or evolutionary norms.
2. Did group members conform to the norms because of normative or informational pressure? What happened if someone did not follow the norms (rules)?
3. What roles emerged in the group? For instance, who assumed a task role, a socioemotional role, the joker role, the leader role? Did members assume gender-stereotypical roles? Why or why not?

InfoTrac College Edition Search Terms

To do research for your papers and assignments, use InfoTrac that's provided free with new copies of this book. Go to: http://infotrac.thomsonlearning.com and enter the following search terms:

- Group Norms
- Psychogenic Illness
- Conformity Research
- Social Impact Theory
- Hate Groups

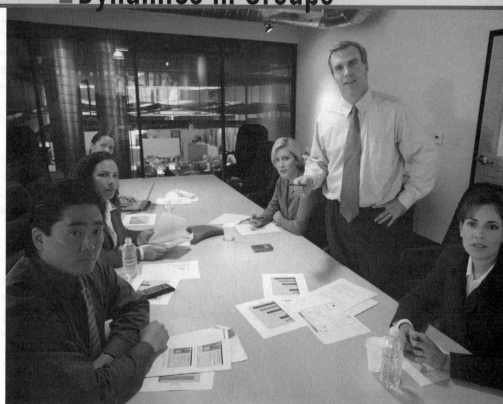

© Steve Chenn/CORBIS

Most people desire respect and influence in groups. In other words, they seek status and power. In this chapter, you will learn to look at groups through the group structure lens of status.

Chapter 3 discussed how group members occupy different roles in the group. The focus of this chapter is on how the roles in a group are not all equally valued, nor are their occupants. Think about it. Isn't it true in most groups that some members enjoy more respect, their opinions and behaviors are more influential (they are more powerful), and they get more attention than other members? Although you may like to think that in principle, people should be equal, in reality they are not. Most groups have a hierarchical status structure—an unequal distribution of rights, privileges, and opportunities and an unequal distribution of respect and popularity (Meeker, 1994).

Status Basics

Defining Status

Status

A group member's standing in the hierarchy of a group based on the prestige, honor, and deference accorded him or her by other members.

Status refers to an individual's standing in the hierarchy of a group based on the prestige, honor, and deference accorded him or her by other members (Lovaglia & Houser, 1996). Most theorists agree that in face-to-face groups, status has three major components: (1) asymmetrical amounts of attention, (2) differential amounts of respect and esteem, and (3) differential amounts of influence in the group. In other words, higher-status individuals are more prominent or visible and receive more attention in the group, are more respected and held in higher regard, and are allowed more control over group decisions and processes (Anderson, John, Keltner, & Kring, 2001).

Status system

The distribution of power and prestige among a group's members, including the "chain of command."

The **status system** of a group reflects the distribution of power and prestige among its members, including the "chain of command" (Forsyth, 1999; Moreland & Levine, 1995). Status may be earned (**achieved status**), or it may be bestowed upon individuals by virtue of their having some characteristic that a group has designated as prestigious and valuable (**ascribed status**). People may have titles, degrees, or specializations that lead the group to assign them high status. Also, people differ by gender, race, wealth, beauty, age, reading ability, dialect, and other characteristics, and these distinctions often have great social significance in groups (Webster & Hysom, 1998), affecting member status. Status is *contextual,* meaning that it is defined with reference to a particular group (Anderson et al., 2001). It is likely that your status varies from group to group, and what helps you to attain high status in one group may be irrelevant to your attaining status in another.

Achieved status

Status that is earned.

Ascribed status

Status given to individuals by virtue of their having some characteristic that a group has designated as prestigious and valuable.

Formal and Informal Status Hierarchies

A group's status system or hierarchy is often reflected in its official structure. For instance, most work organizations are separated into groups, each with a hierarchical structure with relatively few high-status positions and many more low-status positions. Groups generally make clear through pay and employment benefits the relative status of different jobs. Often, you can tell who has high status by the role the person occupies in the group. This role is frequently indicated by the title of the group member's position (such as father, department chair, or clerical assistant).

Educational degrees such as PhD or MD are also used as indications of status. Indeed, we are so accustomed to using titles as an indication of others' status that we may automatically grant high status to those with a title and behave deferentially toward them (Cialdini, 2001). Strangely enough, prestigious titles even lead us to perceive those who hold them as taller (Higham & Carment, 1992). It is as if metaphorically looking up to someone causes us to believe that we literally look up to him or her as well. It seems to work the other way also; literally looking up to someone seems to translate into perceiving him or her to have high status. According higher status in the group to those larger in size may possibly be a remnant from our animal past when status was determined by size and strength (Cialdini, 2001).

A group's status structure may be easily identifiable by the formal or official structure of the group. However, not all groups have formal structures (official roles and titles spelled out by the group or organization), and even those that do often have an informal structure as well. In contrast to formal structures, informal structures exist without ever being explicit described or resting on any formal agreement (Cartwright & Zander, 1968). For instance, even a friendship group often has a leader, an established way of communicating among group members, and status differences among members. Members of a workgroup may officially hold the same status, but in practice the group implicitly agrees that some members have more status than others. Or a member may hold the formal role of leader but have low status in practice if the person is not well respected and has little influence over the group.

Status Markers

Status markers
Nonverbal and verbal behaviors that signify status, such as strong eye contact and commanding and interrupting others.

Because examining the formal status structure provides an incomplete picture of the group's status system, it is useful to observe group members for evidence of **status markers.** Typically, high-status members act differently than those who are lower in status. High-status members are the ones that stand up straighter, maintain eye contact, speak in a firm voice, speak the most, and criticize, command, and interrupt others (Harper, 1985; Skvoretz, 1988; Weisfeld & Weisfeld, 1984). They engage in more domineering and directive behaviors than members with lower status, are evaluated more positively, and have more self-esteem (Levine & Moreland, 1990; Ridgeway & Berger, 1988). They are also allowed to deviate from the group's norms without consequence more than low-status members (Hollander, 1958, 1960), and have greater freedom to express negative emotions

---

Apply It! ••• **Identifying Formal and Informal Status Structures**

Choose a group that you have been a member of that had both a formal and an informal status structure, such as a paid job, a sports team, your family, or a volunteer group (for example, student government or community group). Analyze the relative status of group members according to the formal and informal structures of the group. Describe the "official" and "unofficial" status differences among members.

BOX 4-1 / ASSESSING YOUR STATUS BEHAVIOR IN GROUPS

Instructions: Answer True or False for each item.

1. I am usually one of the quieter group members.
2. I tend to make and maintain eye contact when I talk with others.
3. I do not have a loud or strong voice.
4. I am usually one of the most talkative group members.
5. I tend to avert my gaze (look down or away) when I talk to others.
6. I am quick to offer my ideas in a group.
7. I usually choose to sit in an inconspicuous location.
8. I have a strong, steady voice.
9. I am slow to offer my ideas in a group.
10. I am likely to situate myself so that I receive the group's attention—for instance, by choosing a place at or near the head of the table.

Scoring:

Answering True to odd-numbered items is indicative of behaviors more typical of those likely to be assigned a low status by the group. Count the number of odd-numbered items for which you answered True. Answering True to even-numbered items is consistent with exhibiting behaviors more consistent with higher status. Count the number of even-numbered items for which you answered True. What does this tell you about your status behavior in groups?

such as anger (Ridgeway & Johnson, 1990). As you probably know, high-status members can often "get away" with things that lower-status group members cannot. **Box 4-1** gives you the opportunity to consider whether your verbal and non-verbal behavior communicates to others that you are a high-status group member.

Earned Status

Individuals may earn higher status in a group by helping the group to achieve its goals and by making personal sacrifices for the group (Levine & Moreland, 1990). Members who make the group look good and function well are often rewarded with high status. For instance, my student Brett earned high status on the university water polo team because he scored a lot of points during games and had a personal style that fostered group cohesion and motivation to work as a team. The group felt that he was an important part of the team's making it to the national finals. A nursing group will reward a nurse who regularly works extra hours to help her unit keep its reputation for quality care, by according her higher status. A software designer who comes up with the ideas for the design group's most successful software packages will have high status.

Status Dues Systems

Status dues system
What the group requires of members before they are awarded a higher status.

Most groups have a **status dues system.** A status dues system is what the group requires members to "prove" before they are awarded a higher status. Higher-status members may have had to put in a certain amount of time as low-status members, demonstrate certain skills, or occupy a series of low-status roles before being awarded higher status.

As you read earlier in this chapter, status is contextual and depends on the particular group. Likewise, the path to earning higher status varies depending on the group, but if you pay attention and identify a senior group member willing to mentor you, it will become clear how to earn status in the group. My student, Marie, worked in a restaurant where status was awarded based on how much alcohol, appetizers, and desserts a server sold. As a new employee unfamiliar with the different wines and liquors, her sales and status were low, but she expected this to change once she learned more about the restaurant's offerings. My student, Eric, earned high status in his fraternity by doing everything he was told to do by higher-status fraternity members when he was a pledge.

Climbing the Status Ladder and Paying Status Dues

Many groups require members to work their way up a status hierarchy or status ladder before they are allowed to occupy a role designated as high status. In such groups, attaining high status requires that you first occupy a series of roles in the group, each higher in status than the one before. As a lower-status member, it is often expected that you pay your "status dues" by occupying low-status roles for a particular period of time before you are granted the rights accorded to higher-status members. In a college fraternity, for instance, it is explicitly spelled out that pledges (aspiring and new members) have fewer privileges and must defer to more senior group members. What these status dues consist of, whether they are clearly spelled out, and how long they must be paid, all vary depending on the group. However, paying status dues generally includes taking orders from more senior group members, making few suggestions and going along with the suggestions of senior members, and limiting one's participation in meetings (as well as other, more general "brown-nosing" behavior such as ingratiating oneself to senior members).

Apply It! ••• **Your Experience With Status Dues Systems**

Think of the groups you have been a member of. Identify any status dues that had to be paid and what happened to new group members who failed to understand the group's status dues system.

Status Violations

Status violation

When low-status members engage in behaviors that are inappropriate given their rank and face resistance from higher-status members.

Those who engage in behaviors that are not in keeping with their status are said to have committed a **status violation.** When low-status members engage in behaviors that are inappropriate given their rank, they are likely to be labeled "presumptuous," "uppity," or "aggressive" and to face resistance from senior members (Ridgeway & Berger, 1988). For example, others may resist status violators by ignoring them, talking over them, or commanding, shouting, or glaring at them. I am reminded of a case in which a young professor found that older, established group members were resistant to her promotion. One finally told her that the problem was that her level of participation in faculty meetings was inappropriate for a junior faculty member and that she needed to stop acting as though she were equal to the senior professors. Likewise, one of my students told me that when he was a high school baseball player, there was a rigidly enforced status system. When the team went on the bus to a game, only the higher-status varsity players were permitted to wear their hats on the bus. The varsity players took the hats of status violators and spat in, sat on, and crumpled them. The hat would be so damaged that the player could not play because his uniform was now incomplete.

In groups with status dues systems, newer members cannot behave as equals to more senior group members, regardless of any special talents or skills needed by the group that the new member possesses. Senior members often feel that they have paid their dues and earned their status and are reluctant to grant it to those who have not jumped through the same hoops. As junior group members, they looked forward to the day when they would be the ones in the high-status position with low-status members showing them deference. New members that intentionally or unintentionally circumvent the status process may be rejected and have an even lengthier climb up the status ladder. Again, it is in your best interests to pay attention and obtain mentoring from a senior group member so that you can avoid missteps and expedite the status progression process.

Ascribed Status

The idea that we earn our status is appealing because it suggests that high-status group members are deserving of their high status, and this seems fair and just. However, although we might like to think that high status is always earned and deserved, our experiences tell us otherwise. Think back to some of your group experiences. Have you ever found yourself puzzling about how a given individual had high status while other, more deserving individuals did not? Indeed, as with many other things in life, the assignment of status is not always fair, and all status is not earned. Groups often ascribe or assign status to members before they have earned it, or fail to award it to those who do not look the high-status part.

The Rapid Development of Status Systems in Groups

There is some evidence that status systems develop very quickly in groups, almost within moments of the group's formation (Bales, 1950; Barchas & Fisek, 1984; Levine & Moreland, 1990). Obviously, in such cases, members have not had a chance to earn their status. In workgroups, student groups, friendship groups, and roommate groups, status systems develop quickly. In newly forming groups, the individuals assigned high status by the group often receive this distinction merely by looking and acting as though they have high status. Status markers such as a firm handshake, direct eye contact, and a confident air all communicate that one should be respected (Leffler, Gillespie, & Conary, 1982). Verbally speaking clearly and loudly without tentativeness will also contribute to others' perceptions that you are of high status (Lee & Ofshe, 1981). Telling people what to do, interpreting others' statements, confirming or disputing others' claims, and summarizing and reflecting on the discussion also communicate that one has high status (Stiles, Lyall, Knight, Waung, Hall, & Primeau, 1997). Dominating the conversation and shifting the discussion to things you know about may also help (Dovidio, Brown, Heltman, Ellyson, & Keating, 1988; Godfrey, Jones, & Lord, 1986). The highest-participating member—that is, the one who talks the most—typically becomes the highest-ranked member in a short time (Bales, 1970). Unsurprisingly perhaps, the personality trait of extroversion is related to higher status in groups (Anderson et. al, 2001). This is because extroverts are more socially skilled than introverts and draw more attention to themselves and their skills and abilities.

Ethological Approach to Status

Ethological approach to status

Suggests that the physical strength and size of members influences their status in the group.

Several theories attempt to explain the rapid development of status systems. One theory, the **ethological approach to status,** focuses on the strength of members as a factor in determining their relative status in the group (Mazur, 1985). Ethologists study nonhuman animals in their natural habitats and try to determine the role that various behaviors serve in animal survival. Ethologists often assume that humans behave in ways similar to other animals. For example, many nonhuman animals can be observed engaging in dominance contests. Ethologists believe that humans do this also. They suggest that stronger members (determined by size, musculature, facial expressions, and other personal characteristics) are assigned high status in the group.

Some theorists suggest that status contests, in which members negotiate their status places through verbal acts, gestures, and postures, are common in email discussion groups, social gatherings, and meetings (Owens & Sutton, 2001). For instance, some members may interrupt others in order to redirect the group's activity in a direction that will enhance their social standing. By rolling their eyes or aggressively shaking their head in disagreement when others talk, members may attempt to discredit other contenders for high status. Even behaviors like arriving late to a meeting or leaving early can be "status moves," in the sense that they communicate "I have more important things to do and have graced the group with my presence." Ridgeway (1987) suggests that dominance struggles are relatively rare but when they do occur, nonverbal dominance behavior, along with the amount of support "contestants" receive from other group members, determines the status winner.

Expectation States Theory

Expectation states theory

Proposes that groups make status assignments based on expectations of each member's ability and potential to contribute to the group.

Performance expectations

Assumptions about the ability of other group members to contribute to the group's goals, often based on status characteristics.

Status characteristics

Personal characteristics, such as skills, experience, or demographic factors, that influence performance expectations.

Specific-status characteristics

Skill- or experience-related status characteristics.

Expectation states theory (EST) offers an alternative explanation regarding the determination of status in human groups. According to EST, status is determined by the expectations that group members have of each member's ability and potential to contribute to the group (Berger & Conner, 1974; Berger, Rosenholtz, & Zelditch, 1980; Meeker, 1994; Ridgeway, 2001a, b; Ridgeway & Berger, 1988). These are called **performance expectations.** According to the theory, members almost immediately make assumptions about the ability of other group members to contribute to the group's goals. Performance expectations are often based on **status characteristics**—personal characteristics that influence group members' beliefs about one another (Lovaglia & Houser, 1996). Status characteristics may be skill or experience related (**specific-status characteristics**), or they may be visually obvious features such as age, ethnicity, gender, or attractiveness (**diffuse-status characteristics**). Specific-status characteristics are qualities that are specifically related to performance on the task at hand (such as skills, training, or special abilities). For instance, you may be assigned status in the group based on having a certain educational degree or job experience that is directly relevant to the task. In contrast, diffuse-status characteristics usually carry expectations for competence in a wide variety of situations (Lovaglia & Houser, 1996). The influence of diffuse-status characteristics on performance expectations is due to stereotypes. If you are a 20-year-old blonde female, other group members may have lower performance expectations for you than they do for a 35-year-old Euroamerican male.

A number of studies support the argument that status characteristics are accompanied by differential evaluations, which lead to differential expectations and inequalities in interaction (Driskell & Mullen, 1990; Knottnerus, 1997; Webster & Foschi, 1988). More specifically, performance expectations are important because they affect the extent to which members look to other members

Diffuse-status characteristics

Demographically derived status characteristics, such as age, ethnicity, gender, or attractiveness.

for contributions (termed "action opportunities"); they affect perceptions regarding the value of members' contributions (called "performance outputs"); and they affect who wins in the case of a disagreement ("influence"). In other words, if group members start with a low performance expectation for you, it will be harder for you to gain status in the group. You will not be given as many opportunities to contribute; your contributions may not be positively evaluated; and when a disagreement arises between you and a member for whom others have a higher performance expectation, the group may side with the other member.

Task cues

Behaviors that provide information about a member's actual or potential performance on the task and thereby influence performance expectations.

Performance expectations are also influenced by **task cues**—interactional behaviors that provide information about a member's actual or potential performance on the task (Rashotte & Smith-Lovin, 1997). For instance, task cues include differences in eye contact, verbal response time, voice volume and tone, and maintenance of gaze while talking (Berger et al., 1986; Ridgeway & Berger, 1988). These behaviors are taken as evidence of members' abilities to contribute to the group. For instance, members who participate readily and "sound better" will be judged more competent and awarded higher status.

Task cues may be especially influential in a newly formed group in which, at the outset, there is an absence of performance expectations. In such cases, expectation states theorists say that members will engage in "power and prestige behavior" in an effort to establish their place in the status hierarchy (Berger & Conner, 1974; Ridgeway & Berger, 1988). As they discuss the task, members will ask and be asked for task contributions, will offer task contributions, will give and receive evaluations of contributions, and will have their ideas accepted or rejected by others. Inequalities among these behaviors will influence the development of performance expectations for each member and, consequently, will influence status. By noticing behaviors such as who defers to whom, whose participation seems to be most valued (or devalued), and who gets greater rewards for like effort, members eventually arrive at an agreement on the group's status order (Owens & Sutton, 2001). Figure 4-1 summarizes these processes.

Gender, Ethnicity, and Status

Status Characteristics Theory

Status characteristics theory

A branch of expectation states theory that focuses on how status hierarchies in groups will form consistent with statuses that members possess in society at large.

Status characteristics theory is a branch of expectation states theory that focuses on how external status differences among members determine the distribution of power and prestige within a group (Knottnerus, 1997). The theory suggests that in task-oriented groups, a status hierarchy will form consistent with statuses that members possess in society at large (Lovaglia & Houser, 1996).

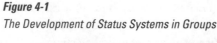

Figure 4-1

The Development of Status Systems in Groups

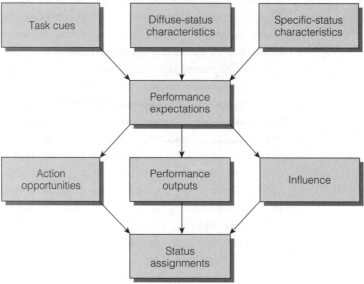

Status generalization

The tendency for group members to use diffuse-status characteristics to assign status in the group, even when the characteristics are irrelevant to the situation.

Status characteristics theorists are particularly interested in **status generalization**—the tendency for group members to use diffuse-status characteristics to assign status in the group, even when the characteristics are irrelevant to the situation. If members of a jury presume that males are more rational than females, that they know more about law, and therefore that they will be more valuable to the group, then status generalization based on the status characteristic of gender has occurred (Webster & Foschi, 1988). In other words, diffuse-status characteristics are believed to have a strong influence on performance expectations (what a member is expected to contribute to the group), and performance expectations influence status assignments. Status generalization happens quickly and appears to operate outside of the realm of conscious awareness (Webster & Foschi, 1988). Furthermore, as Webster and Foschi note, status generalization often occurs in the absence of any real evidence that the status characteristic is indeed relevant, and the outcomes of status generalization are often undesirable because they may result in discrimination and prevent the full use of member potentials.

Those who study status generalization point out that when we look at status in small groups, we often find that higher-status members come from a gender and ethnicity category designated as higher in status by society. Status characteristics theory suggests that this occurs because group members may automatically assign higher status to members from these groups. Remember, status generalization happens when status distinctions that exist in the outside world are "imported" into the group and are allowed to determine status in the group (Webster & Foschi, 1988).

In most societies, gender, ethnicity, age, and socioeconomic status (economic class) are status characteristics associated with general expectations for superior (or inferior) overall ability or ability in specific tasks. The diffuse-status characteristics that are high and low in status vary based on culture, but in virtually every culture, some ethnic groups are ascribed higher status than others, and it is likely that these larger social differences in status affect status hierarchies in small groups. Table 4-1 provides a list of groups that are ascribed high status and low status in a variety of countries.

Cross-culturally, gender is another particularly consistent status characteristic. Simply, membership in the male or female group is, in most parts of the world, an important determinant of status and power. For instance, in most societies, social rules confer greater property rights on men, give greater political power to men, designate high-status roles as male roles, and sanction men's right to control the lives of women (Burn, 2000).

The higher status afforded to men by virtue of their being men affects the dynamics of mixed-gender groups in that male group members are usually cast in higher-status roles and dominate the group more than do female members. For instance, in mixed-gender groups, males will participate more, be asked to

Table 4-1

Groups Ascribed High and Low Status in a Sampling of Countries

Country	High Status	Low Status
Australia	Whites	Aborigines
Belgium	French	Flemish
Canada	Whites	Native Americans
Czechoslovakia	Slovaks	Gypsies
France	Native French	Portuguese immigrants
Great Britain	English	Irish, Scots
India	Nontribals Brahmins High Caste	Tribal people Harijans Low Caste
Israel	Jews Ashkenazis	Arabs
Japan	Japanese	Koreans
New Zealand	Whites	Maoris
Northern Ireland	Protestants	Catholics
Switzerland	Native Swiss	Immigrants
United States	Whites Northern European Immigrants	Blacks Latinos Native Americans

Source: J. Sidanisus & F. Pratto (1999). Social Dominance. *New York: Cambridge. Reprinted with the permission of Cambridge University Press.*

Apply It! ••• **Diffuse-Status Characteristics and Your Status in Groups**

How have diffuse-status characteristics such as age, gender, ethnicity, and physical appearance affected your status in groups? Have they helped or hindered your status? Do you believe that your diffuse-status characteristics have led people make unfair assumptions about your ability to contribute to the group?

---

participate more, display more confident and assertive nonverbal cues, and be more influential than females who are otherwise similar to them (Ridgeway, 2001). This dynamic is not just true of gender, but applies whenever a group is "mixed"—that is, includes members from groups that society designates as high in status and from groups designated as low in status.

Self-Fulfilling Prophecies and Stereotype Threats

Ridgeway and Balkwell (1997) give the following example. Imagine a person who has high performance expectations for his own Group A and low expectations for members of Group B. He encounters a member of Group B who has no such expectations. However, believing that he is more competent, the person from Group A speaks without hesitation, makes suggestions, and plays an active, assertive, and confident role in the encounter. Furthermore, he pays little attention to the suggestions of the person from Group B, as he assumes that person is low in value. Other group members see that the person from Group B is treated as less competent and lower in status and that the person from Group A displays behaviors associated with high competence and status. They then assume that the person from Group A is more competent and worthy than the person from Group B. Meanwhile, the person from Group B is learning that others believe he is less competent and valuable and may therefore adopt lower performance expectations about her group. This may lead her to be more hesitant and more deferential to people in Group A, thus contributing to the low status and value of Group B. This example illustrates two related phenomena: the self-fulfilling prophecy and stereotype threat.

Self-fulfilling prophecy

When our stereotypes lead us to treat stereotyped members differently and this treatment elicits stereotype-confirming behavior from them.

Self-fulfilling prophecies occur because stereotypes lead to performance expectations that then determine the action opportunities provided to group members. The group does not give stereotyped members the chance to show that the stereotype is wrong, and even creates situations in which the stereotype is confirmed. For instance, take the case of the Korean American woman who worked for a public utility. Unlike her male counterparts, she was not given assignments that would allow her to develop or demonstrate leadership abilities. Then, every time a promotion opportunity came up, she was told that she had not demonstrated leadership skills and therefore was unsuitable for the promotion. When she then asked her manager for assignments to prove her leadership abilities, she was told that she should accept that "some people are chiefs and others Indians," and she "was an Indian." It is likely that management had a stereotype that Asian American women are not leadership material. This led them to deny her the opportunity to prove otherwise. Then they said, "See, she isn't leadership material; she's never demonstrated any leadership qualities." But of course, this was only because of what they did.

Stereotype threat occurs when members are aware that other group members have low performance expectations for them because of their diffuse-status characteristics and this knowledge creates performance anxiety (nervousness) that affects their performance. For instance, in a study by Steele and Aronson (1995), African American students who were told prior to a difficult verbal test that the test would measure intellectual ability performed less well than white students. African American students who were told the test did not measure intellectual ability performed as well as the white students. In another study (Spencer, Steele, & Quinn, 1999), women who were told that a test would indicate whether men or women were better at math performed more poorly than men on a math test; women who were not told this performed as well as men. In Chapter 8, Member Diversity and Group Dynamics, you will learn more about the dynamics of stereotyping and how it influences our reactions to other group members; in Chapter 10, Leadership, you will learn more about status characteristics and their influence on leadership emergence.

Stereotype threat
How awareness of others' stereotypes of us may create performance anxiety and lead to a self-fulfilling prophecy.

Changing Early Status Assignments

Once a status ranking exists in a group, is it fixed? Are you out of luck if you are a member of a group designated by society as low in status, or if the group initially designates you as low in status? Fortunately, early status assignments can be changed. For instance, the relative status of members may change as the group's situation changes and members become more or less valuable (Brown, 1988) or as the group comes to recognize the skills and contributions of members (Watson, Kumar, & Michaelson, 1993).

Low-status assignments based on diffuse-status characteristics such as gender or ethnicity may also change. A number of studies suggest that inequalities generated by a diffuse-status characteristic will be decreased in the presence of a performance characteristic with the opposite evaluation (Knottnerus, 1997). That young blonde female that the group initially assigns a low status because of low performance expectations may eventually earn a high status in the group if she performs at a consistently high level. Another example is the changing performance expectations regarding women in paid work situations. As more and more women enter the paid workforce and demonstrate their competence, the expectations associated with the diffuse-status characteristic of "female" are changing (Rashotte & Smith-Lovin, 1997).

Some theorists argue that although initial status assignments may be modified through contributions to the group, those with initially low status may have difficulty proving their worth (Ridgeway, 1982). Diffuse-status characteristics have their greatest impact in the initial phase of interaction, but because they result in performance expectations that influence the evaluation of contributions from status-advantaged and status-disadvantaged members, they often have enduring effects on status structures (Ridgeway, 2001a, b). This means that if you are a member of a group traditionally low in status, you may have to work that much harder to prove yourself. The burden of proof often lies with the stereotyped person, who must demonstrate that the diffuse-status characteristic is in fact irrelevant (Ridgeway, 2001a, b). Once people have expectations of others, it usually takes repeated exposure to behavior that does not fit their stereotypes before they will change their minds (Mackie, Allison, Worth, & Asuncion, 1992a, 1992b). This may take time as well as finesse, because status-advantaged members may see the efforts of the status-disadvantaged members as status violations. Some research suggests that to overcome resistance, it is especially important to show dedication to the group so that your efforts are not seen as illegitimate and self-interested grabs for power (Ridgeway, 2001a, b; Shackleford, Wood, & Worchel, 1996).

Implications of Earned and Ascribed Status for Enhancing Group Effectiveness

The main moral of the status story told so far is that it pays to avoid creating performance expectations of group members based on diffuse-status characteristics such as age, gender, or ethnicity. It is unfair and risky to assign status based on diffuse-status characteristics. You may award too much status to someone who does not deserve it or, conversely, hinder the contributions of a more deserving member and waste the talents of group members.

Leaders are often in the position of assigning members to roles in the group. Therefore, if you are in a leadership position:

1. Be aware of the tendency to reserve higher-status roles for members of gender and ethnic groups more valued by society.
2. Give all members, not just members from certain groups, the experiences and training needed to earn higher status in the group.
3. Realize that you have a special responsibility to model assigning status on the basis of true merit, not on the basis of stereotypes associated with diffuse-status characteristics.

The material you have read so far also has clear implications for increasing your status in groups:

1. If you are a new group member, be aware that you may have to pay some "status dues" before you are allowed to assume a higher status.

2. Because status is contextual, realize that the path to higher status varies depending on the group. Ask several senior group members you trust about how they earned high status in the group.
3. Enhance others' performance expectations of you, especially if you have diffuse-status characteristics that often lead to the assignment of low status. Tell the group about skills and experience you possess that are relevant to the task. "Strategic expression of a previously hidden expertise can force the group to reassess the individual's value to the group" (Owens & Sutton, 2001, p. 301).
4. Work on your "power and prestige behavior," such as maintaining eye contact, responding promptly, and having a strong and steady voice. These things are taken by others as evidence of your ability to contribute to the group and enhance others' performance expectations of you.

If you have reason to believe that your diffuse-status characteristics lead others to have low performance expectations for you, do not give up and accept a low status role.

1. Remind yourself that you belong as much as anyone else.
2. Work hard to contribute to the group, and over time, you will probably earn higher status in the group.
3. You may have to present your case for higher status to the group's leaders. Be prepared to provide proof that you deserve a status promotion. To maximize the likelihood of success, follow the guidelines for constructive confrontation presented in Chapter 7, Understanding and Managing Conflict.

The Effect of Status Differences on Members and the Group

Status differences in groups are a fact of life but have destructive potential if they are perceived to be unjust, if they are exaggerated, or if the quest for status in the group creates competition among members that interferes with their ability to cooperate with one another.

Why People Desire High Status in Groups

One of the most important goals and outcomes of social life is to attain status in the groups to which we belong (Anderson et al., 2001). After all, people with higher status have more opportunities to influence the group and are indeed more influential (Levine & Moreland, 1990). They are also evaluated more positively than lower-status persons who do virtually the same thing (Humphrey, 1985; Sande, Ellard, & Ross, 1986). Also, individuals' status within the group often influences their personal well-being (Anderson et al., 2001). Because a person's status affects his or her self-evaluations (Levine &

Moreland, 1990), individuals who are lower on the status totem pole may feel worse about themselves. As Brown (1988) notes, by locating ourselves in the status structure, we gain insight into our abilities relative to our peers. Being of low status communicates that we are viewed as less valuable. Kemper (1991) found that status loss was associated with feelings of anger and status gains were associated with feelings of happiness.

How the Quest for Status May Interfere With Cooperation

Many groups are structured such that high-status positions are in short supply and members must compete for them. Unfortunately, this quest for status in a group is not always healthy for group functioning. Some group members may attain their status by using deceptive and manipulative tactics such as putting others down, boasting, or behaving aggressively (Anderson et al., 2001). They may blame and attack others, control access to information, align themselves with powerful others, do favors to create indebtedness, and engage in self-promotion, all in an effort to gain an advantage (Allen, Madison, Porter, Renwick, & Mayes, 1979; Mintzberg, 1983). These methods may work, although sometimes other members catch on and shun manipulators for their selfishness (Kyl-Heku & Buss, 1996).

Political behavior

Actions taken by group members to gain a power or status advantage over others.

The term **political behavior** is often used to refer to actions taken by group members to gain a power or status advantage over others. Political behavior seems to have two sources, one situational and the other personal. Political behavior seems most common when there is competition within the group for scarce resources (including status) and when decision-making procedures are unclear (Beeman & Sharkey, 1987; Gandz & Murrary, 1980). When ambiguity is low because rules are clear, political behavior is reduced. Political behavior isn't all about the situation, though. Some people have a high need for power, a basic desire to influence others and control situations, and some have a high need for achievement, a need to compete, achieve, and excel (McClelland, 1985). These needs can motivate political behavior in the quest for power and status.

Some group members will emphasize status distinctions to boost their own self-esteem—that is, because they want to feel superior to someone else. For instance, in a workgroup, some people demonstrate their higher status by treating those in lower-status positions with disrespect. This behavior may demoralize those in lower-status positions and reduce their satisfaction and commitment to the group (I cannot begin to tell you the number of people I have encountered who have left a job because they felt disrespected by higher-status coworkers). Some members strive for status to the point that they may create arbitrary and unnecessary status distinctions that interfere with cooperation among group members. It is hard to work with someone who you feel disrespects you. You may have had an older sibling who, despite a relatively small age difference, insisted that her or she was higher in status than you were. You may have had a job where an employee with slightly more experience or time on the job clearly believed that you were lower in status.

The bottom line is that the quest for status can pollute a group and put individuals who should be cooperating into competition with one another. For instance, in an effort to enhance their status, members often compete for credit when the group succeeds, and this may create conflict (Leary & Forsyth, 1987). Conversely, because group failures may result in status losses, group members often do their best to pass the blame to other group members. This, too, can create bad blood between group members.

Besides being unfair to individuals and creating some nasty group dynamics, emphasizing status differences can also deprive a group of good suggestions from lower-status members and can permit a group to be misled by higher-status people (Webster & Hysom, 1998). Low-status members are usually reluctant to criticize or disagree with high-status members, and the ideas and opinions of high-status members have more influence and tend to be evaluated more favorably, even when the basis of their status is irrelevant to the decision problem (Yukl, 1998).

Member Dissatisfaction Due to Illegitimate Status Inequities

The very nature of status is such that it is determined relative to other people; therefore, it is not surprising that people almost constantly engage in comparisons to determine their status in the group. For instance, in work organizations, employees often use paycheck size as an indicator of status and are very concerned with others' earnings and trappings of status, such as who has the better workspace, office furniture, and parking space. In a friendship group, who was first told of a significant event in a member's life is processed by members as saying something about the relative status of group members. Even in a family, siblings compare who has the larger room, who has more privileges, who has to do more chores (and which ones), who gets the most help with their education, and so on.

Group members make assessments regarding the deservedness of status assignments. They are very interested in whether those who are higher in status deserve to be, and whether status assignments are fair. Group members' satisfaction and commitment depend partly on members' satisfaction with their place in the group's hierarchy. Low-status members are especially likely to experience dissatisfaction if they believe that their lower status is unfair or unjust. Depending on the group's response to their concerns, the integrity of the group may be helped or hurt.

When you are new to a group, and other group members have more task-relevant skills and experiences and have had more time to demonstrate their value to the group, you are inclined to see your status position as just. You understand that status is something that takes time to earn. However, let's say you have been in the group for a time and feel that you have done what you needed to do to attain a "status promotion." Furthermore, imagine that your expertise, experience, and contributions to the group are similar to those of members who have attained higher status in the group, yet you are still relegated to the same low-status position. How would you feel? What would you do? Equity theory (Adams, 1965) predicts that you would experience underpayment inequity.

Equity theory

Says that people desire equity and decide whether what they receive is fair depending on how it compares to what others receive.

Originally a theory about personal relationships, **equity theory** says that people are motivated to have their inputs and outcomes equivalent to the inputs and outcomes of others. With regard to groups and status, the idea is that we put things in (such as time, energy, and qualifications) and we get things out (such as pay, promotions, and status). To decide whether outcomes are fair based on our inputs, we look at how they stack up against what other group members are putting in and getting out. According to equity theory, **underpayment inequity** occurs when you perceive that what you are getting is unfair relative to what others are getting.

Underpayment inequity

Occurs when people believe that what they receive is unfair relative to what others receive and act to restore equity by increasing their outcomes or decreasing their inputs.

Equity theory predicts that individuals experiencing underpayment inequity generally act to restore equity. They may do this in a number of ways. The most common ways involve adjustments to either inputs or outcomes. For instance, most people probably begin by trying to increase their outcomes by pointing out the inequity. They often assume that once the group or its leaders are aware of the inequity, they will make things right. If that does not work, aggrieved members may pointedly ask for a promotion, for greater acknowledgment of their contributions to the group, or for privileges associated with higher status in the group. If this is unsuccessful, they may make things more equitable by decreasing their inputs—for instance, by reducing their effort. Or they may leave the group and seek a group in which more outcomes will be obtained for the same inputs. Indeed, many groups have lost excellent members because these members did not receive the respect and prestige they felt they deserved.

Fraternal deprivation

The perception that one's group is unfairly given a low status relative to other groups.

Perceptions regarding status-illegitimacy may occur not only at the individual level but also at the group level, when members of a group perceive that in comparison to another group, their group has been discriminated against. This is often called **fraternal deprivation** (Brewer & Miller, 1996; Rubin, Pruitt, & Kim, 1994). Feelings of fraternal deprivation are associated with the perception of social injustice and a desire for social change (Brewer & Miller, 1996). For instance, members of a specific gender or ethnic group will be upset if they believe that they and other members like them are unfairly relegated to a lower status in the group. African American workers at one power company in Georgia noticed that no matter how hard they worked, what credentials they had, and how long they had worked for the organization, white workers were promoted before them. In 2001, they joined to file a lawsuit. If a union represents several job categories and secures a contract that benefits members in one job category more than another, it is likely to face a lot of anger from members of the job category that got less. In one such case, members of a job category who felt underpayment inequity left the union en masse. In a blended family, if one parent's children seem to be treated better than the other's, the poorly treated ones will likely unite in opposition, and the family will never reach its full potential as a group. In all of these examples, a subgroup of members collectively believes that they have been discriminated against because of their subgroup membership. Collective action to attain equity then leads to schisms in the larger group.

Social identity theory, first mentioned in Chapter 1, describes the dynamics of groups such as the ones in the previous paragraph. The theory outlines the process by which a once cohesive group becomes divided into competing subgroups (see Turner & Haslim, 2001). This may happen when subordinated subgroups act collectively to enhance their status in cases where they believe the low status is undeserved and they are denied opportunities within the group to climb the status ladder. According to social identity theorists, maltreated group members come to see themselves as members of a discriminated-against group. This becomes an important social identity for them and a source of "groupness" (similarity of fate and shared goals can create a group through social identification). This subgroup identity overrides their identification with the larger group (called the superordinate group) and is strengthened by the belief that acting collectively in terms of their shared subgroup membership is their best shot at changing things. The cohesiveness of the superordinate group is now threatened by competition between its subgroups and the fragmentation of a shared identity. The moral of this group story is that when members of subgroups raise concerns about inequity, the group and its leadership should take these concerns seriously and make an effort to remedy them.

Status Differences and Enhancing Group Effectiveness

The discussion on the effects of status differences on groups is rich in information that can be used to improve group effectiveness.

1. If you are the leader, do not condone or permit the ill-treatment of lower-status members by higher-status members. Model respect and appreciation for what each member contributes to the group. All members should be treated well, regardless of status differences.

2. Do not make status a scarce resource for which group members must compete. Otherwise, competition and political behavior may interfere with group effectiveness.

3. Use a fair system to award status and its trappings, such as titles, resources, and freedoms. If this is not the case, resentments and hostilities are likely, and the group's integrity will be compromised.

4. In a group in which each member has relevant knowledge and nobody has a monopoly on ideas, it is desirable to minimize the influence of status differences on group decisions (Yukl, 1998). One way is to keep meetings free of obvious status symbols such as insignias, titles, and seating privileges.

Another approach is to develop a norm of mutual respect and appreciation for each person's ideas and contributions, regardless of member status.

5. Do not ignore members who feel they are not receiving the respect and prestige they deserve. Otherwise, their commitment to the group is likely to be reduced, and they may leave the group when they get the opportunity. Acknowledging their value to the group and doing what you can to "right status wrongs" will preserve the group's integrity and members' effort and commitment.

Power

A treatment team at a social service agency is meeting to discuss a client's treatment plan. Dr. Bennington, the psychiatrist and clinic director, argues that the client's medication should be increased. The client's caseworker, Kerry, who has a bachelor's degree in psychology, disagrees but doesn't say anything. After all, the psychiatrist is a medical doctor with years of experience, and that trumps her four years of college. No one else says anything either because Dr. Bennington is the one who hired them and the one who can fire them. In this group, Dr. Bennington is a powerful group member.

Power
The ability of a group member to get other members to do what he or she wants them to do.

Power has to do with influence over the group—the ability of a group member to get other members to do what he or she wants them to do, or think what he or she wants them to think. Lewin (1941) defined it as the maximum force Person A can impose on Person B divided by the maximum resistance B can provide. Group members often differ in how much power they wield in the group. Some are better able than others to get the group to do what they want. Power and status are closely related, in that group members who are high in status generally have more power in the group than members who are lower in status, but even low-status group members have ways of exercising power.

Social power theory
A theory that suggests that a group member's power depends on his or her access to different power bases or sources.

Power Bases

Legitimate power
When a member is seen as having the right to tell other members what to do because of his/her position of authority in the group.

Where do individual group members get their power? **Social power theory,** which originated in a classic paper by French and Raven (1959), identifies five power "bases" or sources. **Legitimate power** has as its base the belief that by virtue of his or her position in the group, a member has the right to exercise authority over other members. Parents generally have legitimate authority over their children, teachers over their students, and supervisors over subordinates. Two bases of power originate in control over rewards and punishments. When people have power over us because they have resources we want, they are said to have **reward power.** For example, when employees do what their supervisor requests because he is the one that decides on their promotions and raises, that's reward power. **Coercive power** is based on others' ability to punish us if we don't

Reward power
When a member has power over other members because he or she controls resources and can administer rewards that other members want.

Coercive power

When a member has power over other members because she or he can deliver punishments to members who do not comply.

Expert power

When a member is able to influence others because of his or her knowledge or expertise.

Referent power

When others take up the suggestions of a member out of respect and liking for that member.

Information power

When a person has power because he or she possesses information that others want.

do what they want. If employees do what their supervisor wants to avoid getting fired or yelled at, that's coercive power. Power may also be based in our belief that someone else knows better than we do. For instance, the team may follow the recommendations of a team member with special training. This is **expert power.** Last, sometimes power has as its base admiration and respect. Called **referent power,** it happens when we do what someone asks because we like or want to be like him or her.

Yukl and Falbe (1991) added three more power bases to the French and Raven model. **Information power** is based on a person's possessing information that others want. **Persuasive power** originates in a person's ability to use rational argument, facts, and persuasion to influence others. **Charisma** is power that originates in an individual's charm or enthusiasm. They also suggest that legitimate, reward, coercive, and information power can be grouped together under the broad heading of **position power,** because they are based on a person's formal position in the group or organization. As Pfeffer (1992, p. 75) says, power "comes from the control over resources, from the ties one has to powerful others, and from the formal authority one obtains because of one's position in the hierarchy." In contrast, expert, referent, persuasive, and charisma power are forms of **personal power,** because they all arise from a person's individual characteristics. These ideas are summarized in Figure 4-2.

The Relationship Between Status and Power

Persuasive power

Power derived from a person's ability to use rational argument, facts, and persuasion to influence others.

Charisma

Power that originates in an individual's charm or enthusiasm.

Position power

Power that is based on a person's formal position in the group; includes legitimate, reward, coercive, and information power.

Personal power

Power that arises from a person's individual characteristics; includes expert, referent, persuasive, and charisma power.

Power bases are helpful in understanding why high-status members are often powerful group members. For instance, high-status members often have position power. They occupy high-status positions of authority and have legitimate power over other members. Their role includes the expectation that they will exercise authority over lower-status members, and lower-status members are expected to comply. Likewise, high-status roles often give their occupants reward and coercive power over lower-status group members. High status may also enhance credibility and thus increase expert power, because members assume the high-status person possesses greater expertise. If their position causes others to look up to high-status members and emulate them, they may also possess referent power.

Not all high-status members have power because of their official role in the group. Many have personal power such as referent power. Some members are granted high status in a group because they are liked and respected by other members. Such high-status members tend to have referent power over other members. The group takes up their suggestions because they like, respect, and identify with the member. Also, a member in a role that is "officially" low in status may have expert power if s/he possesses knowledge or expertise that is needed by the group, or information power if s/he controls access to information. For example, the group member who knows the most about computers may possess expert power if s/he is the only one who knows how to get the system back up

Figure 4-2
Yukl and Falbe's Revised Power Bases Model

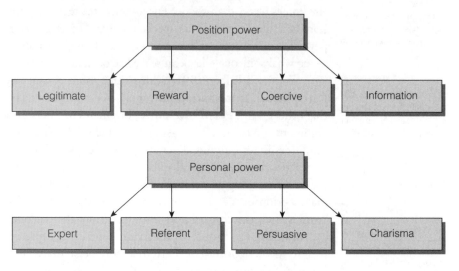

Source: Yukl & Falbe, 1991.

and running when it crashes. Department secretaries and office managers often have considerably more power than their formal position suggests because other members depend on them to obtain needed information and resources.

Influence Tactics

Influence tactics

The specific behaviors that individuals use to wield power and influence others.

What tactics do people use to get group members to do what they want, and which tactics are most effective? A number of researchers have sought to answer these very questions. For instance, Kipnis, Schmidt, and Wilkinson (1980) identified eight categories of **influence tactics:** assertiveness, ingratiation, rationality, sanctions, exchange, upward appeal, blocking, and coalitions. Yukl, Falbe, & Youn (1993) identified nine similar influence tactics. Take a minute to look these over in **Box 4-2.** Influence tactics may also be classified as "soft" or "hard," depending on how much freedom the tactic leaves the target to decide whether to yield or resist (Bruins, 1999). For instance, soft tactics include ingratiation; hard tactics include coercion and pressure.

There are a number of useful guidelines to keep in mind when choosing an influence tactic. One consideration is whether the tactic is consistent with the group's norms and role expectations about the use of the tactic. In other words, the choice of tactic should depend on the situation (Koslowsky & Schwarzwald, 1993). For example, coercive strategies may be acceptable and expected when a

---

BOX 4-2 / INFLUENCE TACTICS

Rational persuasion: The agent uses logical arguments and factual evidence to influence the target.

Inspirational appeals: The agent appeals to the target's values or goals to encourage enthusiasm about the proposal.

Consultation: The agent asks for the target's assistance in planning a strategy, activity, or change, or shows a willingness to alter a proposal for the target's support.

Ingratiation: The agent uses praise, flattery, or friendly or helpful behavior to get the target in a good mood or on his/her side before making a request.

Personal appeals: The agent appeals to the target's feelings of loyalty or friendship when asking for something.

Exchange: The agent promises something in return, an exchange of favors or a share of benefits, if the target helps.

Coalition tactics: The agent gets others on his/her side to help persuade the target, or refers to that support.

Pressure: The agent uses demands, threats, or persistent reminders to influence the target.

Legitimating tactics: The agent refers to his/her right to make the request by saying it is consistent with organizational policies, practices, or traditions.

Source: Yukl, Falbe, & Youn, 1993.

---

military drill sergeant is influencing new recruits but are likely to be unacceptable in most other settings. Your choice should also depend on whether you have the appropriate power bases for a given tactic (Yukl, Falbe, & Youn, 1993). For instance, legitimate power helps in the use of legitimating tactics, and referent power in making personal appeals. In general, higher-status group members use a wider variety of influence tactics because they have more power bases available to them (Schwarzwald & Koslowsky, 1999).

Another consideration is whether a tactic is likely to be effective, given your relationship with the target (Yukl et al., 1993). A number of studies suggest that the status of the agent and the target should affect the choice of influence tactics or strategies (Raven, 1993; Stahelski, Frost, & Patch, 1989; Stahelski & Paynton, 1995; Yukl & Falbe, 1991). Whether the effort is an "upward" influence attempt (a subordinate is attempting to influence a superior), a "downward" attempt (a superior is trying to influence a subordinate), or a "lateral" attempt (peers influencing peers) makes a difference. For instance, using threats or intimidation is unwise when dealing with a higher-status group member who possesses reward and coercive power. Such a person has the power to retaliate and the power to resist. Managers generally view subordinates who use hard tactics in upward influence attempts negatively (Wayne, Liden, Graf, & Ferris, 1997). Rational persuasion is probably the best tactic for upward influence attempts

Apply It! ••• Understanding and Applying Influence Tactics

Look at the influence tactics in Box 4-2. For each one, try to think of a situation in which you have used it. How was your choice influenced by the norms of the group, your relationship with the target, and the perceived costs and benefits of using the strategy? Do you believe that your personality makes you more comfortable with some tactics than with others?

(Yukl et al., 1993), although some research finds that subordinate ingratiation, such as flattery and agreement with the target, is linked to supervisor liking, positive performance ratings, and career progression (Wayne, Kacmar, & Ferris, 1995).

Last, you should think about the relative costs and benefits of using a particular strategy in a given situation. For instance, using ingratiation in an upward influence attempt may harm your relationship with peers if they think it insincere, manipulative, and self-serving at the expense of other group members (Wayne, Kacmar, & Ferris, 1995). Coercive strategies have a particularly high price. Those who use hard strategies tend to reduce others' liking of them, and this reduces their referent power and damages personal relationships (Raven, 1993). Ironically, people often resort to coercive strategies when they feel powerless, but these strategies may backfire because they make targets feel powerless and react by becoming defensive or rebellious (Bugental & Lewis, 1999). Getting people to do what you want by threatening them or pressuring them is also a problem because they tend to do what you want only when you are present and often find ways to rebel—for instance, by doing a substandard job. If you must use pressure, use it in combination with rational persuasion or legitimating, rather than alone (Yukl et al., 1993).

Culture, Gender, and Power

The study of culture, power, and influence tactics is limited and has focused mostly on whether people in different cultures use different influence tactics. Although one study showed that managers all over the world use similar strategies to influence subordinates (Schmidt & Yeh, 1992), other research suggests that culture affects how frequently the various tactics are used (Hirokawa & Miyahara, 1986; Rao & Hashimoto, 1996; Rao & Schmidt, 1995). For instance, in some cultures, such as China, it is very important to allow others to maintain both "self-face" and "other-face"—in other words, to avoid embarrassment and making others feel bad. It is also important to maintain harmony in the group. This means that influence attempts are often subtle and indirect (Krone, Chen, & Xia, 1997). In Japan, a collectivist focus (an emphasis on the group over the individual) and a tradition-based culture leads managers to use legitimating tactics, in which they ask subordinates to comply for the sake of the company or because it is their duty (Hirokawa & Miyahara, 1986). One study found that in India, ingratiation is expected when a subordinate is attempting to influence a superior (Pandey, 1986). There is enough research on this topic to warn us that the tactics that are effective in our culture may not be effective in another culture. However, there is not enough research to make useful recommendations about which tactics to use in a particular culture. Therefore, it is recommended that you observe and ask questions of trusted insiders before plunging ahead with the strategies that work well in your culture. Later chapters on communication, diversity, and leadership all emphasize that if we want to be effective in intercultural contexts, we need to learn what we can about other cultures and adapt accordingly.

When it comes to gender and power, it may be said that, in general, men are more powerful because their greater position power gives them more access to the bases of power. As societies become more gender-equal, this is likely to change, but currently it remains true that men, more often than women, are found in high-status positions that give them greater access to the bases of power described earlier. For instance, men are more likely to have greater reward and coercive power because the social roles that involve control of resources are more likely to be held by men (Eagly, 1987; Johnson, 1976).

Men may also possess more legitimate authority because they are more often found in positions of authority. Even when women occupy such positions, they face more resistance than men when they attempt to assert their authority; their authority is not seen as legitimate (Atwater, Carey, & Waldman, 2001; Butler & Geis, 1990; Carli, 1999; Eagly, Makhijani, & Klonsky, 1992; Rudman & Kilianski, 2000). Men are also likely to possess greater expert power because they are generally considered to be more competent than women, even when there is no objective behavioral or performance evidence to support this perception (Carli, 2001; Ridgeway, 2001a, b). For example, research finds that women have to significantly outperform men to be considered as competent (Foschi, 1996). Males' greater tendency to dominate conversation and interrupt others may also suggest greater competence and enhance their expert power (Tannen, 1995). Because males tend to be more respected than females, they are more likely to be listened to and taken seriously (Atwater et al., 2001). Some research suggests that women possess greater referent power than men because this type of power is not dependent on position power and has its origin in liking (Carli, 1999). Research indicates that women are viewed as warmer and more supportive than men and are better liked (Carli, 2001).

What you just read about gender and power is generally true, but a few other factors affect the relationship. One of these is type of task. For example, although it is generally true that male group members are more influential when the task is considered gender-neutral or masculine, female members are more influential if the task is considered feminine (Carli, 2001). For example, women may have considerable power in the home in regard to child-care tasks. The gender composition of the group—that is, the number of females relative to the number of males—also makes a difference. When a group has close to equal numbers of females and males, females have as much influence as males. However, when females are a numerical minority, they have little influence. Interestingly, when males are in the minority, they still wield influence in the group (Taps & Martin, 1990).

Given these gender differences in access to the bases of power, it is not surprising that corresponding gender differences in the use of influence tactics are found. Research suggests that males are more likely to use hard and direct strategies and females softer, indirect strategies (Bui, Raven, & Schwarzwald, 1994; Hirokawa, Kodama, & Harper, 1990; Steil & Weltman, 1992), because harder strategies are seen as socially unacceptable for females (Buttner & McEnally, 1996; Eagly, 1995; Rudman & Glick, 2001; Tepper, Brown, & Hunt, 1993). After reviewing the research on gender and influence tactics, Carli (1999) concluded that unless women possess legitimate or expert power, they use more indirect and less assertive influence tactics than males, and rely more on interpersonal agreeableness and warmth to influence others.

The Implications of Power for Increasing Group Effectiveness

Research links career advancement and access to resources to the effective use of power (Carli, 1999). Effective group members and leaders understand the subtleties of power. They are aware of who has power over whom and why, and the most effective uses of the power sources available to them. They use their power in a way that respects the rights of other group members and for the good of the group. They choose their influence strategies based on the situation and do not rely too heavily on one power base or influence tactic. That said, here are some more specific suggestions for increasing group effectiveness.

1. Enhance your expert power by demonstrating your knowledge and expertise and making other members aware of your credentials, but be honest. Your power will be eroded if others find you do not have the expertise you said you did. Also, be aware that unscrupulous group members may sometimes exaggerate their expertise in order to enhance their power. Sometimes it is a good idea to check out group members' expertise before acting on the basis of their recommendations.
2. Being likable can increase referent power. Being friendly, warm, positive, and interested in others may help. Those who do a good job and act with integrity are also more likely to possess referent power. Of course, you should be on the lookout for the occasional Machiavellian group member who uses his or her charm to manipulate and deceive others to gain more power in the group.

3. Because the use of coercive power reduces referent power and increases resistance, avoid the use of coercive power even if it is available to you as an option.

4. Pay attention to others' responses to your directives. If they resist doing what you tell them, it may be because you have exceeded the limits of your legitimate power and have violated a norm. The solution is to clarify the roles of group members and who has the "right" to tell whom what to do.

5. When socializing new group members, be explicit about the chain of command and the areas in which he or she is "allowed" to exercise authority.

6. Remember that people in officially low-status positions may actually have considerable power because they are often the key to your getting information or resources you need. They frequently have reward or coercive power in that they can do things efficiently for you or slow your work up. For this reason, it generally pays for you to be respectful and gracious when making requests of them.

7. Norms regarding what is an acceptable influence tactic may vary based on culture, the group, and even personal preferences. For instance, some group members hate to be "wined and dined," while others practically demand it. It is best to learn what you can about the group and about individual members and to adjust influence tactics accordingly.

8. Handle group members who seem to have a high need to dominate the group and others at the expense of the group and other members, by emphasizing norms of cooperation and by adopting group decision-making practices that prevent domination by a few members. The group's leader should explain privately to such members that their behavior is harming their status and power in the group because the group resists them.

Concept Review

Status Basics

- **Status** refers to individuals' positions in a hierarchy of power relations within a social group. In face-to-face groups, status has three major components: (1) asymmetrical amounts of attention, (2) differential amounts of respect and esteem, and (3) differential amounts of influence in the group.

- The **status system** of a group reflects the distribution of power and prestige among its members, including the "chain of command."

- Status may be earned (**achieved status**), or it may be bestowed based on the possession of some characteristic that a group has designated as prestigious and valuable (**ascribed status**).

- A group's status hierarchy is often reflected in its official structure (official member roles and titles).

- To identify high-status members, it is also useful to examine **status markers** such as nonverbal behavior, verbal behavior, and the influence that members have on the group.

Earned Status

- High status may be earned by helping the group to achieve its goals and by making personal sacrifices for the group.
- The path to earning higher status varies depending on the group.
- Earning status often requires that members "work their way up" a status hierarchy to the point where they occupy a role designated as high in status. High-status members are often those who have been in the group the longest.
- Many groups have a **status dues system,** implicit or explicit norms requiring that members occupy a low-status role (and behave accordingly) before they are granted the rights of the higher-status members. A **status violation** occurs when lower-status members act as if they had higher status before they have paid their dues.

Ascribed Status

- Status systems develop very quickly in groups, almost within moments of the group's formation.
- Individuals assigned high status by the group often receive this distinction merely by looking and acting as though they are of high status.
- The **ethological approach to status** suggests that stronger humans (determined by size, musculature, facial expressions, and other personal characteristics) are assigned high status in the group.
- **Expectation states theory** suggests that status is determined by the expectations that group members have of each member's ability and potential to contribute to the group (**performance expectations**). Performance expectations are based on personal characteristics that may be skill or experience related (**specific-status characteristics**) or visually obvious such as age, ethnicity, gender, or attractiveness (**diffuse-status characteristics**).
- Performance expectations affect the extent to which members look to other members for contributions (termed "action opportunities"), perceptions regarding the value of members' contributions (called "performance outputs"), and who wins in the case of a disagreement ("influence").
- In a newly formed group without performance expectations, expectation states theorists say that members will engage in "power and prestige behavior" in an effort to establish their place in the status hierarchy.

Gender, Ethnicity, and Status

- Women and members of traditionally underrepresented or undervalued groups are often assigned a low status in mixed groups. This is explained by **status characteristics theory,** a branch of expectation states theory that focuses on how external status differences among members determine the distribution of power and prestige within a group.
- **Status generalization** happens when status distinctions that exist in the outside world are "imported" into the group and are allowed to determine status in the group. In most societies, gender, ethnicity, age, and socioeconomic status are status characteristics associated with general expectations for superior (or inferior) ability.
- Groups often create **self-fulfilling prophecies.** Their stereotyped beliefs lead to the differential treatment of group members such that some group members are not given the opportunity to make valuable contributions to the group. Their expectations lead them to create a situation in which their beliefs are proven correct.
- Members of social categories designated as low in competence and value are aware of this designation, and this knowledge may create an apprehension (nervousness) that may affect their performance (**stereotype threat**).
- The relative status of members may change as the group's situation changes and members become more or less valuable, or as the group comes to recognize the skills and contributions of members.
- Although initial status assignments can change through contributions to the group, those with initially low status may have to work that much harder to prove their worth.

The Effect of Status Differences on Members and the Group

- Most people prefer to be higher in status, but the quest for status can pollute a group and put individuals who should be cooperating into competition with one another. Assessments regarding the deservedness of those with higher status are common, and bitterness and dissatisfaction are often the result.
- Emphasizing status differences can also deprive a group of good suggestions from lower-status members and can permit a group to be misled by higher-status people.
- Individuals who feel they deserve to be higher in status given their contributions to the group are not usually content to accept their lower status. **Equity theory** says that people are motivated to have their inputs and outcomes equivalent to the inputs and outcomes of others and will act when they experience **underpayment inequity.** Typically, they will try to increase outcomes, or decrease inputs.

- Perceptions regarding status-illegitimacy may occur at the group level when members of one group perceive that in comparison to another group, theirs has been discriminated against (**fraternal deprivation**). According to social identity theorists, maltreated group members come to see themselves as members of a discriminated-against group, and this becomes an important social identity for them and a source of "groupness." The cohesiveness of the superordinate group is now threatened by competition between its subgroups, and the fragmentation of a shared identity results.

Power

- **Power** has to do with influence over the group, the ability of a group member to get other members to do what he or she wants them to do, or think what he or she wants them to think.
- French and Raven identified five bases, or sources, of power. **Legitimate power** has as its base the belief that by virtue of his or her position in the group, a member has the right to exercise authority over other members. People who have power over us because they have resources we want are said to have **reward power. Coercive power** is based on others' ability to punish us if we don't do what they want. **Expert power** originates in a person's expertise or knowledge. Power arising out of admiration and respect is **referent power.**
- Other researchers have added the following power bases: **Information power** is when a person has power because he or she possesses information that others want. **Persuasive power** originates in a person's ability to use rational argument, facts, and persuasion to influence others. **Charisma** is power that originates in an individual's charm or enthusiasm.
- Legitimate, reward, coercive, and information power can be grouped together under the broad heading of **position power** because they are based on a person's formal position in the group or organization. Expert, referent, persuasive, and charisma power are forms of **personal power** because they all arise from a person's individual characteristics.

The Relationship Between Status and Power

- High-status members tend to have more access to the bases of power. They often have position power. They occupy high-status positions of authority and have legitimate power over other members.
- High-status roles are also associated with reward and coercive power. High status may also enhance credibility, thus increasing expert power because members assume the high-status person possesses greater expertise. Members often look up to high-status members and emulate them, so they may also possess referent power.

Culture, Gender and Power

- Similar strategies to influence others are used cross-culturally, but culture affects how frequently the various tactics are used. For instance, in Chinese culture, where saving face and group harmony are paramount, influence attempts are often subtle and indirect.
- Males tend to have more position power than females because they are more likely to be found in official high-status roles. This gives them more access to the bases of power. Also, because of gender stereotypes, male authority is seen as more legitimate, and males as more competent.
- Some research suggests that women possess greater referent power than men because this type of power is not dependent on position power and has its origin in liking.
- Male group members are more influential when the task is seen as gender-neutral or masculine; female members are more influential if the task is seen as feminine.
- When a group has close to equal numbers of females and males, females have as much influence as males. However, when females are a numerical minority, they have little influence. When males are the minority, they still have influence in the group.
- Unless females possess legitimate or expert power, they use more indirect and less assertive influence tactics than males and rely more on interpersonal agreeableness and warmth to influence others.

Skill Review

Enhance Your Status

- Be aware that you may have to pay some "status dues" before you are allowed to assume a higher status.
- Enhance others' performance expectations of you. Tell the group about skills and experience you possess that are relevant to the task.
- Work on "power and prestige behavior" such as maintaining eye contact, responding promptly, and having a strong and steady voice.
- If you have reason to believe that your diffuse-status characteristics lead others to have low performance expectations for you, remind yourself that you belong as much as anyone else. Work hard to contribute to the group, and over time you will probably earn higher status in the group.

Use Power Wisely

- Avoid the use of coercive power.
- Enhance your expert power by demonstrating your knowledge and expertise and making other members aware of your credentials.

- Increase your referent power by being friendly, warm, positive, and interested in others.
- Get clear on the legitimate authority associated with your role in the group. When socializing new group members, be explicit about the chain of command and the areas in which they are "allowed" to exercise authority.
- Remember that people in officially low-status positions may actually have considerable power. Be respectful and gracious when making requests of them.
- Consider that norms regarding what is an acceptable influence tactic may vary based on culture, the group, and even personal preferences. Learn what you can about the group and about individual members, and adjust influence tactics accordingly.

Enhance Group Effectiveness

- Avoid creating performance expectations of group members based on diffuse-status characteristics such as age, gender, or ethnicity.
- Be aware of the tendency to reserve higher-status role for members of gender and ethnic groups more valued by society. Develop clear and objective ways to assign status. Give all members the experiences and training needed to earn higher status in the group.
- Do not condone or permit the ill-treatment of lower-status members by higher-status members. Model respect and appreciation for what each member contributes to the group.
- Do not make status a scarce resource for which group members must compete.
- Use a fair system to award status and its trappings, such as titles, resources, and freedoms.
- In a group in which each member has relevant knowledge and nobody has a monopoly on ideas, minimize the influence of status differences. Keep meetings free of obvious status symbols such as insignias, titles, and seating privileges, and emphasize a norm of mutual respect and appreciation for each person's ideas and contributions.
- Do not ignore members who feel they are not receiving the respect and prestige they deserve. Acknowledge their value to the group, and do what you can to "right status wrongs."
- Emphasize norms of cooperation to handle group members who seem to have a high need to dominate the group and others at the expense of the group and other members.

Study Questions

1. What are the "status basics" described at the beginning of the chapter?
2. How can you identify high-status group members?

3. How can individuals earn high status in a group? What does it mean to say that you may have to pay "status dues"?
4. According to the ethological approach, how does status develop in groups?
5. How does expectation states theory explain how status is determined in groups? How do performance expectations influence the assignment of status?
6. What is status characteristics theory, and what is status generalization?
7. What is a self-fulfilling prophecy, and what is a stereotype threat? How do these perpetuate the lower status of individuals from certain groups?
8. Can early status assignments change? How can individuals enhance their status?
9. How may the quest for status pollute a group? What can be done to prevent this?
10. What does it mean to say that our perceptions of our status are influenced by social comparative processes? What happens when we compare ourselves to other group members and come to believe that our status is lower than is fair?
11. What happens in a group when some members come to believe that they and other members of their subgroup are unfairly denied the opportunity to climb the group's status ladder?
12. What are the sources or bases of power described by French and Raven?
13. What is the relationship between status and power?
14. What are influence tactics? What factors should guide the choice of influence tactic?
15. What do we know about culture, gender, and power?

Group Activities

Activity 1: Observe Status and Power Dynamics in a Decision-Making Group

A five-person group of students sits in a circle in the middle of the classroom (sometimes this is called a "fishbowl"). They are told that they are a student government committee that is to create a policy on professor–student dating at the university. They have 45 minutes to come up with a draft policy. The rest of the students form a large circle around them and quietly observe the status and power dynamics in the group. When discussion time is up, the larger group should break into groups of five and consider the following: (1) Identify the most influential group members; that is, which members' ideas were most likely to be taken up by the group? (2) Comment on the status markers displayed by group members (eye contact, body posture, firmness of voice, amount of participation). (3) Status characteristics theory suggests that in task-oriented groups a status hierarchy forms consistent with the statuses that members possess in society at large. Did this hold true for this group? (4) If the "fishbowl" group were to meet again to complete the policy, what recommendations would you make to them to improve group effectiveness?

Activity 2: Analyze Status Case Studies

With your group, analyze the following cases using chapter concepts.

CASE 1 This past summer I was one of 200 college undergraduates selected to participate in Disney's summer college program. The program requires working in the park doing regular minimum-wage jobs and taking professional Disney University classes. Little did I know when I arrived that I would be a program "rookie." Fortunately, I was blessed with three great roommates, all third- and fourth-year returnees to the program. As I whined about having to do such menial jobs as street sweeping and guest control during parades and fireworks, my roommates laughingly assured me that they had all began that way their first year and that you have to start at the bottom to get to the top. They told me that the first year you get the worst positions, the second year you get to pick, and by the third or fourth year, you can walk into an excellent corporate-style internship job experience. They also reminded me that every Disney CEO or department head I have met started his or her career on Disneyland's Main Street or in Fantasyland.

CASE 2 I recently began working at an engineering firm. My position normally requires a bachelor's degree that I am six months from finishing, but I persuaded the interviewers that I could do the job. They hired me at a salary that is higher than most of those in my job category, even though my peers have college degrees. I think it helped that I am bilingual and worked for a successful engineering firm. Also, maybe it helped that I "look the part" of the successful engineer—I am Euroamerican, 30 years old, six feet tall, with a short haircut and glasses, and look very professional. The supervisors had high expectations of me and immediately gave me high-level projects. They obviously have faith in me and think that I deserve to be treated well. Oddly though, my coworkers are unfriendly toward me and are reluctant to share information I need to complete my assignments. I am not sure what I have done wrong and what I can do to become more accepted.

Activity 3: Study the Relationship Between Target and Influence Tactics

Each group member makes three lists: (1) How I Get My Way With My "Superiors" (boss, coach, parents, or teacher), (2) How I Get My Way With My Romantic Partner, and (3) How I Get My Way With My Peers (or coworkers). Together, the group classifies responses according to the nine influence strategies discussed in Box 4-2. What differences were seen in the influence tactics used, based on who the target was?

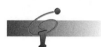

InfoTrac College Edition Search Terms

To do research for your papers and assignments, use InfoTrac that's provided free with new copies of this book. Go to: http://infotrac.thomsonlearning.com and enter the following search terms:

- Social Status, Psychological Aspects
- Social Status, Research
- Status Characteristics
- Social Power Theory
- Influence Tactics

Chapter 5 Communication in Groups

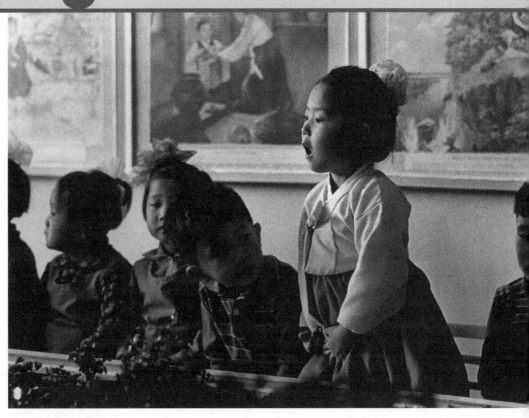

© Miroslav Zajic/CORBIS

People often say that their group has "communication problems," or that their group's problems could be solved if there was "better communication." After reading this chapter, you will know more about what healthy group communication looks like and how to promote it. You will understand how to increase verbal and nonverbal effectiveness and how to stand up for yourself in a group without hurting other members. You will have learned about the challenges of communicating with group members from other cultures and how this may be done more effectively. You will recognize the role of communication structure in group effectiveness.

Communication is the transmission of information and understanding between group members. Communication is central to groups. As we saw in Chapter 1, for a collection of people to be a group, there must be interaction and

Communication
The transmission of information and understanding between group members.

influence. These are accomplished through communication. Communication may also be viewed as part of a group's structure (Cartwright & Zander, 1968). In most groups, there is a predictable direction and flow of messages between members. For example, members communicate with some members more than they do with others, and some individuals in the group receive more communications than others do. Communication is also linked to group effectiveness. Members must communicate to exchange information, solve problems, and coordinate their efforts. Failures in communication can lead to misunderstandings and conflict, poor use of member skills and resources, and wasted time. For tasks requiring interaction and coordination, communication is central to making our intentions known to others, requesting and providing information, inviting others to share thoughts and suggestions, directing others to take actions, and managing social relations among group members (Orasanu, Fischer, & Davison, 1997). Finally, because group work includes a relational dimension, how members communicate with one another influences their satisfaction with the group (Anderson & Martin, 1999).

Communication as Part of Group Structure

Communication structure

A group's established communication network, the pattern of information sharing in the group.

Do you talk equally to all members of the groups you are a part of? Do all members participate equally? What is the pattern of information sharing in the group—who tells what to whom? These questions pertain to a group's **communication structure.** Most groups have an established communication network that is part of the group's structure (Cartwright & Zander, 1968). This network includes the communication channels in the group and who communicates with whom.

Centralized and Decentralized Communication Networks

Centralized communication network

A communication structure in which members must go through a central person to communicate with one another and one member is the principal source and target of communication.

Research on communication networks consistently shows that one of the most important features of a network is its degree of centralization (Brown & Miller, 2000; Shaw 1964, 1978). In a **centralized communication network,** members must go through a central person to communicate with one another, and a single person within the group is the principal source and target of communication (Brown & Miller, 2000). Members who talk a lot and have dominant personalities often become the center of the network (Bales, Strodtbeck, Mills, & Roseborough, 1951; Brown & Miller, 2000). Contrast this with a **decentralized communication network,** in which information can flow between members without going through a central person and there is a more or less equal distribution of communication and access to information (Foushee, 1984; Tushman, 1979). Overall, research suggests that for simple tasks requiring only the collation of information, centralized networks

Figure 5-1

Examples of Centralized and Decentralized Communication Networks

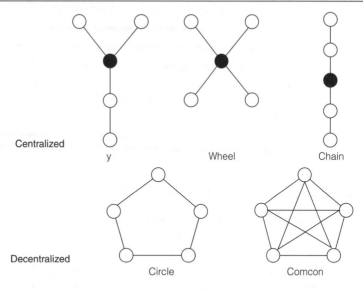

Centralized

y   Wheel   Chain

Decentralized

Circle   Comcon

In centralized networks, messages pass through a central person (indicated here by the filled in circle). Decentralized networks give members the opportunity to communicate equally with one another.

Decentralized communication network

A communication structure in which information flows between members without going through a central person and communication and access to information are more or less equally distributed.

emerge, whereas decentralized structures appear when tasks are complex and require more extensive information processing (Brown & Miller, 2000; Hirokawa, 1990; Watson & Michaelsen, 1988).

For groups to operate effectively, their members must be able to communicate easily and efficiently (Shaw, 1971). Early research suggested that hierarchical and centralized communication networks such as the "wheel," the "Y-shape," and the "chain" were most effective (see Figure 5-1). Leavitt (1951) concluded that a centralized network such as the wheel or Y-shape was the most efficient for solving problems, whereas the circle was least efficient in terms of time to solution, number of errors, and number of communications. Later, researchers discovered that this is only true when the task is a relatively simple one and communication is needed mainly for the collection of information (Brown & Miller, 2000; Hirokawa, 1990; Shaw, 1971). Simple, routine tasks with established procedures for completion have low information-processing requirements and do not require or benefit from multiple communications among multiple group members (Brown & Miller, 2000; Hirokawa, 1990).

For complex tasks, especially ambiguous and uncertain tasks requiring not only information but also analysis, decentralized communication networks such as the circle, and "comcon" are more effective than centralized networks (Brown & Miller, 2000; Shaw, 1964, 1978). In this case, one person would likely be over-loaded with information, or what Shaw (1964) called "saturated" (Davies, 1996; Shaw, 1964). Decentralized communication structures are also advisable because when communication is centralized, morale in the group drops, and ultimately, productivity is negatively affected (Bavelas, 1950). As Shaw (1964, 1971, 1978) noted, in centralized networks such as the wheel and chain, one person makes most of the decisions and sends and receives most communications. This person is usually more satisfied than members who occupy more peripheral communication positions in the group. In general, group members prefer an active role in the group, and being left out of the "communication loop" is unsatisfying.

Formal and Informal Communication Networks

Formal communication network

A layered communication network officially designated by the group or organization.

Communication networks may also be categorized as formal or informal. Communicating with the president of your university probably requires that you go through specified channels. You probably cannot just dial the president's number and reach him or her directly. At the very least, you will have to talk first with the administrative staff, who will probably follow particular guidelines to decide whether and how to relay your message. Most organizations have such hierarchical (layered) **formal communication networks** and channels. For instance, it might be standard practice for the executive director to convey a policy change via memo to the supervisors, who convey it via phone call to the shift leads, who share it with the line staff at a weekly meeting.

Informal communication network

A group's unofficial communication network.

Not all groups have formal communication networks, but all groups have **informal communication networks.** Early in the life of the group, an informal communication structure tends to form based on participation rates, with one or a few members sending and receiving a majority of communications (Davies, 1996). This structure tends to mirror status and attraction patterns in the group (Forsyth, 1999; Shaw, 1964). In other words, higher-status members tend to be more central in the communication structure, sending and receiving more messages, and the patterns of communication in the group usually reflect members' liking for one another in that members who like one another communicate more frequently.

Grapevines and Gossip

Grapevine

The channel through which gossip, rumors, and other unofficial information travels through the group.

Informal communication networks often arise to make up for shortcomings in the formal network. Such is the case with **grapevines**—the name for the channels through which gossip, rumors, and other unofficial information travels through the group. Grapevines are often a source of information for those who are left out of the formal communication loop because of their lower status. The clerical staff at my university has a well-functioning grapevine. I am often amazed by what clerical staffpeople know from the staff grapevine. Sometimes they have information well before it makes its way through the formal communication channels. My neighborhood, in a new housing tract built by a developer, also has a grapevine. The male neighbors have bonded through the sharing of information passed along the grapevine. They talk over the fence in their backyards, at the community mailbox, and when taking out the trash. They talk about who has what problem with their house, how the developer is dealing with resident complaints, and various strategies used to get the developer to act. Information is passed from one person to another until all group members are updated.

Gossip

Communications about other group members that may or may not be factual.

Rumor

Unsubstantiated gossip.

not supported by evidence

Gossip and rumors also travel through the group via the grapevine. **Gossip** can be defined as news about the affairs of another, or as any hearsay of a personal nature, be it positive or negative, spoken or in print (Rosnow & Fine, 1976). Although gossip and **rumor** are often treated as the same, they can be distinguished in that the basis of rumor is always unsubstantiated, whereas gossip may or may not be based on a known fact (Rosnow & Fine, 1976). Gossip and rumor are frequently considered forms of female communication, and males are rarely said to gossip. However, recent research indicates that although we may be less likely to label what males do as gossip, they in fact gossip about as much as females (Harrington & Bielby, 1995; Johnson, 1994; Nevo & Nevo, 1993). For instance, the men in my neighborhood talk about the personal qualities of the developer's employees and why particular employees have left. They also share information about the people they have seen looking at the houses for sale and what they know about who is moving in. I have never heard what they do call gossip, but I think that if women engaged in the same conversations, their communication would almost certainly be labeled gossip.

Gossip has the potential to both create and destroy social bonds in the group. To be trusted with gossip builds member bonds because it "indicates who is trustworthy and who is not" (Merry, 1984, p. 291). We can feel closer to another member who trusts us enough to share secret information. However, we all know that gossip and rumor can be damaging to a group and to individual members. For instance, mistakenly treating a rumor as fact can lead the group to make a poor decision. Gossiping about other group members may cause damage to their reputations and to member relationships if there is the perception that confidences were violated or that the gossiper's intention was to harm. This can contribute to conflict and to member dropout.

Despite these problems, gossip is common, and many find it hard to resist. This is because it serves a number of different functions. For instance, we often seek information about others via gossip for purposes of social comparison (for instance, employees may gossip about salaries), and hearing others' woes can make us feel better about our own situation (Festinger, 1954; Suls, 1977). There is also a certain thrill obtained from gossip because of its forbidden nature. Producers of gossip gain power and status from being able to "manage the news," while consumers of gossip receive personal pleasure from being "privileged insiders" (Rosnow & Fine, 1976, p. 88). Embedded in gossip we often find information about group norms and values. In other words, hearing some members gossip about the behavior of other members, we learn what is acceptable and unacceptable in the group.

Sharing gossip and secrets about other group members can even enhance the stability of relationships by discharging tension and enlisting the listener's help in dealing with the other person (McGoldrick, 1998). Gossip may also provide information about other group members that is relevant to group functioning but preserves member dignity. For instance, you may know that one member is dealing with his partner's cancer diagnosis. When other members gossip about his declining performance, you share your insider information, and the complaining members understand and "cut him slack." Gossip may also fulfill social needs, bringing members together for social interaction and giving diverse members something in common to talk about. In my experience, groups often use gossip to alleviate boredom. In sum, gossip is not all bad. Sometimes we need to talk about other group members, and doing so can contribute to group cohesion, create stronger group identification, and clarify group boundaries (Gluckman, 1963; Nevo & Nevo, 1993).

Communication Structure and Improving Group Effectiveness

Communication structures and practices often evolve to serve the needs of the group at that time. But they may become entrenched and outlive their usefulness when tasks change. Or, in the case of gossip and rumor, they may be destructive to the group. Here are some suggestions for using what you have learned about communication structure to enhance group functioning.

1. Review your group's communication structure. For example, if the structure is centralized and central members are overwhelmed because of task complexity, or if members are dissatisfied with being left out of the communication process, decentralize. If the structure is decentralized when a more centralized structure would be more efficient, centralize.
2. Manage gossip and rumors so that they do not harm the group. Keep others informed, because people "left in the dark" will talk with one another to try to figure out what is going on.
3. Foster a cooperative group culture in which gossip is more likely to be benign and done carefully to avoid damage to members and their reputations. In a competitive group, gossip and rumors are more likely to be intended to harm others.
4. Leaders should also pay attention to the amount and type of gossip that occurs in the group and confront gossiping members if gossip threatens to ruin the group or harm individual members. Rumors should be addressed immediately.

Apply It! ••• **Create an Interaction Diagram of a Group**

Observe a group meeting and create an "interaction diagram" following the guidelines described by Beebe and Masterson (1994). Draw a circle for each member of the group, and arrange them in the same relative positions as those in which group members are seated. Use arrows between members to represent communications sent from one member to another. Use a short crossmark near the tip of the arrow to represent each occurrence. If a member sends a message to the entire group, draw an arrow from the person to the center of the group. Who is the most vocal member of the group? Is communication centralized or decentralized?

5. Members should remember that they are under no obligation to participate in gossip. If others' gossip makes you feel uncomfortable, offer a neutral response such as "uh-huh" or a more assertive "I am really not comfortable talking about this."

6. Check out information obtained from the grapevine before sharing it as fact or making a decision based on it. Ask people where they got it, and since people tend to embellish (exaggerate), ask them exactly what was told to them.

Verbal and Nonverbal Communication

As was said earlier, communication is the transmission of information and understanding between individuals. People send messages, and people receive messages. Ideally, the message received is the one sent, but the complexity of communication means that this is not always the case. Accurate communication is challenging because so many modes of communication operate simultaneously; because senders and receivers do not always agree on what words, tones, and gestures mean; and because people do not listen well.

Verbal Communication, Nonverbal Communication, and Paralanguage

Verbal communication
The way we communicate using words.

Nonverbal communication
The way we communicate using body language such as gestures, body orientation, touching, personal distance, paralanguage, and facial expressions.

Group members talk, and what they say, how they say it, and what they are doing while they talk all matter. Our words, our **verbal communication,** are obviously an important part of our communication. A little later in the chapter, you will read about the types of verbal communication that promote cooperation and the types that create a hostile group climate. Equally important is **nonverbal communication**—the way we communicate using body language such as gestures, body orientation, touching, personal distance, paralanguage, and facial expressions.

Nonverbal behavior is loaded with information. It often tells us about the relative status of group members because higher-status members tend to make more eye contact, stand closer, touch more, and assume more prominent physical locations in the group such as sitting at the head of the table. It is also often meta-communicative, serving to qualify verbal behavior. Nonverbal communication may also communicate information that is too embarrassing or sensitive to state directly. Because it frequently occurs without conscious awareness, it is less subject to censorship than verbal behavior, so emotional messages often "leak" out nonverbally (Mehrabian, 1972). For instance, you cannot always control those looks of disappointment, frustration, disgust, or hurt that cross your face, and these expressions communicate a great deal to those who observe them. Likewise, you may not realize that you are yawning or staring off into space, thereby communicating to others that you are bored. Similarly, your messages are often communicated unintentionally via **paralanguage,** a form of nonverbal communication that includes voice pitch, rate, quality, and tone as well as nonword communications such as "tsking" and sighing. Think, for instance, about all the different ways you can say "Oh" and what each variation communicates.

Paralanguage
A form of nonverbal communication that includes voice pitch, rate, quality, and tone as well as nonword communications such as "tsking" and sighing.

Culture affects nonverbal communication. For instance, a nod in Japan means only that I am listening, whereas in the United States, it means that I agree. Gender also affects nonverbal communication. Women tend to smile more, and men tend to engage in more nonverbal dominance behavior (Dovidio, Ellyson, Keating, Heltman, & Brown, 1988; Wood, 1994). Research also suggests that females are better at reading nonverbal messages (Hall, 1998). However, many researchers believe that this is because people, regardless of gender, are sensitive to nonverbal signals when they are low in power, and women usually have lower power and status than males (Tavris, 1992). Such sensitivity makes sense because to survive, "subordinates" must be able to read and respond appropriately to the behavior of powerful others.

BOX 5-1 / COMMUNICATING VIA EMAIL

Communication through email is increasingly common. Early on, users discovered that the medium often resulted in miscommunication. The lack of face-to-face contact and the absence of the spoken word reduced the amount of information sent and received—there were only words. It did not take long for users to develop a system of nonverbal communication in which symbols, called "emoticons," could be used to convey emotions that could not otherwise be communicated. For instance, writing in all capital letters is sometimes used to signify a loud tone of voice, LOL means "laughing out loud," and ROTFL means "rolling on the floor laughing." Here are some common emoticons:

:-) smiling or agreeing	:-(frowning or sad
:-D grinning	;-) winking or joking
:-[pouting	:-O surprise

Apply It! ••• Analyzing Your Nonverbal Communication at a Recent Meeting

Think about the last group meeting you attended. Did you use gestures when you communicated, and did these help convey your message? Did your tone of voice accurately reflect your feelings? How was the volume of your voice? Did you look up, scan the group, and make eye contact? When other group members spoke, what did your nonverbal behavior communicate? Did you smile, frown, grimace, nod your head, shake your head, close your eyes, stare into space, lean forward, or away? Where did you locate yourself in the room, and what did this communicate? Can you identify some areas for improvement?

Nonverbal communication in the group is especially interesting when you consider that although only one person may be speaking, all other members are communicating nonverbally at the same time. They open their eyes wide and raise their eyebrows when surprised. They may wrinkle their brows in confusion, raise their top lip to indicate disgust, or roll their eyes or shake their heads in disagreement. They may smile at a good idea or nod their heads in agreement. They may lean forward and orient their body toward the speaker or lean away and stare off into space. A lot is communicated nonverbally at any given time in the group; for this reason, it is good to get in the habit of scanning the group whether you are the speaker or a listener.

Congruent Communication

Congruent message
When the verbal and nonverbal content of a message are consistent and match.

Incongruent message
When the verbal content and the nonverbal content of a message are mixed and suggest different things.

When verbal and nonverbal messages match and are perceived to be communicating the same message, we say that the message is **congruent** (Satir, Banmen, Gerber, & Gomari, 1991). Congruent messages are easier to understand because the information is consistent; we do not have to figure out which message to believe. However, many times the verbal content says one thing, yet we receive a different impression from the nonverbal content. In other words, the message is **incongruent.** "It's okay," a member says, with teary eyes and a quivering voice, giving you the distinct feeling that it is not okay. Or a member says he supports a group decision, but he has pulled away from the table and has his arms crossed over his chest. Incongruent communications are often confusing, because we aren't sure which message to listen to or whether our mind is playing tricks on us. Was the contradictory message really communicated? Or is my interpretation merely the projection of my own desires or insecurities? When in doubt about a message, ask for clarification. For example, you could say, "I know you said X, but somehow I'm getting the impression that you feel Y." Often such statements can bring about a meaningful discussion.

You may run across a group member who regularly delivers mixed messages—messages that could be taken in several different ways. For example, such a person might say something about your performance in the group that feels hurtful but is couched as a friendly joke so you don't really know which way to take it. Although some people deliver mixed messages to hurt others and avoid taking responsibility for it, most often people who do this are fearful of conflict yet want to communicate their dissatisfaction or disapproval. If you take it well, they might own it, but if you do not, they can deny it is what they meant. Also, in some groups and cultures, it is normative to deliver feedback in this indirect fashion. It allows everyone to save face. Unfortunately, some people will consciously or unconsciously ignore subtle messages they do not like, placing the burden on you to send the message directly. Others do not hear these subtly delivered messages because they simply do not have the ability to decode them, whether because of cultural differences or because they lack the skills to do so.

Guidelines for Effective Verbal and Nonverbal Communication

You just learned about the multiple levels of communication. Here are some guidelines for using this information to send the messages you want to send, and to receive the messages others intend to send.

1. Try to communicate congruent messages (messages in which verbal, nonverbal, and paralanguage do not communicate contradictory messages).
2. Ask for clarification if you feel you are receiving a mixed message.
3. Consider your listeners, and adapt your message to increase the likelihood they will receive the message you intended to send.
4. Be sensitive to others' comfort level regarding touch and personal distance by reading their nonverbal cues. Touching and decreased personal distance may be experienced as dominating, intimidating, disrespectful, and even as sexually harassing.
5. Be aware that even if you are not speaking, you are communicating nonverbally. Work to send the messages you want to send.

Group Communication Climate

Group communication climate

Whether the context in which group communication occurs is cooperative and supportive or defensive and competitive.

Group communication climate refers to the context in which group communication occurs. This context affects how the group works together. Which group would you prefer to be a member of—Group A, in which the majority of communications are devoted to supporting one another and the group's work, or Group B, in which members are defensive and competitive with one another? In Group A, communication occurs in a context of cooperation and joint problem solving. In Group B, communication occurs in a context of competition and battle.

Supportive (Cooperative) and Defensive (Competitive) Communication Climates

Cooperative or supportive climate

A communication climate in which members feel free to communicate honestly and the communication is directed toward the group's work.

Competitive or defensive climate

A communication climate in which members distrust one another and communication is competitive.

Do members trust one another and view their relationships as primarily cooperative ones in which they work together to solve group problems and achieve group goals? In such a **cooperative or supportive climate,** members feel free to communicate honestly, and the communication is directed toward the group's work. Or is there a **competitive or defensive climate** in which members distrust other members, viewing them as competitors? In this climate, members engage in guarded or defensive communications in order to protect themselves or get what they want.

A supportive climate promotes cooperation, and a defensive climate promotes competition. In a defensive climate, members' communications are oriented toward defending themselves against negative comments, resisting members' attempts to control the group, trying to get others to care, trying to gain the respect they deserve, and trying to put others in their place. When members are defensive, energy is diverted that might have been better devoted to promoting the group and its tasks, and the bonds of trust in the group are broken. In a supportive climate, communications in the group promote the group's well-being and task accomplishment. Members feel safe sharing ideas and say things that indicate they care about the group, the task, and other members. Feedback is constructive, and the climate is one of mutual respect and flexibility in problem solving.

A cooperative communication climate has a number of benefits. A cooperative group communication climate leads to increased cohesion and increased productivity (Johnson & Johnson, 2000). When cooperation is high, people work harder and longer at group tasks (Tyler & Blader, 2000). Cooperative behaviors lubricate the group's social machinery, reducing friction and increasing coordination of member efforts (Podsakoff, Ahearne, & MacKenzie, 1997; Tyler & Blader, 2000). Members are more satisfied in groups with supportive, cooperative communication climates (Anderson & Martin, 1999; Bormann, 1990).

Given the importance of a cooperative climate, it is worth the time to consider carefully what people do in groups that can lead to either a supportive or a defensive communication climate. A classic article by Gibb (1961) identified six categories of member behaviors that influence whether a climate is supportive or defensive:

1. **Evaluation versus description.** In a defensive group climate, members respond to ideas they do not like with negative judgmental reactions that make the ideas' originator feel criticized and defensive. These evaluative responses erode trust and cohesion. For instance, after one member makes a suggestion, another might say "That's ridiculous, that would never work." Evaluative responses may also be nonverbal such as eye-rolling or head-shaking. Depending on the person, evaluative responses may lead members to retreat from the group

or to vociferously defend their idea, even if they originally were not very committed to it. In the supportive group climate, bad ideas may be rejected, but this is done neutrally, without suggesting that the person who offered the idea is an idiot. The receiver simply responds with a description of what s/he thinks, feels, or observes. For instance, saying "I like your idea in theory, but I don't see how we could implement it in time" is a way of rejecting the idea while maintaining a feeling of support.

2. **Control versus problem orientation.** A defensive climate is also likely when one or more members attempt to manipulate or control the group to get their way. A control orientation can be seen in a number of different group member behaviors. For instance, a member may try to get his or her way through a condescending suggestion that he or she knows what is best for the group and they do not. A member may also try to bully the group by dominating the group's discussion time until they cave in. Some members intimidate the group by yelling or appearing physically threatening. Many members will resist the manipulator's efforts to control the group, taking up a lot of valuable group time. Some members will retreat from the group out of fear of the controller. In contrast, in the supportive climate, no one member is trying to impose his or her will on the group, and there is a sense that the group is working together to solve a problem.

3. **Strategy versus spontaneity.** Similarly, a defensive climate is likely when members believe that other members are manipulating the group in order to get what they want. If some members feel deceived, and that other members are acting for personal gain and not for the good of the group, they are likely to become defensive and resistant. In contrast, in the supportive climate, members act honestly, without deception, and no one tries to direct the group based on hidden or selfish motivations.

4. **Neutrality versus empathy.** If some members do not seem to care about the group, its task, and its members, a defensive climate may result. For instance, members who are obviously not paying attention in a group meeting, who locate themselves in a corner of the meeting room, or who are unresponsive detract from the group. When a member is indifferent to what others have to say, it signals a detachment from the group that interferes with cohesion. In a supportive climate, members are involved and present, not just physically but interpersonally. Members care about other members and what they have to say.

5. **Superiority versus equality.** When some members act in a superior manner, it is likely to create defensiveness as the put-down members feel demoralized and withdraw, or try to defend their honor. In the supportive climate, members feel valued and appreciated and trust that they will not be made to feel inferior.

6. **Certainty versus provisionalism.** Defensiveness is also likely when some members are not open to the ideas of others and act as though they already have all the answers. This type of obstinate certainty is belittling and aggravating. We

---

Apply It! ••• **Identify Supportive and Defensive Communication Climates**

Choose three groups you are a member of. Analyze each to determine whether there is a supportive or defensive group climate. In what way do your responses in the groups contribute to the groups' climates?

---

need to trust that the group is one in which we will be listened to and our input valued. In the supportive climate, members are open-minded. Their attitudes are provisional, and they are willing to change them depending on other members' input.

Confirming and Disconfirming Responses

In a supportive communication climate, members' responses to one another are confirming and encourage the sharing of ideas. Because members feel understood and validated, they are more likely to commit fully to the group. Unfortunately, in many groups, members feel disregarded or rejected by the responses of other members, causing them either to withdraw or to become more obnoxious in an effort to be heard. Observations of effective and ineffective groups suggest that in effective groups, communications are likely to include more **confirming responses,** such as the following (Sieberg & Larson, 1971):

Confirming responses

Supportive responses that encourage the sharing of ideas.

1. **Direct acknowledgments.** An acknowledgment such as "That's really something for us to consider" makes it clear that a member's message was heard.
2. **Adding to the information given by the other.** Saying, for instance, "I have something to add that suggests Donna is right" reinforces a member's message.
3. **Supportive responses.** A response such as "I can see why this matters so much to you" shows caring and understanding.
4. **Clarifying responses.** A response such as "Tell me more about that—I want to understand what you're saying" shows that the listener wants to hear what the sender has to say.
5. **Expression of positive feelings.** An example would be "I really like your idea."

These confirming responses make senders feel valued.

In ineffective groups, in contrast, communications are more likely to include **disconfirming responses,** such as the following (Sieberg and Larson, 1971):

Disconfirming responses

Unsupportive responses that make members feel disregarded or rejected.

1. **Impervious response.** An impervious response occurs when there is no acknowledgment of what a member has said. Being ignored in this way makes members feel "small" and rejected.

2. **Interrupting response.** When members interrupt one another while they are talking, the interrupted person feels dismissed and frustrated.
3. **Irrelevant response.** If a member says something and a second member responds by changing the subject or saying something completely unrelated, the second response is considered irrelevant.
4. **Tangential response.** A response is classified as a tangential response when the responder makes brief reference to the previous message but then immediately takes the conversation in another direction. A typical example is "Yeah, but . . ."

All of these disconfirming responses make people feel devalued, disrespected, and unimportant. Therefore, they are detrimental to cooperation and group effectiveness.

Suggestions for Fostering a Supportive Communication Climate

You just learned that members' responses to one another play an important role in creating a cooperative or competitive group climate. Here are some ways to use this information to improve your group behavior.

1. Avoid responding to others judgmentally. Express disagreement without suggesting that the other person is unintelligent or uninformed. Never use the word "stupid" (or any equivalent word) in responding to a group member.
2. Do not insist that your ideas are the only ideas that have merit. Show a willingness to consider other perspectives.
3. Do not attempt to manipulate the group to get your way. Behave honestly and openly in the group.
4. Participate in the group. Remember that if you act indifferent to the group and its members, they are likely to feel rejected.
5. Confirm others by adding to their ideas, asking them for clarification, and expressing understanding or support. Show them that you want to hear what they have to say.
6. Avoid disconfirming responses, such as changing the subject, giving a response that shows no acknowledgment of other members' contributions, or following another member's comments with responses such as "Yeah, but . . ."
7. Do not interrupt others. If you accidentally do so, catch yourself and say "I'm sorry, I interrupted you. Please finish what you were saying."
8. If you find yourself responding defensively in response to another group member, analyze your response to determine what made you feel defensive. Consider talking with the member who triggered your response and explaining why you reacted the way you did. The confrontation guidelines described later in this chapter may be useful for this purpose.
9. If you are a group leader and recognize that your group displays a defensive rather than a supportive climate, consider educating the group about supportive communication. Lead a discussion, and help the group agree to the adoption of supportive communication norms.

BOX 5-2 / EVALUATING YOUR ASSERTIVE TENDENCIES

Review the following scenarios and consider how you would likely respond.

1. What would you do if a coworker was consistently late and you had to cover for her or him?

    a. Try to ignore it. (passive, unassertive response)

    b. Calmly and directly tell the person that this creates a problem for you and from now on you need him/her to be there on time. (assertive response)

    c. Raise your voice, angrily telling the person that you'll make sure the boss hears about it if s/he doesn't straighten out. (aggressive response)

2. What would you say if a group member suggested a course of action for the group that you disagreed with?

    a. Say nothing. (passive, unassertive response)

    b. Speak up, acknowledging the merits of the other position but simply and directly expressing your concerns. (assertive)

    c. Loudly argue your point to get your way. (aggressive response)

3. How would you respond if another group member insulted you?

    a. Suffer the hurt in silence, possibly complaining to others about it later. (passive, unassertive response)

    b. Tell the person that you do not like to be talked to in that way. (assertive response)

    c. Say something equally mean or meaner back to the person. (aggressive response)

Are you more passive, assertive, or aggressive? What are the advantages and disadvantages of your tendency? Now consider the consequences of the three different responses (passive, assertive, aggressive). Which type is most likely to promote the health of the group and good working relationships between the members?

Assertive Communication

You will not always agree with other group members. Sometimes they do things that make you feel uncomfortable. On occasion, you may feel disrespected by the actions of another member. You may find yourself in a situation in which the group is about to undertake an action you disagree with, or simply do not want to participate in. How you handle these situations affects your relationships with other members and your commitment to the group. Take a minute to read **Box 5-2** before continuing. It will help you think about the different ways people can respond in these situations.

Unassertive (Passive), Aggressive, and Assertive Behavior

Many people are unassertive and passive when others displease them. Unassertive people fear others' anger or emotion, or believe that nice people should defer to others and not complain. Therefore, they keep their concerns to themselves.

People who are nonassertive deny themselves, allow others to choose for them, feel inhibited, hurt, and anxious, and do not achieve their goals (Alberti & Emmons, 1995). They do not speak up for themselves and do not deny the unreasonable requests of others. For instance, I know a young man who got a prominent tattoo he did not like because his tattoo artist designed it especially for him. He felt he could not say no and hurt the artist's feelings. A woodworker I knew shared a studio with some other woodworkers and became increasingly upset with the others for borrowing his tools. Rather than say anything, he suddenly moved out one weekend. The group had no idea why.

By holding back, unassertive people deny themselves full participation in the group. Although their hearts may be in the right place and they may believe that they are preserving group harmony, their dishonesty often hurts the group in unexpected ways. By not letting others know how they think and feel, unassertive group members do not let us wholly know them, and this prevents their full membership in the group. There are also times when the unassertive member's input could have prevented the group from making a mistake or would have contributed to a better product or decision.

Another problem is that although in some cases unassertive people can successfully let go of a concern, in other cases they cannot. The way unassertive persons handle this situation is to grow increasingly distant from the group, possibly even leaving it. They may also become so irritated that they engage in passive–aggressive behavior such as refusing to support others' ideas, turning in work late, or being distant and unfriendly. These negative behaviors are often efforts to get the group to figure out that a problem exists. It is also common for unassertive persons to eventually overreact to some minor transgression or impulsively (and ineffectively) confront when they can keep it in no longer.

When displeased in the group or with other members, a member can also respond either aggressively or assertively. Aggressive people forcefully speak their minds and may shout at others or bully others—for instance, by putting them down—to get their way. Aggressive people enhance themselves at the expense of others, choose for others, and lead others to feel hurt, defensive, and humiliated (Alberti & Emmons, 1995). Aggressive people prevent others from participating as equals in the group and contribute to defensive and competitive group climates. They may get what they want, but their behavior hurts others and interferes with group cohesion.

Assertive behavior
Behaviors oriented toward asserting one's own rights, opinions, or boundaries in a way that also respects the rights of others.

In contrast to both passive and aggressive behavior, **assertive behavior** "promotes equality in human relationships, enabling us to act in our own best interests, to stand up for ourselves without undue anxiety, to express honest feelings comfortably, and to exercise personal rights without denying the rights of others" (Alberti & Emmons, 1995, p. 6). Assertive behavior is self-expressive, honest, direct, firm, and respectful of the rights of others. It is simple and unblaming, tactful and diplomatic. It contributes to a cooperative, open communication climate in which members can express their ideas responsibly. Assertive behavior also prevents some of the problems associated with passive or aggressive behavior. Passive and aggressive behaviors diminish some members because they communicate that the interests of some members count more than do the interests of other members. Passive and aggressive behaviors cause damage to member relationships because they create hurt, anger, and withdrawal in the group.

Assertive behavior often takes practice and requires changes in both verbal and nonverbal behavior. Simple and straightforward words are used to say what you need to say, but *how* the message is conveyed is equally important. For instance, a relaxed and steady gaze, and occasionally looking away, enhances direct communication. Looking down or away communicates a lack of confidence and status. Conversely, staring too intently may threaten the other person. An active and erect posture, while facing the other person directly, bolsters the assertive message, whereas a slumped, passive posture does the opposite. A level, well-modulated, conversational tone is best for communicating an assertive message. One should not be too loud or soft, or sound whiny or angry. Also, assertive messages are communicated with a smooth, nonhesitant flow of speech.

Gender and Assertiveness

In the 1970s, when discussions of assertiveness first became popular, it was believed that women especially could benefit from assertiveness training. This is not surprising because the traditional female gender role has a relational focus, encouraging other-centeredness and to some extent submissiveness, especially to males. Conversely, the traditional male role, with its emphasis on competitiveness, is more compatible with assertive and aggressive responses. In general, high-status people are more assertive than low-status people are (Twenge, 2001), and the higher status of males relative to females in most societies (as evidenced by the greater educational, economic, and political opportunities afforded men) has also contributed to their greater assertiveness and aggressiveness (Burn, 2000). For instance, women's assertiveness in the twentieth century rose and fell in concert with their status in society, and most recent studies in the United States find no gender differences in assertiveness (Twenge, 2001). However, members of groups or societies that emphasize traditional gender roles may encounter social penalties for straying from these gendered expectations. Groups or group members with traditional ideas about gender may even label assertive women as aggressive, and assertive men as passive.

Culture and Assertiveness

Culture affects assertiveness in several ways. As mentioned previously, your culture may have different expectations regarding passive, assertive, and aggressive behavior depending on whether you are female or male. Also, cultures vary in power distance—the amount of respect and deference less powerful (subordinate) members are expected to give to more powerful (superior) members (Hofstede, 1980, 1991). In high power distance cultures, it is considered inappropriate to assert oneself when interacting with elders and those in authority. It is also important to consider that effective assertive behavior may differ depending on culture (Cheek, 1976; Comas-Diaz & Duncan, 1985; Yoshioka, 2000; Zane, Sue, Hu, & Kwon, 1991), especially as you are likely to find yourself working in groups with diverse members. In some cultural contexts, being effectively assertive may require more indirect, subtle language than in other cultures. For example, in comparison to other groups, Asian Americans and Latin Americans are often more understated and more respectful to others when asserting themselves (Comas-Diaz & Duncan, 1985; Zane, Sue, Hu, & Kwon, 1991). Also what is assertive in one cultural context may be perceived as aggressive in another. For instance, Cheek (1976) notes that the language of African Americans is spoken with vigor and energy, at a relatively high volume, and may be perceived as aggressive outside of that cultural environment.

Yoshioka (2000) found that assertive responses differ based on culture, mainly in terms of the intensity of the language used. Hispanic, African American, and Euroamerican women were asked to respond to six scenarios. Their responses were judged as unassertive, assertive, or aggressive by a female "judge" from their culture who was regarded as assertive in her community. For the Hispanic group, *simpatia* (avoidance of conflict) and *personalismo* (promotion of a personal quality in interactions) were recurrent themes in assertive responses, whereas African American and Euroamerican women were more likely to make explicit reference to consequences or obligations on the other person's part that impelled compliance. **Box 5-3** provides an example from Yoshioka's study.

BOX 5-3 / EXAMPLES OF CULTURALLY ACCEPTABLE ASSERTIVE RESPONSES

Here are sample responses from Yoshioka's (2000) study, showing how what was considered assertive depended on culture.

Vignette: You and this guy are friends. One day, you get into an argument. He gets really mad and shoves you hard. Then right away he says he's sorry. He hasn't been smoking, drinking, or doing anything. If you had to stand up for yourself and tell him that he can NOT do it again, what would you say?

A Euroamerican woman: "You can't be treating me this way. Otherwise our relationship will not work."

An African American woman: "Let me tell you, sorry ain't good enough. You don't push on me. Anytime you push on me, I am going to push you right on back. Don't take me for granted. We're supposed to be friends so you might as well leave me alone 'cause it can't go this way no more. It's over."

A Hispanic woman: "Esta bien acepto tu disculpa, pero que por favor nunca vuelva a suceder eso, porque eso si que no se lo voy a permitir." ("It's okay, I accept your apology, but please don't let that ever happen again because I won't permit it.")

Message matching
The idea that message senders should tailor their message to the target so that the intended message will be understood.

Because culture affects what is considered a passive, aggressive, or assertive communication, Cheek (1976) recommends that we engage in **message matching.** Message matching means that as *senders* we consider various verbal options in relation to the particular target person and select the most appropriate and effective assertive message so that it is more likely that the message we intend is the one received. Message matching also requires that as *receivers* we take into account the sender's culture so that we hear the message that was intended. Many people resist this more flexible approach, preferring to see their own cultural practices as correct and demanding that others toe their cultural line. Unfortunately, this type of thinking reduces their intercultural communication competence. You will learn more about intercultural communication later in the chapter.

It should also be noted that message matching applies at the individual level as well. Personality and style differences are such that, for optimal communication effectiveness, we should tailor our message to the individual and consider individual differences when receiving messages as well. In other words, an assertive message from one group member may sound very different than an assertive message from another. Likewise, you may send a message intended to be assertive that may be heard as assertive by one member and as aggressive by another.

Communicating and Resolving Differences

Constructive confrontations
Calm, well-prepared confrontations that involve clarifying and exploring the issues and the feelings of the participants, and mutual problem solving.

Chapter 7 focuses specifically on conflict and its resolution, but communication oriented toward conflict resolution between group members is relevant here as well. Sometimes you need to talk with a group member about a difficult issue that threatens your relationship, interferes with the group's work, or makes it hard to work together. It is best to do this thoughtfully rather than impulsively so that you can clearly express your view of the conflict and at the same time issue a sincere invitation to the other person to do the same. This is the heart of constructive confrontation. **Constructive confrontations** involve clarifying and exploring the issues, the needs of the participants, and their feelings (Johnson & Johnson, 2000). Effective confrontations do not involve uncensored expressions of thoughts and feelings; they are not about getting mad and dumping on someone after months of keeping quiet. On the contrary, planning and tact are what make truth-telling, and truth-hearing, possible in difficult situations and about the toughest subjects (Lerner, 1989). Diplomacy is almost always more effective than unbridled expressions of anger.

Confrontations work best when you are calm and have thought carefully about how to present the conflict. In fact, it is often a good idea to write it down and rehearse the confrontation so that you have the words in mind. Define the conflict in a small and specific way. Do not drag out everything that has ever bothered you about the person or the relationship. That's called "gunny-sacking" or "kitchen sinking" (as in everything but the kitchen sink) and is bound to overwhelm the person and cause defensiveness.

It is often good to start by saying that the relationship or person is important to you but this "thing" is getting in the way of continued closeness or cooperation and that you wouldn't do something so difficult if the relationship weren't important to you or if you didn't think it was important for group effectiveness. Then, present the conflict as a mutual problem to be solved. What can *we* do? For example, "I've always enjoyed working with you and expect we'll be working together for at least another ten years. That's why I feel we have to talk about a few things that have been making our work together harder than I think it has to be. I'd like to tell you what it looks from my side, and then I'd really like to hear what it looks like from yours. Then together, I am hoping that we can come up with some solutions." Or, "We've been friends forever and I want to keep it that way. But I am finding myself avoiding you right now because I'm feeling resentful about a few things. I know this is not good for our relationship, so I'd like us to talk about it and hopefully come to a joint understanding so that we can get our friendship back where it used to be." Above all, stay as calm as you can, because anger is likely to be met with anger, intensity only breeds more intensity, anxiety only more anxiety, and so on. People tend to return what is given to them, good or bad. If you have a competitive confrontation stance, so will others; if you have a cooperative stance, they will mirror that. In the intimate relationship confrontation, it is especially important to remain calm. As Lerner (1989) points out, to get at the emotional truth may actually require not acting too emotional.

Think about your contribution to the conflict, and take your share of responsibility for it. Chances are you do bear some of it, and if you take your share, other people are more likely to reciprocate by taking theirs. "Jill, I bear some responsibility for this situation because I didn't clearly communicate the job expectations." "I apologize for not telling you sooner that this was a problem for me. You couldn't be expected to know without my telling you."

Frame the conflict in terms of issues and actions, not personalities. "It is so inconsiderate of you to leave early when you know I'll have to stay late to finish your work" is an example of a statement likely to create defensiveness and an attack on you. (Who wouldn't react negatively to being called inconsiderate?) In contrast, imagine the reaction you'd get with this approach:

> I know I've been less friendly than usual, and I think I owe you an explanation. It's because I've felt mad at you but was scared to talk to you about it. Then I realized it's not fair to be mad at you without even talking to you about what's going on, so here it is. For the last two months, you've left early at least twice a week, and I've had to stay late to finish all the work. This is a problem for me because I need to get home to help my kids with their homework, get them their baths,

and put them to bed at a decent time. The first couple of times you left early, I thought "no big deal," but when it started to be a regular thing, I started feeling angry about it. I want us to have a good working relationship because I've always liked working with you, so I'm hoping we can figure something out together.

Present your definition of the issue, but make an effort to hear the other person's. As Harriet Lerner (1989) pointed out, it is a huge challenge to get to a place where our wish to understand the other person is as great as our wish to be understood. Go in with an open mind and a willingness to understand the other. It may take a while, but it is the key to true conflict resolution. Try to see it from the other side. Taking the perspective of the other increases an understanding of the other person's intentions and reduces perceptions of threat (Richardson, Green, & Lago, 1998).

Minimize the likelihood of defensiveness by not attacking other people's self-concept. This means thinking about what kind of person they like to see themselves as and making sure that you do not attack it. For instance, if it is important to them to be a considerate person or an intelligent person, then it is important for you to choose your words so as not to suggest otherwise. State things such that they are able to save face if possible. Even if you think they should be ashamed or should feel guilty, remember that if you shame or guilt them, defensiveness will likely ensue and prevent constructive dialogue. In the scenario above, you might help the person "save face" by adding "I really think of you as a considerate person, so I realize you didn't know this was a problem for me." One of my students confronted a boss who was driving the employees crazy by micromanaging their work. When confronting the boss, he expressed admiration for the boss's dedication to the job and his professionalism so that the boss didn't feel that this important part of himself was under attack when my student expressed his concerns.

Psychologists often tell us to use "I" statements in such situations. "I" statements begin with "I am/I feel/I hear/I think" and so on (Satir et al., 1991). The general pattern is to say "I felt _____ when you did _____." My student said something like

> I understand that your high standards and dedication are what make you check up on our work so much, and I appreciate where you are coming from, but I feel that you may be interfering with our work by interrupting us so frequently and requiring we get approvals on everything. I think we're as committed as you are to customer service. I feel that we are trustworthy and that you don't have to check up on us quite so often. I really believe the unit would operate more efficiently if we were given a little more responsibility for our work and didn't have to get your approvals on so many things.

Notice the absence of blaming "you's," such as "*You* make us feel . . ." "If *you* would only do things differently, we would be more productive." "*You* should trust us." "*You* shouldn't make us get so many approvals." People hear "I" messages much more easily than "You" messages.

If others act "attacked," gently assure them that that is not your intent. For instance, "I can see that you're upset and feel that I'm saying you're not a good lover/father/sister/brother/employee/coworker/boss. That's not at all what I mean. I'm just hoping that we can come up with a solution that works for both of us so that we can both accomplish our goals." If they attack you, do not "take the bait" by getting angry and counterattacking. This will get you off track and aggravate the conflict. Say something like "I can see that you're upset, and that's understandable, but if we stay focused, I think we can work this out." If you know the person very well, try to anticipate his or her defensive maneuvers and be prepared with responses to gently defuse them.

What do you do when a group member confronts you with your behavior? When someone approaches you with a problem that this person has with you or something that you did, do your best to use the Four R Method (Donohue & Kolt, 1992):

1. *Receive* the other's comments without interruption or defensiveness. Listen for emotion. Before solutions can be discussed, emotions need to be aired.
2. *Repeat* the comments to reflect the emotion, and in the process validate the person's right to have an emotional experience.
3. *Request* more information about the problem.
4. *Review* options, and decide on the best approach.

Communication in the Diverse Group

Communication conventions vary depending on age, culture, and sometimes gender, and in general, we are less comfortable with people who are different from us. This means that a diverse group membership poses some distinct challenges to group communication.

Apply It! ••• **Practice Constructive Confrontation**

Apply the guidelines described above to constructively confront someone. In preparing, you should consider (1) how you will begin, (2) what you will say to take your share of responsibility, (3) the person's self-concept and how to avoid making him/her feel defensive (and what you will say if it happens), (4) what words you will use to stick to specific behaviors, (5) how you will present the situation as a mutual problem to be solved, and (6) a good time and location.

Effects of Diversity on Group Communication

Several studies suggest that diversity reduces the frequency and quantity of communication between group members (Smith et al., 1994; Wagner, Pfeffer, & O'Reilly, 1984). Homogeneity on demographic traits (member similarity) leads to a shared language among members that increases communication frequency and integration of the group (Weirsema & Bantel, 1992). We are more motivated to communicate with similar individuals because of the rewards of ease and consensual validation. We may avoid communication with dissimilar others because of the effort it takes and our general discomfort with them. This affects the cohesion of the group because increased rates of social interaction are associated with the formation of positive feelings between members, which in turn affect individuals' attitudes toward the group as a whole (Tolbert, Graham, & Andrews, 1999).

Group member differences also make the possibility of miscommunication more probable and in this way may contribute to coordination difficulties and even to conflict. As you learned earlier, miscommunication occurs when the receiver gets a different message than the sender intended. Cultural differences affect the sources of miscommunication, including the differing experiences of the sender and receiver, the meanings and interpretation of specific words, and the encoding and decoding of messages (Tung, 1997). Even when we are communicating in the same language, miscommunications may arise from unfamiliar accents or the use of slang common to one culture but not to another. Communication errors may also arise from cultural differences in acceptable communication styles. We also may not understand the subtleties and innuendoes associated with other cultures. For instance, I was once on a committee where I had to work with a person from New York City. There was quite a bit of awkwardness as I adjusted to her direct style and New York accent and she adjusted to my southern accent and more polite, indirect style. At first, my inclination was to see her as bossy and rude, and hers was to see me as submissive and indecisive.

Isomorphic attribution
When we interpret the behavior of others in the same way they intended it.

Ideally, we want to give the same meaning to the behavior of others that they intend to give. This is called an **isomorphic attribution** (Triandis, 1994). Cultural differences in communication, however, give rise to a greater occurrence of nonisomorphic attributions, ones in which the intended message is not the one received. Misunderstandings and discomfort can easily arise as a result of language differences, cultural differences in the appropriateness of eye contact, the extent to which gestures are used and what they communicate, how closely people stand to one another, and how much touching is acceptable. Albert (1996) reviews the research on such differences between Latin American cultures and North American cultures. For example, when a student lowers her eyes when talking to a teacher, North Americans interpreted this as disrespectful and Latin Americans viewed it as a show of respect. Communication through gestures is more common in Latin American than in North American cultures, and Latin

Americans generally stand and sit much closer to others than is customary in North America. The amount of touching is also much greater among Latin Americans, but it is highly dependent on the relationship and context. Gestures also differ. In Brazil, former United States President Nixon created quite a stir when he used an American gesture meaning "okay" (thumb and index finger in a circle) that is used by some people in Brazil to make a sexual proposition (Triandis, 1994).

Sometimes we realize that our message is not understood or that we do not understand someone else's message, and appropriate clarifications are made. A Dutch copilot may ask an American pilot what was meant by her comment "Keep your eyes peeled" and receive the amplification he needs to avert disaster. However, because we are generally unaware of the ways in which our communication is shaped by our culture, we often do not provide sufficient information to establish mutual understanding (Orasanu et al., 1997). Sometimes it is only later, when something is not done in the expected way or by the expected time, or when we feel angry and misunderstood, that we realize miscommunication occurred.

Sometimes our greater comfort with members similar to us causes us to talk more to similar others. If group members interact with one another on the basis of subgroup identities, they may be exclusionary in their communications and may even exhibit open bias toward those who are not in their subgroup (Larkey, 1996). This exclusion, and the general challenges of communicating with members from different backgrounds, may restrict the group's ability to get valuable input from minority members. Imagine a meeting of a project team in which five members share social category membership (they are the same gender, ethnicity, and culture) and direct their ideas and comments to one another, and not to the three other members, each from a different social category. This exclusion of the minority members from the group's discussion may restrict the ideas and options considered by the group. It may also lead minority members to feel unwelcome and to leave the group.

Intercultural Exploration as a Solution to Cultural Miscommunications

Intercultural exploration

A process of sharing cultural assumptions and values that is intended to avert or clarify misunderstandings and misperceptions that arise out of cultural differences.

Kimmel (1994, 2000) suggests that we are subject to misunderstanding people from other cultures because of basic and unconscious differences in communication, cognition, perception, and reasoning. When the communications and behaviors of "foreigners" do not fit with our mindset, we are likely to attribute them to undesirable character traits such as arrogance or unreasonableness, instead of considering the meaning of their actions in cultural context. Kimmel recommends that we engage in a process of **intercultural exploration,** as follows:

1. Identify the major cultural assumptions and values that guide our perceptions and behaviors in the negotiations.
2. Communicate these as part of the negotiations; encourage the other negotiators to communicate their major cultural assumptions and values.

3. Move toward creative and collaborative problem solving. The point is to avert or clarify misunderstandings and misperceptions and to create a microculture (a developing relationship) where there are commonalties in meaning, norms of communication and behavior, and shared perceptions and expectations.

Modesty and graciousness are also central parts of intercultural exploration.

Kimmel (2000) tells the story of several American professors who traveled to India to teach. The professors were popular teachers at their American universities, where they were appreciated for their knowledge, humor, and informality (they joked freely, dressed casually, and invited much student participation). However, the Indian students had trouble with the professors' style. In India, professors dress and behave formally and do not consult with the students. Both the professors and the students were miserable. The professors were frustrated that their attempts to involve the students were not working, and the students considered the professors to be incompetent (or why would they constantly ask the students' opinions?). An intercultural communications expert was consulted. He explained to the professors the students' expectations about teachers and suggested that the professors explain their philosophy of teaching to the students. Once they did this, the students and the professors were able to come up with an accommodation that they were all comfortable with. They developed a microculture around this discussion and began intercultural exploration.

Low-Context and High-Context Communication Cultures

Low-context communication

Direct and precise communication where value is placed on providing a clear message through words, common in individualistic cultures.

High-context communication

Indirect communication where the meaning of messages is conveyed by how something is said rather than what is said, common in collectivistic cultures.

Cultures also differ in whether the communication is high context or low context. For instance, in individualistic cultures, **low-context communication** is more typical (Albert, 1996; Triandis, 1994). This means that *what* is said—that is, the verbal content—is where we are to find the message. Low-context communication is direct and precise, and value is placed on providing a clear message through words. In contrast, in collectivist cultures, **high-context communication** is more characteristic (Albert, 1996; Triandis, 1994). This means that the meaning of messages is more likely to be conveyed by *how* something is said rather than what is said. In high-context communication, meaning is often found in the context, such as touching, personal distance, eye contact, gestures, and other nonverbal signals. One must be able to "read between the lines" because communication is more indirect. Triandis (1994) tells the story of a young Indonesian man who wanted to marry a young woman from a higher social class. To explore this possibility, his mother went to visit the young woman's mother. The young woman's mother served tea and bananas. Since tea is not usually served with bananas and is considered a bad match, this communicated to the young man's mother that the young woman's family found the match unacceptable.

Apply It! ••• **Your Experiences With Culture and Communication**

Can you think of instances in which you could have benefited from greater knowledge of another culture's communication conventions? Have you ever left out a group member that you found challenging to communicate with? Have you been the one left out? How did that feel? If you were to make an effort to learn more about another culture's communication conventions, which one would you choose and why?

Communication context is important because it can contribute to misunderstandings and conflict when individuals from low-context cultures interact with individuals from high-context cultures. For instance, imagine a situation in which a person from a low-context culture (LCC) and a person from a high-context culture (HCC) are interacting. The LCC person will communicate primarily with words and pay attention to the words of the HCC person, whereas the HCC person will communicate primarily through context and will pay attention to the context of the LCC person's message. Difficulties in communication would not be surprising in such a situation. Low-context communicators may be frustrated because they are not sure what high-context persons are trying to communicate. Meanwhile, high-context communicators may be shocked and perceive low-context communicators as rude because of the directness with which they express their meaning, or they may fail to grasp the meaning because their attention is on the context, not the words.

Reducing Communication Problems in the Diverse Group

In the diverse group, keep in mind that communication may be more challenging and conflicts more likely. The following suggestions should help.

1. Look out for miscommunications resulting from language and style differences that may interfere with coordination and increase conflict. Problems may be solved more easily if you perceive them as due to honest misunderstandings rather than as intentional acts arising out of arrogance or hostility.
2. Learn about the communication conventions of the cultures of other members so that you can communicate better with them.
3. Avoid slang that may not be understood by some members.
4. Aim for a group culture in which all members are confident that they will be heard, understood, and validated when they share their experiences and perspectives.
5. Watch your language, and encourage others to do so as well. Some things that might be said without a second thought in your culture or subculture may be highly offensive to members of other groups and may erode trust and cohesion in the group. Rather than defensively labeling others as overly sensitive, seriously consider changing your language. See **Box 5-4** for examples.

BOX 5-4 / WORDS THAT HURT: SENSITIZING YOURSELF TO LANGUAGE

What all of these examples have in common is the unintentional damage that they can do to the group. Such comments reduce trust between members and, by communicating that other members are inferior or undesirable in some way, reduce members' commitment and cohesion.

1. A group member does not respond immediately when a question is directed at him. The one asking the question becomes frustrated and says "What are you, deaf and dumb?" The other replies, "Well, actually I am hearing impaired, and by the way, we are as intelligent as hearing people." • Labels matter, and words and terms such as *handicapped, lame, crippled,* and *deaf and dumb* are offensive to many persons with disabilities. Because disabilities are not always evident, you can embarrass yourself and damage your image by making such comments.

2. The group discovers that before they can accomplish their task, they have to fill out a lot of paperwork. One group member says "That is so gay!" by which he means "That is so stupid." Another group member who is gay, but has not yet shared this with other members, no longer feels welcome in the group and retreats. • If you are heterosexual, the odds are good that you will be in groups with lesbian, gay, or bisexual members (LGB persons), even if you do not know it. In general, the way the word *gay* is used in the example and jokes about homosexuals are experienced by LGBs as offensive and as evidence of prejudice. Heterosexuals who are not actually prejudiced against homosexuals often use this type of language unthinkingly.

3. Group members are talking about what they did over the weekend. One says "I went to the flea market and got a good deal on a DVD player once I jewed the guy down." Another group member, who is Jewish, is offended that a fellow group member would say something so prejudiced against Jews. A group member is telling how her sister gave her an old VCR but then demanded it back. She describes her sister as an "Indian giver." The comment reminds a Native American group member that negative stereotypes of Indians still persist, even among Euroamericans he thought were culturally sensitive. He avoids the person who made the comment. • These two examples illustrate how many slang words and phrases originate from times of prejudice and are used unthinkingly and without regard to their origin. However, to some people they are offensive, as they are bitter reminders of the discrimination their group has faced.

4. A non-Hispanic group member uses the term "Beaners" in a joke that makes fun of Hispanics. His group at home loved the joke. What he doesn't realize is that several members of this group are of Hispanic heritage. Although they don't say anything, they are hurt and think that both the speaker and the others who laugh are idiots. Later, one of the Hispanic members confronts the offender and says "I was uncomfortable when you told that 'Beaner' joke because my father is from Mexico." The offender replies, as if giving a compliment, "Wow, you really don't look or act like one of 'them.' " • Many people unthinkingly adopt prejudicial language from their own social group and harm their relationship with other group members. Furthermore, suggesting that someone is not representative of their social category is not usually taken as a compliment, but rather as evidence of your prejudice and ignorance.

BOX 5-4 (cont') / WORDS THAT HURT: SENSITIZING YOURSELF TO LANGUAGE

5. At a group outing to the park, a white group member comments that a black group member must be a good basketball player. The black member comments bitterly, "Yeah, and I am a good dancer too," and thinks the white member is ignorant. An Asian American group member is offended when she is referred to as Oriental by another group member, assumed to be good at math by another, and asked by a third if she knows karate. "Rugs are oriental; I am not a rug," she says. "I am Asian American. Not all Asians are good at math, and no, no one in my family knows martial arts." • Individuals from identifiable social groups often tire of having assumptions made about them based on narrow stereotypes of their social category. Their commitment to the group may be reduced by such comments unless it is clear that other members are interested in learning about their culture.

6. A blonde group member is repeatedly subjected to blonde jokes. When she doesn't laugh, she is accused of not having a sense of humor. "It's not that I don't have a sense of humor," she replies. "It's just that I've heard all of these jokes before, and I'm sick of having to prove that being blonde has no correlation with intelligence." • People who do not like jokes made about a group are often told they have no sense of humor, but this fails to acknowledge that jokes play a role in perpetuating stereotypes of different groups. Jokes can also make people feel unwelcome because they are reminders that they are members of a negatively stereotyped group.

7. A group leader uses the word "girl" to describe female members, talks about finding a "chairman" for a committee, refers to the "lady engineer," and talks about how many "man-hours" and how much "manpower" it will take to accomplish a task. He doesn't understand why female members of the group tend to leave after only a short time. They feel demeaned by his use of the word "girl," and excluded and made to feel unwelcome by his language. • Sexist language can have the effect of excluding some group members and suggesting that certain jobs are appropriate only if you are of a particular gender. Although some will not notice or care about gendered language, it is better to avoid it. For instance, we can use *chairperson* instead of *chairman,* talk about *staff-hours* instead of *man-hours,* and call adult females *women* rather than *girls.*

8. A biracial professional (her mother is white, her father black) joins a group of black professionals. The conversation turns to race, and many disparaging things are said about white people. She feels very uncomfortable and withdraws from the group, expecting them to reject her once they find out her mother is white. • Many people are multiracial, or do not appear or behave as we expect people from a particular social category to look or act. When we make exclusionary comments, we may not realize that members of that group are present and that our behavior has alienated them.

Concept Review

Communication as Part of Group Structure

- Most groups have an established communication network that is part of the group's structure. This network includes the communication channels in the group and who communicates with whom.
- In a **centralized communication network,** members must go through a central person to communicate with one another, and a single person within the group is the principal source and target of communication. In a **decentralized communication network,** information flows between members without going through a central person, and communication and access to information are more equally distributed.
- For simple tasks requiring only the collation of information, centralized networks are effective. Decentralized structures work best when tasks are complex and require more extensive information processing.
- Most formal groups have official or formal communication networks and channels, but all groups have informal communication networks, not formally designated by the group, that evolve over time.
- An important part of a group's informal communication structure is the **grapevine,** or the channels through which gossip, rumors, and other unofficial information travel through the group. Gossip is common because it serves multiple functions. It may have positive or negative effects on the group depending on how it is managed and whether the group is cooperative or competitive.

Verbal and Nonverbal Communication

- The words we say are known as **verbal communication,** but as much or more is communicated nonverbally. **Nonverbal communication** is the way we communicate using body language such as gestures, body orientation, touching, personal distance, and facial expressions. **Paralanguage** is part of nonverbal communication and includes voice pitch, rate, quality, and tone as well as nonword communications such as "tsking" and sighing.
- Nonverbal behavior often tells us about the relative status of group members and is meta-communicative, serving to qualify verbal behavior. Nonverbal behavior is also less subject to censorship than verbal behavior and often "leaks" emotional messages.
- Culture and gender affect nonverbal communication.
- When verbal and nonverbal messages match, the message is **congruent;** when they are contradictory, the message is **incongruent.** Congruent messages are easier to understand. Incongruent messages happen when people

are not ready to take responsibility for their feelings or when they come from a culture in which it is normative to deliver feedback in this indirect fashion.

Group Communication Climate

- **Group communication climate** refers to the context in which communication occurs. In a **cooperative or supportive climate,** members feel free to communicate honestly, and the communication is directed towards the group's work. In the **competitive or defensive climate,** members distrust other members, view them as competitors, and engage in guarded or defensive communications in order to protect themselves or get what they want.
- A cooperative climate leads to increased cohesion and increased productivity because people work harder and longer at group tasks. Members are more satisfied in groups with supportive, cooperative communication climates.
- Gibb (1961) identified six categories of member behaviors that influence whether a climate is defensive or supportive: evaluation versus description, control versus problem orientation, strategy versus spontaneity, neutrality versus empathy, superiority versus equality, and certainty versus provisionalism.

Assertive Communication

- People who are nonassertive or passive do not speak up for themselves and do not deny the unreasonable requests of others. By holding back, they deny themselves full participation in the group. Rather than assert themselves, unassertive people sometimes distance themselves from the group, even leaving it. They may also become so irritated that they engage in passive–aggressive behavior or overreact to some minor transgression when they can keep it in no longer.
- Aggressive people forcefully speak their minds and may shout at others or bully others to get their way. Aggressive people prevent others from participating as equals in the group and contribute to defensive and competitive group climates. They may get what they want, but their behavior hurts others and interferes with group cohesion.
- **Assertive behavior** is self-expressive, honest, direct, firm, and respectful of the rights of others. It is simple and unblaming, tactful and diplomatic. It contributes to a cooperative, open communication climate in which members can express their ideas responsibly. Assertive behavior often takes practice and requires changes in both verbal and nonverbal behavior.
- High-status people are more assertive than low-status people. The higher status of men relative to women in most societies has contributed to their greater assertiveness and aggressiveness. However, most recent studies in the United States find no gender differences in assertiveness.

- Some cultures have different expectations regarding passive, assertive, and aggressive behavior depending on gender. Also, cultures vary in power distance. In high power distance cultures, it is inappropriate to assert oneself when interacting with elders and those in authority. In some cultural contexts, being effectively assertive requires indirect, subtle language, and what is assertive in one cultural context may be perceived as aggressive in another.
- Because of cultural differences, **message matching** is recommended. Message matching means that senders select the most appropriate and effective assertive message given the receiver, and receivers take into account the sender's culture.
- **Constructive confrontations** involve clarifying and exploring the issues, the needs of the participants, and their feelings. Confrontations work best when confronters are calm, have thought through how to present the conflict, take their share of responsibility, and frame the conflict in terms of issues and actions, not personalities.

Communication in the Diverse Group

- Diversity can reduce the frequency and quantity of communication between group members. This affects the cohesion of the group because increased rates of social interaction are associated with the formation of positive feelings between members, which in turn affect individuals' attitudes toward the group.
- Cultural differences make miscommunication more probable and in this way may contribute to coordination difficulties and conflict.
- The general challenges of communicating with members from different backgrounds may restrict the group's ability to get valuable input from minority members. Minority members may feel unwelcome and leave the group.
- **Intercultural exploration** is a process in which we identify the major cultural assumptions and values that guide our perceptions and behaviors. We communicate these when there is a problem, move toward creative and collaborative problem solving, and create a microculture in which there are commonalties in meaning, norms of communication and behavior, and shared perceptions and expectations.
- Communication context is important because it can contribute to misunderstandings and conflict. **Low-context communication,** more common in individualistic cultures, is direct and precise, and value is placed on providing a clear message through words. **High-context communication** means that the meaning of messages is more likely to be conveyed by *how* something is said rather than *what* is said. It is more common in collectivistic cultures.

Skill Review

Consider Communication Structure

- Review your group's communication structure and alter it if needed.
- Manage gossip and rumors so that they do not harm the group. Confront gossiping members if gossip threatens to ruin the group or harm individual members.
- Check out information obtained from the grapevine before sharing it as fact or making a decision based on it.

Improve Verbal and Nonverbal Communication

- Communicate congruent messages, and ask for clarification if you receive a mixed message.
- Consider your listeners, and adapt your message accordingly.
- Be sensitive to others' comfort level regarding touch and personal distance by reading their nonverbal cues.
- Be aware that even if you are not speaking, you are communicating nonverbally. Work to send the messages you want to send.
- To create a supportive communication climate, express disagreement without suggesting that the other person is unintelligent or uninformed. Show a willingness to consider other perspectives. Do not attempt to manipulate the group to get your way. Behave honestly and openly in the group. Participate in the group.
- Confirm others by adding to their ideas, asking them for clarification, and expressing understanding or support.
- Avoid disconfirming responses such as changing the subject, giving a response that shows no acknowledgment of other members' contributions, or following another members' comments with responses like "Yeah, but . . ." Do not interrupt others.

Increase Assertive Behavior

- Work to communicate assertively, not passively or aggressively.
- Use a relaxed and steady gaze, looking away occasionally. Face the other person directly, and use a level, well-modulated, conversational tone with a smooth, nonhesitant flow of speech.
- Realize that culture affects assertiveness, and use message matching to select the most appropriate and effective assertive message. Consider culture when receiving assertive messages.

■ Look out for miscommunications resulting from language and style differences that may interfere with coordination and increase conflict. Problems may be solved more easily if you perceive them as due to honest misunderstandings rather than as intentional acts arising out of arrogance or hostility.

Confront Constructively

■ Confront when you are calm and have thought carefully about how to frame the conflict.
■ Define the conflict in a small and specific way.
■ Think about your contribution to the conflict, and take your share of responsibility for it.
■ Frame the conflict in terms of issues and actions, not personalities. Use "I" statements such as "I am/I feel/I hear" and so on.
■ State the issue in such a way that the other person is able to save face.
■ Go in with an open mind and a willingness to understand the other side.

Improve Intercultural Communication

■ Learn about the communication conventions of the cultures of other members so that you can better communicate with them.
■ Avoid slang that may not be understood by some members.
■ Aim for a group culture in which all members are confident that they will be heard, understood, and validated when they share their experiences and perspectives.
■ Use culturally sensitive language, and encourage others to do so as well.

Study Questions

1. What is communication structure? How do centralized and decentralized communication networks differ, and when is each one most likely to be effective?
2. What are formal and informal communication networks? What factors determine the nature of the informal network?
3. Why is gossip so common in groups? What positive functions may it serve? How can it be prevented from becoming destructive to the group?
4. What are verbal and nonverbal communication? How do culture and gender affect nonverbal communication? What does it mean to say that a message is congruent or incongruent? Why do some people deliver incongruent messages, and how should you handle them?

5. What is a supportive (cooperative) group communication climate, and what are its benefits? What is a defensive (competitive) climate, and how does it negatively affect the group?

6. What six member behaviors influence whether a climate is supportive or defensive? What types of responses are confirming, and what types are disconfirming?

7. How do passive, aggressive, and assertive behaviors differ, and what effects do they have on a group? How do gender and culture affect assertiveness?

8. What are the main features of the constructive confrontation? What is the Four R Method for responding to others' complaints about our behavior?

9. How does diversity in groups affect communication?

10. What is intercultural exploration?

11. What is an isomorphic attribution? How can understanding cultural differences increase isomorphic attributions?

12. What difficulties might a person from a low-context communication culture experience in communicating with a person from a high-context communication culture?

 Group Activities

Activity 1: Demonstrate Centralized and Decentralized Communication Networks

In a five-person group, arrange your chairs or desks to correspond to each of the communication networks depicted in Figure 5-1. After each configuration, talk about how communication would occur with this structure while remaining in the configuration and communicating accordingly. Who would talk to whom? Which member is the center of the network? For what types of tasks might this structure work well? Can any group member think of a real-life example of the network?

Activity 2: Share Experiences of Electronic Communication and Miscommunication

In a small group, have a discussion about the "emoticons" you commonly use in email communication. Next, discuss the perils of e-communication in the absence of nonverbal communication, and share experiences in which miscommunications have occurred. Last, share the communication norms and conventions of Internet communication. For instance, what are the norms of any e-groups you regularly participate in? What are the communication norms around "instant messaging"? What does your group recommend to enhance e-communication?

Activity 3: Receive Feedback on Confirming and Disconfirming Responses

With your group, review the difference between supportive and defensive climates and confirming and disconfirming responses, and make sure all members understand what types of behaviors fall into each category. Each person should take notes. After that, look at the list below of various causes of death. Your small group is to rank-order the list from the most deadly in the United States annually to the least deadly. While your group does this, members are to be on the lookout for disconfirming responses and those that contribute to a defensive climate. Each time you observe such a response, you are to say "Flag on so-and-so for [type of disconfirming or defensiveness-creating response]." After the group is done rank-ordering the list, they should discuss what happened in the group.

Causes of Death

Heart attack
Car accidents
Breast cancer
Asthma
Drownings
Accidental shootings
Homicide
Lung cancer
Earthquakes
AIDS
Hepatitis

InfoTrac College Edition Search Terms

To do research for your papers and assignments, use InfoTrac that's provided free with new copies of this book. Go to http://infotrac.thomsonlearning.com and enter the following search terms:

- Nonverbal Communication
- Assertiveness (Psychology)
- Gossip
- Intercultural Communication
- Electronic Discussion Groups

6 Group Development

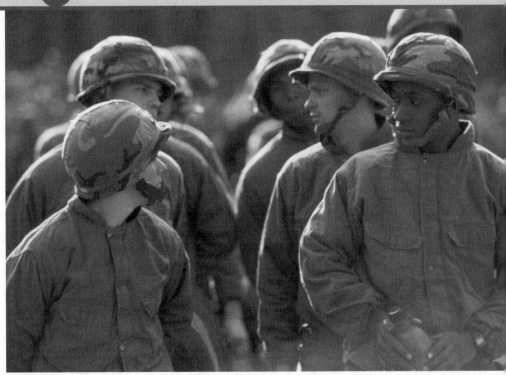

© Leif Skoogfors/CORBIS

This chapter focuses on how groups develop over time (group development) and how new members join and learn about groups (group socialization). A group's development story starts with a collection of individuals who come together to accomplish some task (such as a workgroup) or who end up talking because they are in close proximity (such as a friendship group). Over time, this collection of individuals comes to feel more and more like a group. They develop their own culture and ways of doing things and perceiving things. Depending on the group, they have conflicts. They may disagree about what needs to be done and how to do it. They may become angry at one another if someone behaves inconsiderately or violates the group's norms. They will ignore the conflict or work it out. The story ends when members leave because of unmanageable conflict, life changes, or task completion. For instance, a friendship group may break up because members leave for college, get involved in romantic relationships, or get divorced. A workgroup, such as a committee, a group of summer camp counselors, or a therapy group, may end when the job is done. Sometimes, the group goes on but changes as longtime members experience growth and change, new members replace old members, the group expands, or it splinters. A new employee joins a workgroup. Your sisters and brothers marry, and their spouses join your family group for holidays. In such cases, these new members are socialized into the group and may influence the group as much as it influences them.

Most people agree that group beginnings are often awkward, a tight-knit group is something special, group endings are frequently sad, and being a new member in an established group is typically stressful. These topics are addressed in the study of group development.

Group development
How groups change over time as members interact, learn about one another, and structure relationships and roles within the group.

Group development involves changes in groups over time as members interact, learn about one another, and structure relationships and roles within the group (Mennecke, Hoffer, & Wynne, 1992; Moreland & Levine, 1988). The study of group development began with Bales (1950). Recall that Bales developed an observational rating system of groups known as IPA (Interaction Process Analysis). Using IPA, Bales attempted to chart the actions and reactions of members in a group over time in an effort to identify group phases. Although he was only moderately successful, his work stimulated similar efforts. Hare (1973) summarizes this early research on group development.

Sequential stage theories of group development
Theories suggesting that groups progress through a series of stages in a particular order.

There are dozens of theories of group development. The majority of these are **sequential stage theories of group development** suggesting that groups progress through a series of stages in a particular order. Like stage theories of individual development, group development theories often assume that there are certain developmental tasks to be accomplished at each stage in order to move from earlier to later stages. Also, just as some stage theories of individual development suggest that individuals may become fixated (stuck) in early stages of development, some group development theories assume that some groups become fixated in earlier stages and never move on to later stages. For example, a group that remains in the superficial, polite early stages of development may not grapple with issues that would lead to greater depth in the relationships between members or to quality decision making. A group unable to resolve conflicts may never get to the point where they are able to work productively. Theories of individual development frequently assume that ideally individuals become more mature and develop their unique potentials as individuals. Likewise, some group development theorists think of groups as developing toward maturity. For instance, in a classic article on group development, Bennis and Shepard (1956) suggest that a mature group is one that "knows what it is doing" and can resolve its internal conflicts, overcome obstacles to valid communication, and mobilize its resources.

The Basic Group Development Model (Tuckman)

Tuckman's theory of small group development

The basic sequential model that postulates five stages: forming, storming, norming, performing, and adjourning.

The best-known sequential stage theory of group development is **Tuckman's theory of small group development,** and most other theories of group development resemble the basic Tuckman model. It focuses on "zero history groups"—that is, new groups whose members have little or no experience together. Tuckman (1965) analyzed 50 articles that chronicled the progression of small groups. The groups included therapy groups, T-groups (human relations training groups), and social and professional groups, some from real-world settings and some brought together for the purposes of studying groups. Tuckman, like Bales (1953), theorized that group members must simultaneously work to complete tasks and relate to one another interpersonally. Tuckman (1965) initially identified four stages of group development—forming, storming, norming, and performing—and later added a fifth stage, adjourning (Tuckman & Jensen, 1977). In the following sections, you will learn about Tuckman's descriptions of these stages, as well as possible variations, and consider ways of facilitating a group's development in each stage.

Forming (Orientation)

Imagine the polite cautiousness the following scenarios would probably inspire in you and the others in each newly formed group:

You meet for the first time with four other students with whom you will complete a group project.

On your first day of basic training as a new military recruit, you meet the other new recruits in your unit.

You are a member of a newly formed support group for people who have recently lost a loved one.

You meet for the first time with seven other managers to solve a distribution problem.

It is the first time you and your partner hang out with the couple who live next door.

You are a child whose mother has just married a man with two children, and it is the first week of your all living together.

Forming stage

The first stage in the basic model of group development, in which member participation is hesitant and dependent on the leader and rules.

These examples represent groups in the **forming stage.**

Tuckman (1965) characterized the forming stage as a stage of "testing," or "hesitant participation," as group members try to figure out what interpersonal behaviors are acceptable in the group. Group members are "dependent" in the sense that they rely on a group leader (teacher, supervisor, or take-charge member) for guidance and structure. In this stage, people also tend to adhere to any formal norms or guidelines evident in the situation, for these provide safety. There is an effort to define the task and how the group will tackle it.

This includes a discussion of both relevant and semi-relevant issues, the discussion of peripheral problems, and complaints about the institutional environment in which the group operates. The specifics of this stage depend on the setting, which determines what must be oriented to and how.

Researchers have not studied what factors determine how long the forming stage lasts, but it is safe to say that it depends on the membership, leadership, and task of the particular group. For instance, the interpersonal style of some individuals has the effect of creating a group environment that is more relaxed. Such individuals act as "group catalysts" in the sense that their extroversion and efforts to draw everyone into a group conversation hasten the group's progression through this stage. Another factor affecting the length of this stage is the group's task. Some groups do not have time to stay in this stage for very long. They must quickly get past any awkwardness and move on to the business of task production. Conversely, groups that have as their purpose an emotional task, such as a therapy or family group, may proceed cautiously for quite some time.

Storming (Conflict)

Look back at the list of examples of groups in the forming stage. How long would it take before members of these groups drop their guard, censor their behavior less, get on one another's nerves, and disagree about who should do what and how? You can imagine the students disagreeing about the best way to tackle the assignment, the blended family disagreeing about family rules and rituals, the managers at odds with one another about whether drastic measures are needed to solve their distribution problem. People cannot hide their unique personalities and perspectives for long, nor are they very good at overlooking others' imperfections (unless they are madly in love). To do these things requires a level of concentration and self-monitoring that cannot easily be kept up. It is also true that group members must get down to the work of real engagement with one another if they are to develop as a group and accomplish group tasks. But as they engage, they are likely to have conflicts, or "storm."

Storming stage

The second stage of the basic model of group development, in which members may disagree about what to do and how, the leadership, and their roles in the group.

The **storming stage** is one of intragroup conflict (conflict within the group). Group members become aggravated with one another and with the leader. Tensions arise as individuals move away from the earlier, polite stage and show themselves. Resentments and hostilities may also occur as individuals resist the demands of the task and working with others and try to change things to fit their personal agendas. Leadership struggles are common in this stage as individuals jockey for position. Frequently, warring factions represent each side of a polarized issue. For instance, some seek to remain dependent on the leader, whereas others do not; some wish to stick with the familiar, whereas others want to take more risks.

It is important to realize that storming may not occur as dramatically as its name suggests. For instance, it may be somewhat understated in organizational cultures where professional demeanor is expected and agreement emphasized. It may also be more modestly expressed in groups where conflict is avoided and harmony valued. Similarly, storming may be subtler in groups from collectivist cultures, such as Japan or India, that emphasize ingroup harmony and where communication is more indirect.

The sequential model does not say how long groups storm or what leads them to stop, although it does imply that it ceases when issues, such as how to approach the task and who will do what, are resolved. As in other development stages, what happens here depends on a number of factors specific to the group. For instance, the presence of a leader or other individual who has the skills to direct the conflict in constructive rather than destructive ways may reduce the time spent in this stage. Individuals who state their differences in assertive rather than aggressive ways will also move the group toward conflict resolution, whereas aggressively expressed differences are likely to escalate the conflict. Contrary to the model, storming does not always occur. Short-term groups may have to get right down to business, and some groups are not together long enough to storm. Conflict may also be absent if members do not care enough about the group to bother to become involved in conflict or are so fearful of conflict that they avoid it. Storming may also occur repeatedly in the group. Not only may new conflicts arise, but earlier conflicts may resurface if not fully resolved.

Norming (Structure)

Norming stage

The third stage of the basic model of group development, characterized by group cohesion and the emergence of structure, roles, and "we-feeling."

The **norming stage** is the calm after the storm. Tuckman (1965) describes it as a stage of group cohesion in which members accept the group and the idiosyncrasies of individual members. The emotionality of the storming stage is followed by a sense of "pulling together" and being more sensitive to the concerns of individual members. The members feel a part of the group and accept the group's norms. Structure, roles, and "we-feeling" emerge. Although members have alternative interpretations of the task and how to accomplish it, the emphasis is on harmony. Members put aside conflicts or develop norms to handle them.

Group cohesion

A multidimensional concept that includes a sense of we-ness and belongingness, members' liking of the group and one another, and teamwork.

The norming stage is focused on **group cohesion,** a concept with a long history in group dynamics (see, for example, Festinger, Schacter, & Back, 1950; Lewin, 1943). Definitions abound. Lewin (1943) and Festinger and his collaborators (1950) saw it as the forces that bind the group together. You probably think of group cohesion as group unity or how close-knit the group is. Indeed, many theorists look at group cohesion as a sense of we-ness and belongingness (Dion & Evans, 1992; Fine & Holyfield, 1996). Variations on this theme include defining cohesion as the extent to which members feel a part of the group and desire to remain in the group (Bollen & Hoyle, 1990; Evans & Dion, 1991; Langfred, 1998). Some definitions stress attraction—that members of cohesive groups like one another (Lott & Lott, 1965) or like the group (Carron, Widmeyer, & Brawley, 1985; Dion, 1990; Zander, 1982). Still other definitions emphasize teamwork (Carron, 1982; Guzzo, 1995). For instance, Carron (1982, p. 124) defines cohesion as "a dynamic process that is reflected in the tendency for a group to stick together and remain united in pursuit of its goals and objectives."

The definition of group cohesion has been debated widely (see Wood, Kumar, Treadwell, & Leach, 1998, for a review) and largely resolved by viewing group cohesion as a multidimensional concept (one that has a number of components). As Forsyth (1999) points out, binding social forces, a sense of unity, attraction to other members and the group itself, and the group's ability to work as a team are all components of cohesiveness, but not all cohesive groups exhibit all of these. For instance, the cohesive sports team is likely to exemplify different aspects of cohesiveness than is a friendship group or a therapy group.

Performing (Work)

Performing stage

The fourth stage of the basic model of group development, in which the group focuses on task accomplishment.

You are a member of a student project group. You have spent time getting to know one another a bit, and defining the task and how to accomplish it. Now it is time to plunge ahead and do it. Your group has reached the **performing stage.** There comes a time in the life of most groups when it is time to focus on getting the job done. The performing stage is when group members get down to the business of task accomplishment. According to Tuckman (1965), in the performing stage, the interpersonal structure developed in earlier stages becomes a tool of task accomplishment. Interpersonal problems are left in the past, and group energy is channeled into the task. The focus is on successful task completion. Group members work cooperatively to appraise the task realistically and solve it.

Adjourning (Dissolution)

Adjourning stage

The final stage of the basic model of group development, in which members begin to disengage from social, emotional, and task activities.

Have you ever pulled back from participating in a group that was ending to avoid the emotion associated with saying good-bye? Have you picked fights with anyone to make it easier to leave? These behaviors are common in the **adjourning stage.** Adjourning is about the group's ending. According to Tuckman, members begin to disengage from social, emotional, and task activities in the group in order to cope with the group's termination. When groups end, members often feel sadness and anxiety. They are likely to pull back and participate in less intense ways, in anticipation of the ending of the group.

Ideally, the adjourning stage provides for personal and professional growth, but because most groups end abruptly without providing the chance for good-bye or review, this opportunity is often lost. Sometimes people are reluctant to show emotion, and they avoid saying good-bye. However, despite the difficulties, telling group members what they meant to you and wishing them well is usually a positive experience. Task groups often work up until deadline, leaving little time for reflection and review. This too is unfortunate, because group members miss the opportunity to learn from mistakes and reward effort and achievement.

Improving Group Effectiveness With the Basic Model

The beauty of the Tuckman model is that it offers a clear and simple model of group development that applies to many groups (Moreland & Levine, 1988). Knowledge of the stages is both useful and comforting. If you are able to identify what stage your group is in, you can do things to ease the group's passage through it, or find comfort in knowing that what your group is doing is normal given the group's stage of development.

One way to facilitate the forming stage is to use "icebreakers"—activities that stimulate interaction among new group members and foster movement through the forming stage. For example, an icebreaker activity was used on the first day of a retreat for a group of HIV-positive clients. Participants were instructed to state on a large piece of paper three things about themselves (I am . . .). Then, silently, they held up their paper as they walked around in a circle reading everyone else's. In the next stage, participants made a comment to every other member about his or her statements. In another icebreaker activity, participants took turns saying their name, something about themselves, and when they were infected with the virus. Icebreaker activities are used in a variety of settings, such as the university, alcohol and drug treatment programs, the military, management workshops, recreational settings such as camps, and fraternity and sorority houses. Even the family member who gets distant relatives at a family gathering to play a game together is using an icebreaker activity of sorts.

Storming is common in groups, and conflict and conflict resolution are discussed at length in Chapter 7. However, for now you should know that most group dynamics scholars agree that well-managed, constructive conflicts can motivate needed change in individuals and in the group's approach, lead to increased liking and trust, and increase satisfaction with the group.

If you wanted to foster "norming" and cohesiveness in a group, how would you go about it? Part of cohesion is members' liking for one another. Research in social psychology indicates that we like those who like us (Aron, Dutton, Aron, & Iverson, 1989; Curtis & Miller, 1986), we like those who are similar to us (Byrne, Clore, & Smeaton, 1986), and we like those who are familiar (Bornstein & D'Agostino, 1992). Because familiarity is fostered by physical proximity, Zander (1982) suggests that to foster cohesiveness, offices, seats, or workspaces should be situated in such a way that persons are within easy reach of one another.

You can promote similarity among group members by assembling persons who are already alike in terms of purpose, background, training, experience, or temperament (Zander, 1982). In a diverse group, a leader may have to help group members feel more alike by emphasizing shared goals and creating shared experiences. Shared goals also promote group cohesiveness because they provide a sense of unity. Therefore, it often makes sense to emphasize goals that members have in common and, when composing a group, to choose members with similar goals. Unity is also enhanced by a shared identity. Separation of the group from other units helps members perceive the group as a distinct entity. Do this by giving the group its own physical space, tools, equipment, resources, or task (Zander, 1982). Zander suggests giving the group unique characteristics such as a name, logo, flag, or uniform which leads to distinctiveness.

Social identity theorists note that the creation of an outgroup (an enemy) also has the effect of building group solidarity (Tajfel, 1981). As Turner and Haslam (2001, p. 38) put it, "We can define ourselves as a distinct we-group on the basis of our shared interests in contrast to others." For example, I have seen a diverse group of students on one dormitory floor united by viewing another floor of students as rivals. I have seen workers in one unit build cohesion by seeing another unit as the enemy. I have seen workers build solidarity by seeing management or a coworker as the enemy, and students who bond at the expense of a teacher. Identifying or creating comparisons between ingroup and outgroup that make the ingroup look good and the outgroup look bad builds cohesion. It makes the group distinctive and gives diverse members something in common (antipathy for the designated enemy and a belief that their group is superior). Although this "us versus them" mentality may bring the group together, it can contribute to destructive conflict between groups, something we will talk about more in later chapters. It can also be harmful to those individuals who are chosen by the group to be the enemy. Many groups pick on relatively weak and powerless group members and build solidarity at their expense. Many of my students have shared that conversations about an odd brother or sister are a source of cohesion in their families. Members of groups that build solidarity in this way often report some guilt and rationalize that if the person does not know about it, then it is not so bad. However, it may still have the effect of stereotyping that individual unfairly, and it may contribute to the exclusion of the individual from the group.

Remember that part of cohesion is members' commitment to the group. Zander (1982) suggests that to increase commitment to the group, leaders should help members identify individual needs that they may be able to satisfy in the group, and increase the group's ability to meet them. Because people frequently look to groups to satisfy belongingness needs, satisfaction of this need usually enhances commitment. When group members feel that they are known and valued as individuals, and feel safe to be themselves, they provide other members with the same courtesy. Feeling that the group is committed to them, they become more committed to the group, and vice versa. This combination of knowing and accepting others and being known and accepted by them builds cohesion. This may happen naturally if members are together for a long time, but it may also be promoted by providing opportunities for social interaction, such as parties, or by group activities that require group members to share things about themselves (self-disclosure activities).

Giving members a chance to make sacrifices for the group also increases commitment to the group (Zander, 1982). When people freely choose to put time, money, or effort into a group, they need to believe that it was worth it; otherwise they feel foolish (Cialdini, 2001). This is why people who have had to work hard to join a group—for instance, a fraternity, sorority, or exclusive club—are especially committed to the group. It is also why some religious organizations request that followers give most of their material wealth to the organization. Having freely chosen to do so, members need to believe it was worth it.

The performing stage goes smoothly if the group has the resources it needs, member skills are matched to team tasks, the work of members is well coordinated, and members are committed to group goals and do their jobs. Much of this book is focused on enhancement of the performing stage. A supportive communication climate, constructive conflict resolution, good leadership, teamwork, and effective decision-making strategies are all topics covered in other chapters that are relevant to the performing stage.

Good-bye rituals are often helpful in facilitating the adjourning stage. For social groups, this often means a good-bye party or event where the members have one last group experience together and reminisce about their experiences together. Although it may sound trite, such rituals provide "closure," a sense of completeness that makes it easier to move on. People who do not do this often express regret.

Workgroups should also take the time to formally adjourn. Workgroups frequently have going-away luncheons and parties for those who have found other jobs or are retiring. But a member's departure is not the only time the workgroup should take time to formally adjourn. An evaluative learning session as a final phase of a task group provides members with an opportunity to make the good-bye more effective personally and professionally (Keyton, 1993). Too often, workgroups complete their work in a frantic, harried fashion, leaving little time for interaction and reflection that could be carried to subsequent group assignments (Keyton, 1993). Keyton emphasizes that workgroups that are disbanding upon task completion should also take the time to

1. Review what was accomplished.
2. Assess output compared to objectives.
3. Review the process and procedures that were used.
4. Facilitate the ending of group relationships.
5. Recognize and celebrate group accomplishments.

Keyton (1993) notes that how these issues are dealt with depends on the members' relationships with one another, as well as whether the experience was

Apply It! ••• **Trace a Group's Development With the Basic Model**

Think about a friendship group or roommate group you were part of, and trace the group's development through the stages of the basic model. How well did the model fit your group's development? Can you identify any problems with the model after trying to apply it?

positive or negative. For example, when group members are of similar status in terms of authority and responsibility, they tend to be more willing to conduct an honest assessment of what happened in the group. Members may not see the need for evaluation when an experience was positive, but evaluation is still important so that the sources of success can be identified and repeated in the future. In the case of negative experiences, members may avoid evaluation in order to avoid conflict and to leave an unpleasant situation as quickly as possible. However, it is important to explicitly identify factors that led to the negative experience so that critical problems may be avoided in the future.

The Integrative Model of Group Development (Wheelan)

The Tuckman model is often criticized for suggesting that groups must move through all stages in a particular order and because it is limited to zero-history groups. In reality, group development is ongoing, even in long-term groups. As group development theorist Wheelan (1994) points out, groups may skip stages or revisit them because, like individuals, groups may fluctuate widely depending on the forces and circumstances affecting the group at a given time. Changes in the membership, leadership, or external demands may result in the revisiting of earlier stages. Also, groups can get stuck in a stage. For instance, they may spend so much time fighting that they cannot perform, or so much time dealing with the emotional aspects of the group's life and making people feel good that they don't focus on the work.

Integrative model of group development
A revised, expanded version of the basic group development model that emphasizes that group development is ongoing and cyclical.

After reviewing decades of work on stage theories of group development, Wheelan (1994) has proposed an **integrative model of group development** with five stages. Although this model bears many similarities to the basic Tuckman model, it also has some important differences. One is that its stages apply to more than just the zero-history group. Wheelan's model also offers more details about what happens in the stages, emphasizes the ongoing and cyclical nature of group development, and recognizes that groups can get stuck in a stage or go backwards.

Observational studies and analyses of group discussions support the five stages proposed by the integrated model of group development (Verdi & Wheelan, 1992; Wheelan & Krasick, 1993; Wheelan & McKeage, 1993). The fol-

BOX 6-1 / WHEELAN'S INTEGRATIVE THEORY OF GROUP DEVELOPMENT

Stage	Characteristics	Studies
Dependency & Inclusion	Tentativeness and politeness, dependence on the leader, individuals attempt to identify acceptable behavior.	Babad & Amir, 1978; Bales, 1950; Bennis & Shepard, 1956; Bion, 1961; Caple, 1978; Dunphy, 1964; Hill, 1974; Mills, 1964; Rogers, 1970; Slater, 1966
Counterdependency & Fight	Struggles regarding authority, power, and status, clarification of values. If conflicts are resolved well, group becomes more trusting and cohesive.	Bennis & Shepard, 1956; Bion, 1961; Mann, Gibbard, & Hartman, 1967; Tuckman, 1965; Yalom, 1975
Trust & Structure	Open negotiation regarding roles, goals, group structure, and division of labor.	Lundgren & Knight, 1978; Mills, 1964; Slater, 1966; Wheelan, 1990
Work & Productivity	Increased task focus and open exchange of feedback.	Bennis & Shepard, 1956; Bion, 1961; Slater, 1966; Tuckman, 1965
Termination	Distinct end point of group with possible disruption and conflict, potential for expression of positive feelings and separation issues.	Braaten, 1974–1975; Dunphy, 1964; Farrell, 1976; Gibbard & Hartman, 1973; Lundgren & Knight, 1978; Mann et al., 1967; Miles, 1971; Mills, 1964; Slater, 1966; Yalom, 1975

lowing sections describe the stages in some detail. **Box 6-1** summarizes the stages, along with the early studies from which they are derived.

Stage One: Dependency and Inclusion

Dependency and inclusion stage

Stage 1 of the integrative model of group development, in which members are dependent on the leader and concerned about being accepted.

Dependency on a leader and concerns about the safety of the group and whether the individual will be accepted as a member characterize the **dependency and inclusion stage.** Individuals new to a group are anxious and tense. Worrying about whether they will be accepted and not yet knowing the group's rules, they rely on the leader for protection and structure and are very solicitous toward him or her. Members make efforts to get to know one another and determine the rules. However, this is done very tentatively and politely as members fear being perceived as deviant and fear being excluded or attacked.

Stage Two: Counterdependency and Fight

Counterdependency and fight stage

Stage 2 of the integrative model of group development, in which members conflict as they express their goals and ideas about group structure.

The hallmark of the **counterdependency and fight stage** is conflict—between a single member and the leader, among members, or between members and leaders. The group's task is to decide how to operate and what roles members will play. Issues of power, authority, and status are present at this stage. Feeling confined by their dependence on the leader, members seek to become more independent. They begin to express their goals and ideas about group structure. Coalitions begin to form, comprised of members with similar ideas and goals. When these splits occur, conflict arises. The leader is attacked by some and defended by others.

Paradoxically, conflict unites the group and helps individuals to feel safe. Conflict is the way that the group arrives at a unified direction from divergent points of view. It is also a way for members to establish trust. It lets them know that they will be accepted and not abandoned, despite differences with other members, and permits greater intimacy and collaboration. Wheelan and Hochberger (1996) note that groups that avoid this stage may remain dependent, uncertain, and incapable of true collaboration, unitary action, or productive work.

Stage Three: Trust and Structure

Trust and structure stage

Stage 3 of the integrative model where the group lays the foundation for task accomplishment by organizing itself.

Once members feel more secure and trusting of each other and their leader after the successful resolution of conflict, they begin to more openly negotiate group goals, organizational structure, procedures, roles, norms, and divisions of labor. In this **trust and structure stage,** the group is "designing itself." The group lays the foundation for task accomplishment, which increases the group's ability to work effectively and productively. As relationships become more defined, role assignments can be made based on competence and talent, rather than fantasy or wishes for safety or power.

Stage Four: Work and Productivity

Work and productivity stage

Stage 4 of the integrative model of group development, in which the group turns ideas into products.

Wheelan defines work as an idea that ends with a product. To work, there must be free communication. If members withhold information or feedback from the group for fear of reprisal, the product will suffer. Because work occurs in a time-bound frame, awareness of the time available is required for work to occur. Good use of available resources such as information, member expertise, and materials is also essential. According to Wheelan (1994), efficient groups in the **work and productivity stage** rarely spend all of their time working on tasks. Instead, they spend up to 40 percent of their time on group maintenance activities such as socializing and dealing with interpersonal issues.

Stage Five: Termination

Termination stage

Stage 5 of the integrative model of group development, in which the group ends in some form as members leave or tasks are completed.

According to Wheelan, there are endings associated with every group. Temporary groups may be in the **termination stage** when the job is done or members go their separate ways. In continuous groups, such as families or institutional groups, there are various endings as some members leave or tasks are completed. In functional groups, at each ending point, group members evaluate their work together, give feedback, and express feelings about one another and the group. Impending termination may result in regression to earlier stages, and conflict and negativity may reoccur. Sometimes, members discuss their reactions to the termination of the group.

The Integrative Model and Improving Group Effectiveness

Wheelan (1994) emphasizes the importance of the leader in Stage 1. It is up to the leader to act in ways that facilitate an open discussion of values, goals, tasks, and leadership, so that differences of opinion can emerge and the group can move to the next stage. In particular, the leader must create a climate in which members feel competent in their skills and safe sharing ideas. To move successfully through Stage 2, both leaders and members must act in ways that allow conflicts to be resolved cooperatively for the good of the group. They either compromise, finding a solution somewhere between opposing positions, or problem solve until a solution that satisfies the needs of both parties is found. If they are unable to resolve the conflict themselves, then a third party, such as an outside mediator, is brought in.

The group's task in Stage 3 is to "consolidate the gains in trust and cohesion and to forge a more efficient social structure that will support group goal achievement and productivity" (Wheelan, 1994, p. 85). In other words, an effective group in Stage 3 takes the time to plan. The group cooperates to develop the specifics of how the group will accomplish its goals. Roles and tasks are assigned on the basis of member abilities, and task-oriented subgroups are created. Wheelan provides a long list of factors, based on research on group productivity, that enhance Stage 4 (Work). A sampling of these factors appears in **Box 6-2**. Finally, Wheelan recommends debriefing sessions, in which members share their concerns over the group's ending and discuss the group's accomplishments, to help with Stage 5.

Membership Change and Group Development

Several theories of group development have focused specifically on development in the long-term group as a result of membership change. As Arrow and McGrath (1993) note, when the membership of a group changes—whether the change

BOX 6-2 / HALLMARKS OF A SUCCESSFUL STAGE FOUR GROUP

- Members are clear on and agree on group goals.
- Members are clear on and accept their roles and status.
- The group's communication structure matches the task.
- The group has an open communication structure where all members are heard.
- The group norms encourage high performance and quality.
- The group is cohesive and cooperative.
- The group has the technical and human resources necessary for the task.
- The group has effective conflict resolution strategies.
- The group spends enough time planning, making decisions, and solving problems.
- The group has enough time to develop into a mature working unit and do its work.

Source: Based on Wheelan, 1994

Apply It! ••• **Assess Your Group's Stage of Development**

In 1996, Wheelan and Hochberger reported on the creation and validation of the Group Development Questionnaire (GDQ). This instrument has four 15-item scales that correspond to the first four stages of group development (dependency and inclusion, counterdependency and fight, trust and structure, work and productivity). Each scale measures the presence or absence of the behaviors characteristic of a particular stage of group development. Wheelan and Hochberger (1996) hope that the GDQ will stimulate more research on group development and that the GDQ may be eventually used as a diagnostic tool to help work teams become more effective. Sample items from the GDQ are shown in **Box 6-3.** Choose three different groups you are a member of. Look at the items, and identify the stage of development each group is in.

---

involves the arrival of new members, temporary absences, permanent departures, turnover and replacement, or guests—other aspects of the group's functioning are bound to change as well.

Group Socialization

Group socialization

Changes in the relationship between the group and each of its members.

Group development refers to changes in the group over time, but as Moreland and Levine (1988, 1995) note, as time passes, changes also occur in the relationship between the group and each of its members. They refer to these changes as **group socialization.** Three psychological processes—*evaluation, commitment, and role transition*—are used to analyze group socialization.

> **BOX 6-3** / SAMPLE ITEMS FROM THE GROUP DEVELOPMENT QUESTIONNAIRE

Group Development Stage	Sample Items
I. Dependency & Inclusion	1. Members tend to go along with whatever the leader suggests. 2. There is very little conflict expressed in the group. 3. We haven't discussed our goals very much.
II. Counterdependency & Fight	1. People seem to have very different views about how things should be done in this group. 2. Members challenge the leader's ideas. 3. There is quite a bit of tension in the group at this time.
III. Trust & Structure	1. The group is spending its time planning how it will get its work done. 2. We can rely on each other. We work as a team. 3. The group is able to from subgroups, or subcommittees, to work on specific tasks.
IV. Work & Productivity	1. The group gets, gives, and uses feedback about its effectiveness and productivity. 2. The groups acts on its decisions. 3. This group encourages high performance and quality work.

Source: Wheelan & Hochberger, 1996

Evaluation involves judgments by the groups and individual members about the rewardingness of the individual–group relationship and of alternative relationships. These evaluations affect the level of commitment of the member and the group to one another. For instance, as the perceived rewardingness of their past, present, and future relationships increases, the group and the individual become more committed to one another (Moreland & Levine, 1988); conversely, if the perceived rewardingness of alternative relationships increases, commitment decreases. A role transition occurs when the relationship between the individual and group is altered as a result of changed levels of commitment. Evaluation occurs at various points throughout the relationship and produces further changes in commitment and role transitions.

To illustrate, imagine a group of roommates who initially evidence a high level of commitment to a group member, and she to them. This high level of commitment originates in the group's belief (evaluation) that he will be a good roommate, as he is fun to be with and easygoing. Likewise, the roommate expects his relationship with the group to be a good one and plans to live with the group until he graduates (commitment). Let's say, though, that it turns out that this roommate is messy and keeps hours at odds with the rest of the group. This creates problems for the member and the group, and the relationship changes (role transition) as they reevaluate the rewardingness of the relationship, especially when the member becomes aware of an alternative living situation and the group becomes aware of a potential roommate who appears to be a better fit.

Moreland and Levine (1988, 1995) suggest that individuals pass through five stages of group membership, separated by four role transitions (see Figure 6-1 for a graphical depiction of the model). The first stage, the **investigation phase,** is characterized by the group's effort to recruit new members and potential new members engaging in "reconnaissance," looking for a group that fits their needs. Both the group and the individual have their own *entrance criteria* (EC) that must be met in order to choose the other. For instance, a first-year student at a university may search for a fraternity that does a lot of community service and relatively little partying, and fraternities are searching for members that fit the culture of their group. Similarly, a business may seek to recruit a new manager with particular qualifications, and a manager seeking to change jobs evaluates different businesses in an effort to find one that fits her needs. In these cases, the

Investigation phase

The first phase of group socialization, in which the group recruits new members and potential members look for a group that fits their needs.

Figure 6-1

Moreland and Levine's Model of Group Socialization

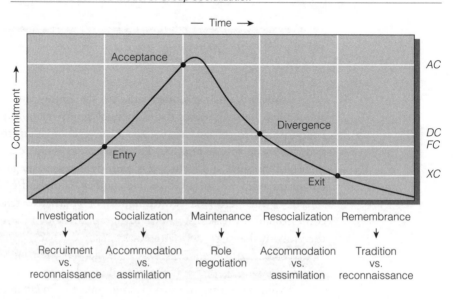

Source: Moreland & Levine, 1995.

role transition of *entry* occurs if the evaluations of both parties result in high commitment levels—in other words, if they appear to meet one another's needs. According to Moreland and Levine, an induction ritual such as a party or ceremony often marks entry.

Socialization phase

The second phase of group socialization, in which the new member tries to change the group while the group attempts to change the person.

In the second stage, the **socialization phase,** the new member tries to change the group to better meet his or her needs while the group attempts to change the person so that s/he can contribute more to the achievement of the group's goals. In other words, the group and the new member are still "checking each other out" to see if things are going to work out, and both have *acceptance criteria* (AC) that must be met before the member becomes fully part of the group. For instance, a new secretary may request that she be able to come in earlier and leave earlier so that she can pick her child up after soccer practice. She also requests an ergonomic workstation. Her manager, meanwhile, explains to her that the early morning hours are well covered in the office and that she is needed in the late afternoon. However, the manager says that they will be able to provide her with the desired workstation and provides her with a catalog from which to choose one. If the secretary agrees, and the group and the secretary are able to agree on additional requests, then each has met the other's acceptance criteria, the role transition of *acceptance* occurs, and the person becomes a full group member. Once acceptance occurs, the member often gains access to information that is only known by full members of the group.

Maintenance phase

The third phase of group socialization, in which the person and the group try to reach an agreement that satisfies the goals of both parties.

During the third or **maintenance phase,** the person and the group negotiate as they try to find a specialized role that maximizes the person's satisfaction and the achievement of the group's goals. Both the group and the member have their own *divergence criteria* (DC). This "bottom line," if not met, reduces the commitment of the group to the person or the person to the group. For instance, a new faculty member and her department may negotiate regarding the classes she is to teach. It is important to her that she teach courses in her area of specialization, and it is important to her department that she teach some introductory courses. If role negotiations succeed and they are able to reach an agreement that satisfies the goals of both parties, then the commitment levels of both parties remain high. If negotiation fails, then the commitment level falls, and it is likely that the member will become marginalized (excluded in some way from the group). This role transition of *divergence* is often marked by behaviors such as giving the person the cold shoulder and excluding the person from group activities—for instance, not inviting them to go to lunch with the group.

Resocialization phase

The fourth phase of group socialization, in which a member again tries to change the group and the group tries to get the member to accept things the way they are.

The fourth stage of group membership is the **resocialization phase.** Again, the member desires changes in the group (accommodation) while the group tries to get the person to go along with the way things are (assimilation). Once more, both the member and the group have their bottom lines—in this case, their *exit criteria* (XC). For example, let us say that a company has established new and higher productivity goals, and an employee resists the new standards and fails to meet them. His manager tries to get him to accept the standards and increase his productivity (assimilation). He tries to get his manager to see that the standards are unfair and that he should not have to meet them because he was hired under different standards (accommodation). If a resolution takes place (he or the manager budges), then the *role transition of convergence* occurs and the person regains full membership in the group. However, if the commitment levels of both fall to their respective exit criteria (for instance, neither budges), then the role transition of *exit* occurs, and the person becomes an ex-member.

Remembrance phase

The final phase of group socialization, in which group membership ends and the person and the group evaluate their experience.

Group membership ends with a **remembrance phase,** in which both the person and the group evaluate their experience. Both the member and the group may reminisce about the member's time in the group. Remembrances about the ex-member may become part of the group's lore. In some cases, ex-members retain some contact with the group, and some low level of mutual commitment continues. For instance, an employee who leaves because he can make more money elsewhere may maintain contact with his ex-coworkers for several years. However, in time, these commitment levels fall; the person seldom thinks about the group, and the group all but forgets about the member.

Although Moreland and Levine (1988, 1995) distinguish between group socialization and group development, they note that they might influence one another. For example, they suggest that it is highly unlikely that the socialization activities of maintenance, resocialization, and remembrance would occur in the forming stage of group development because the group norms that guide the socialization process have not yet been determined. They also point out that groups may accept more accommodation and less assimilation when a group is ending and that resocialization can detract from the group's development if it diverts too much of the group's time away from task activities.

Member Change and Group Development

Many groups are ongoing groups that face membership changes as some members leave and others join. Recently, group dynamics scholars have begun to consider how these changes affect group development. Depending on the extent of the membership change and the types of members added or lost, the group may form, norm, and storm all over again. Performance is also likely to be affected by membership change.

Arrow and McGrath (1993, 1995) point out that groups vary in the extent to which membership changes, why it changes, and how new members join. These factors make membership change and its effects on groups complex. This area of study is still in its infancy, and most of the work on this topic has focused on identifying the factors that might influence the effects of member change. Future research may study the specific effects of these factors.

According to Arrow and McGrath (1993, 1995), some groups have continuous membership flux, whereas others have a fixed and stable membership, and this affects how member change impacts the group. Groups with a fixed and stable membership (closed groups), especially those that operate as teams, are more affected by membership changes than are "open" groups whose members are somewhat interchangeable. A group's openness/closedness depends on the group's purpose and the social-organizational context in which it operates. For instance, the Supreme Court has a closed, fixed-size membership, and members are expected to serve until death or incapacitation. At that point, elaborate procedures are used to replace the departed member. College sororities and fraternities are largely closed but have predictable and periodic member change at the beginning of the year following rigorous screening and at the end of the year when seniors graduate. In contrast, an Alcoholics Anonymous meeting may be open to anyone who is interested, and attendees may vary from week to week.

According to Arrow and McGrath (1993, 1995), how membership change affects the group depends partly on how the change is initiated. In other words, the *impetus* for member change matters. The group may respond differently to the loss of a member depending on whether s/he left because of illness, was fired, or was expelled by the group. Likewise, the group may react differently depending on whether a new member was recruited by the group or was assigned to the group by a boss. *Temporal aspects* of member change and continuity also matter. Temporal aspects include the frequency, duration, regularity, and predictability of membership change. Groups that expect regular member changes are affected less than groups that are unprepared. Timing in relation to the group's development may also make a difference. For instance, changes that occur when a group is still forming will have different effects than changes that occur in a well-established group.

Arrow and McGrath (1993, 1995) also note that the *arithmetic* of member change matters. By this, they mean that the magnitude (size) of member change also makes a difference. The addition or subtraction of a large number of members relative to the group's size will have more impact than a smaller number. Indeed, at a certain point, the loss of old members and the addition of new ones results in a new group. Lastly, *who* changes matters. Members are not interchangeable, and the loss or addition of high-status, central members is more likely to affect the group's development than changes in members who are more peripheral and less important to the group's activity.

Apply It! ••• **Consider the Impact of Member Change on a Group**

Think of a group you are or were a member of that experienced the loss of members. What was the reason for the member change, and how did it affect the group? Was the departure expected or unexpected, and how did this affect the group? How was the impact on the group influenced by who left and how important they were to the group?

Group Development in Specialized Groups

No group development model can predict the development of all groups because group behavior and interaction are influenced by such factors as the task, the members, and time (Menneke et al. 1992). Group development theorists are increasingly aware that the development of particular types of groups may follow their own unique patterns, and they have developed a number of group development models that are specific to particular types of groups. In this next section, you will learn about Worchel's model that examines the development of groups that "spin off" from other groups, Gersick's description of the development of time-limited task groups, and Corey and Corey's description of group development in therapy groups.

Worchel's Developmental Approach to Group Development

Worchel's develpmental approach

A cyclical group development theory that describes the development of groups that "spin off" from other groups because their needs are not being met.

Period of Discontent

Stage 1 of the developmental approach, in which some members feel alienated and estranged from the group.

Precipitating Event

Stage 2 of the developmental approach, in which a distinctive event has the effect of galvanizing disgruntled members.

Worchel, Coutant-Sassic, and Grossman (1992) have added to our understanding of group development by considering how groups and social movements begin and develop. After studying the civil rights movement, the women's movement, professional organizations, community political and environmental action groups, and a variety of other small social, work, and religious groups, they have created a model that describes the development of groups that "spin off" from other groups because their needs are not being met. In contrast to the linear sequential models of group development, **Worchel's developmental approach** is a "cyclical" model. It assumes that groups progress through cycles that are repeated several times throughout the life of the group.

Group members who feel that the group is not meeting their needs characterize the initial period of group formation (Stage 1: **Period of Discontent**). These members feel alienated and estranged from the group and frequently decline to participate in it. Passivity is common among these members, but they sometimes "act out" in an effort to get attention or express their frustration. The length of this period varies depending on how powerful group members respond. For instance, if discontented members' concerns are addressed, then it may be over. However, many typical responses from those in power prolong this stage. These responses include ignoring the situation, appealing to the loyalty and patriotism of the discontented members by emphasizing the sanctity of the group and the individual's history with it, and focusing attention on an outside threat to increase member commitment. Such approaches may work temporarily.

In Stage 2 (**Precipitating Event**), some event brings the discontented members together. This event differs from group to group, but in general, the event is clear and distinctive and symbolizes the issues with which they are concerned. Reactions to the event help identify other members who are alienated from the group and who may comprise the new group. Knowledge that there is a core group of discontented members stimulates activity because if a number of people are interested in change, it now appears that activism may be effective.

Group Identification

Stage 3 of the developmental approach, in which the dissatisfied subgroup breaks off and forms a new group.

Stage 3 (**Group Identification**) is the beginning of the new group. The first concern is clearly distinguishing the new group from its parent group. Clear, extreme, and uncompromising positions on issues relevant to the group are quickly staked out. The group identifies its leaders and structure and specifies norms for members. Enemies (including the parent group) are identified; they are perceived as dangerous, immoral, and corrupt, and competition and conflict with these outgroups are encouraged. Members at this stage demonstrate a high level of commitment and identify strongly with the group.

Group Productivity

Stage 4 of the developmental approach, in which the new group, having formed a clear identity, turns its attention to accomplishing goals and tasks.

Once the group has developed a sense of identity as a separate group, it turns its attention toward group goals and tasks (Stage 4: **Group Productivity**). The group tries to figure out which members have the skills to perform specific tasks and may recruit new members based on their skills. The group may soften its doctrine somewhat and isolate itself less. It may even work with the old group, as long as its independence is recognized. However, periodic conflicts that remind the groups of their separate identities are likely.

Individuation Stage

Stage 5 of the developmental model, in which members shift from a focus on the group to a focus on their own goals and needs within the group.

Next is a stage where group members shift from a focus on the group to a focus on their own goals and needs within the group (Stage 5: **Individuation Stage**). Worchel et al. (1992) suggest that the previous stage draws members' attention to their uniqueness, and this recognition is carried into the fifth stage. Individuals demand recognition, seek fairness in comparison to other members, evaluate their membership in the group, and consider membership in other groups. This process gives rise to Stage 6 (**Decay**), in which the group begins to disintegrate. Members begin to question the value of the group, internal struggles for power occur, and leaders are challenged. Discontent and alienation increase, and the cycle repeats.

Decay

Stage 6 of the developmental model, in which discontent and alienation occur, and the cycle repeats.

The Worchel model is an interesting and useful one, and the dynamic described is one you are likely to see at some point in your experience with groups. You may have already experienced it, for example, in a friendship or roommate group that splits off from another group, or in a family when one part splits off from another. You will see it in organizations as well. Recently, I was amused as my father talked about how he and some members of his model airplane club were considering leaving the club and forming a new club devoted to teaching children about aeronautics. He and these members were increasingly dissatisfied with the direction of the club. My own department acquired a Master's Program in Psychology that had jumped ship from a counseling and education department and a Bachelor's in Child Development program that came to us from a home economics department.

Punctuated equilibrium model

Gersick's group development model focusing on time-limited task groups with specific deadlines.

Gersick's Punctuated Equilibrium Model

The **punctuated equilibrium model** (Gersick, 1988, 1989) focuses on the development of small groups given creative tasks with specific deadlines for their completion. Time-limited task forces or committees and groups to invent new products or strategies are all common. In all of these cases, the groups must progress through the task and pace themselves to fit the work into the time available. Gersick (1989) points out that the development of these groups is different from that of other types of groups.

A field study conducted by Gersick (1988) explored the life cycles of special project groups. Eight naturally occurring teams that had from seven days to six months to complete their task were studied to reveal the developmental phases of time-limited task groups. The teams came from a variety of organizations, including a bank, a hospital, a community fund-raising group, a psychiatric treatment center, and two universities. Using case histories and interviews, Gersick documented what happened in the teams and how they progressed over time. None of the groups studied conformed to the basic developmental model, although there were conflicts and periods of performance. Instead, the groups exhibited what Gersick calls **punctuated equilibrium**—alternating between periods of inertia, in which the group carried on according to plan, and periods of creativity and change.

Gersick reported that by the end of the first meeting, all groups had made decisions about how to approach the task. They stuck with this approach for half of the time allotted for task completion. At the halfway point, the group underwent a major transition, dropping old patterns, reengaging with outside supervisors, and making dramatic progress. Gersick notes that this is a unique time in the group's life. The **transition phase** is the only time when all three of the following are true: members are experienced enough with the work to understand contextual requirements and resources, have used up enough time that they feel they must get on with the task, and still have enough time to make significant changes in product design. In the **final phase,** the group accelerates its production in order to meet the deadline. **Box 6-4** summarizes Gersick's phase model of group development.

Punctuated equilibrium
The idea that time-limited task groups alternate between periods of inertia, in which the group acts according to plan, and periods of creativity and change.

Transition phase
A period in the development of time-limited task groups in which old patterns are dropped, the group reengages with outside supervisors, and dramatic progress is made.

Final phase
The last period in the development of the time-limited task group, in which the group accelerates its production in order to meet the deadline.

Group Development in Therapy Groups

Therapy groups are led by trained psychotherapists or social workers and typically have between six and twelve members. Much of the early study of group development included therapy groups. Some group therapists find it useful to think of the therapy group as developing in stages. These therapists maintain that certain issues and behaviors are characteristic of each stage. The idea is that certain things may be expected at different points in the group's development and that awareness and preparedness can maximize the growth potential of each stage. Furthermore, the progression from one stage to the next is positive and represents growth. For instance, Lewis and Beck (1983) examined group development in therapy groups. Their concern was with how the groups move from an unwillingness to be involved (Stage 1) to using what happens in the group as a source of self-awareness and self-exploration (Stage 7). Corey and Corey (1997)

BOX 6-4 / GERSICK'S PHASE MODEL OF GROUP DEVELOPMENT

First Meeting & Phase 1	Midpoint Transition	Phase 2	Final Meeting & Completion
At the first meeting members display the framework through which they approach their projects for the first half of their calendar time. A period of inertia results where group moves on the course suggested by its initial framework.	Midpoint between the time it starts work and its deadline, the group undergoes change. Sense of urgency about finishing on time. Contacts between organizational contexts lead to reframing of strategy and new agreement about how to complete the task. Little conflict.	Execution of plans created in transitional phase. Interpersonal conflicts likely. A second period of inertia occurs where group moves according to the revised framework.	Focus on preparation of final product for presentation. Discussion of outsider expectations prominent.

Source: Gersick, 1988

and Corey, Corey, Callahan, and Russell (1992) conceive of four group stages: the initial stage, the transition stage, the working stage, and the final (termination) stage. **Corey and Corey's therapy group development model** is briefly described here because it is often used in the training of group therapists.

During the **initial stage,** members are typically anxious about being rejected and revealing themselves. Members wonder whether they will be able to trust other group members to listen and to accept them. Also during this stage, roles, power structures, and alliances emerge, and members watch the leader and other members to determine their expectations. Corey and Corey (1997) provide suggestions for leaders of groups at this stage. These suggestions include ways for members to begin to get to know one another and to explore feelings about the new group.

The **transition stage** is a difficult stage in which members are deciding to invest themselves fully in the group experience and are learning the importance of saying what they feel and think about the group. The group is not yet cohesive enough to delve deeply into members' issues, and the leader must continue to work to create trust and cohesion. Corey and associates (1992, 1997) suggest that defensiveness and other problem behaviors are especially likely during this stage. Conflict between members is also typical. By the end of this stage, with the

Corey and Corey's therapy group development model

A model describing how trust and cohesion develop in the therapy group so that therapeutic progress can be made.

Initial stage

The first stage in the therapy group, in which members are anxious about being rejected and revealing themselves.

Transition stage

A stage in the therapy group in which leaders work to create trust and cohesion and overcome defensiveness.

leader's guidance, members know how to talk about their feelings in the group, have learned how to confront others in a caring and constructive way, and can accept feedback without defensiveness.

Working stage

A stage in the therapy group in which members are willing to self-disclose and to have direct and meaningful interactions with other members.

In the **working stage,** members are usually willing to initiate work or themes they wish to explore. Members self-disclose more and feel safer doing so. They are also willing to have direct and meaningful interactions with other members and to confront and work through conflicts with other group members. Members give and receive direct and honest feedback. The mutual sharing of pain and growth results in an increase in group cohesion during the working phase. Corey et al. (1997) explain that not all groups reach this stage. In some cases, the working stage may never be reached because the initial stage was poorly handled, and members never feel safe enough to move beyond superficial encounters. Participants who are required to attend the group—for instance, by court order—may also merely go through the motions.

Final stage

The termination stage of the therapy group; ideally used as another opportunity for personal growth, learning, or adjustment.

The **final stage,** termination, is especially important in therapy groups for members have shared intimate information and shared in each other's emotional journeys. This makes saying good-bye especially hard, and feelings of loss especially great. Consistent with the goals of these groups, the ending should be used as another opportunity for personal growth, learning, or adjustment. As Corey et al. (1997) note, the more members verbalize their experiences in the group, the greater their chances of integrating and using the lessons they have learned. This normally takes more than the last session. Generally, participants should discuss such things as what they have learned in the group and what they will do with that learning, what they did and did not like about the group, and ways that the group experience could be designed to have more impact.

Dyadic Group Development

The group development models presented so far focus on the development of groups with three or more members, but there are models of two-person group development as well. In this section, you will learn about two theories of dyadic group development: social penetration theory and relational dialectics.

Social penetration theory

A theory of dyadic relationship development suggesting that relationships develop as people gradually engage in reciprocal self-disclosure.

Social penetration theory (Altman & Taylor, 1973) suggests that relationships develop as people gradually reveal more about themselves to each other—in other words, as they self-disclose. Johnson (2000, p. 46) defines **self-disclosure** as "revealing to another person how you perceive and are reacting to the present situation and giving any information about yourself and your past that is relevant to an understanding of your perceptions and reactions to the present." Self-disclosure is critical to relationship development because it enables people to value each other for who they are and to really know one another (Johnson, 2000).

Self-disclosure

The sharing of personal information, perceptions, and reactions with another.

Altman and Taylor (1973) suggest four stages in the development of intimacy, based on increasing reciprocal self-disclosures.

Orientation stage

The first stage of social penetration theory, in which people exchange superficial information about themselves.

Exploratory affective stage

The second stage of social penetration theory, in which more information is exchanged, but it is still not very personal.

Affective stage

The third stage of social penetration theory, in which close friendships develop and some intimate details are exchanged, but some barriers remain.

Stable exchange stage

The final, and rare, stage of social penetration theory in which both people share very private feelings and personal possessions.

1. In the **orientation stage,** people meet and exchange pieces of superficial information about themselves (for example, where they are from, where they work).
2. In the **exploratory affective stage,** people expand the areas about which they exchange information, but when the talk touches on personal levels, they do not intrude and do not reveal personal information about themselves.
3. In the **affective stage,** close friendships develop. People talk about many different aspects of themselves and offer praise and criticism to each other. Some intimate details are exchanged, but some barriers remain.
4. In the **stable exchange stage,** both people allow each other access to very private feelings and to personal possessions. Few relationships reach this level.

Altman and Taylor (1973) also suggest that there is a *reciprocity norm for self-disclosures.* Intimate relationships are based on trust, and trust is furthered if our self-disclosure is reciprocated by a self-disclosure from the other person. If I tell you something intimate about myself and you do not reciprocate, I should infer that you do not want our friendship to progress, and I should stop disclosing. If you do reciprocate my self-disclosure, then our relationship moves to a deeper level of intimacy. Also, in order for self-disclosure to propel a relationship forward, it must be responded to not simply with a reciprocal disclosure, but with evidence that it was heard, understood, and supported (Johnson, 2000).

Although self-disclosure is important for propelling a relationship forward, it should not be rushed. Research suggests that if people begin to reveal intimate information too quickly, we are not attracted to them and are likely to think them maladjusted (Chaiken & Derlega, 1974). If you have ever had a stranger on a plane or at a party disclose very intimate information to you, you know what I mean. You are likely to think "What kind of a person would tell a complete stranger such personal information?" Also, because we are not likely to trust a person who reveals too much too soon to keep our secrets, we are unlikely to reciprocate. We may assume that this information is shared with everybody and therefore not interpret it as signaling a potential special relationship.

Although we must take the risk of self-disclosing if our friendship is to deepen, it is clearly the case that self-disclosure is not always appropriate. Johnson (2000) reminds us that we should only self-disclose when it is appropriate to do so. The following are some of his guidelines:

1. Make sure that your disclosures are not random or isolated acts, but rather are part of an ongoing relationship.
2. Be sensitive to the effect that a disclosure may have on another person. Many people become uncomfortable when the level of self-disclosure exceeds their expectations.
3. Disclose only when it has a reasonable chance of improving the relationship.
4. Continue only if your disclosures are reciprocated.
5. Gradually move disclosures to a deeper level.
6. Keep your reactions and feelings to yourself if the other person is competitive or untrustworthy.

Brehm (1992) also notes that once a relationship is developed, quid pro quo reciprocity of self-disclosures occurs less frequently. In other words, self-disclosure of intimate information is more likely to be followed by expressions of support and care than an immediate reciprocal self-disclosure. When the relationship is ongoing, reciprocation may occur later, on an as-needed basis.

Altman and Taylor's (1973) initial formulation of social penetration theory offered a linear view of relationship development. In other words, it assumed that relationships develop along a straight path. After further study, however, it became clear that dyadic relationships "ebb and flow." Sometimes relationship partners offer deep self-revelations to each other, and at other times only superficial disclosures (Altman, Vinsel, & Brown, 1981). Altman et al. (1981) suggest that there is a *dialectic* between openness and closedness. A dialectic is characterized by tension between opposing yet related forces. The idea is that people cannot sustain complete openness and intimacy over long periods and that the relationship pendulum swings back and forth between self-disclosure and a need for privacy. Johnson (2000) echoes this point when he notes that you do not simply self-disclose more each day. Instead, there are cycles of seeking intimacy and avoiding it. What counts, he says, is the cumulative history of self-disclosure in the relationship.

Relational dialectics

The idea that dyadic relationships constantly change in response to opposing, yet related forces (dialectics).

The development of social penetration theory from a sequential stage theory to a theory emphasizing the dialectical nature of relationships mirrors changes in the study of close relationship development. Early efforts tried to identify a fixed sequence of stages through which close relationships passed, but as Brehm (1992) concluded, evidence for a fixed sequence of stages in intimate relationships is quite weak, and the stages postulated happen at different times in different relationships. Most dyadic relationship theorists now agree that relationships are a process rather than static, fixed entities and that relationships change constantly in response to opposing forces or dialectics. This perspective is called **relational dialectics.**

Openness/closedness dialectic

The relationship tension created by wanting to reveal ourselves and maintain our privacy.

Baxter (1990, 1994) identifies three main relationship dialectics that may be operating in a relationship at any given time. One is the **openness/closedness dialectic** mentioned previously—the tension between revealing ourselves and maintaining our privacy. On the one hand, open disclosure between partners is a necessary condition for intimacy; on the other hand, openness creates vulnerabilities for self, other, and relationship that necessitate information closedness (Baxter, 1990). A second dialectic, **novelty/predictability** involves our desire for excitement and newness in our relationships and the competing desire for security and predictability. Last, the **autonomy/connection dialectic** describes the tension between our desire to be independent and our desire to feel emotionally attached and connected to another person. We must forsake some individual autonomy to be in a relationship; however, if too much is forsaken, the relationship will be destroyed. Conversely, too much autonomy also destroys individual identity in the sense that connections with others are vital to who we are.

Novelty/predictability dialectic

The relationship tension created by our desire for excitement and our competing desire for the comfort of the familiar.

Autonomy/connection dialectic

The relationship tension created by our desire to be independent and our desire to be emotionally connected to another.

Apply It! ••• **Examine Dialectical Pressures in Group Endings**

> Baxter (1986) found that people's accounts of why their relationships ended fit the relational dialectics model. Examine one or more of your now-terminated close relationships. Did the inability to deal with dialectical pressures play a role in the ending of your relationship?

According to Baxter (1990), in the initial stages of a relationship, issues of openness/closedness are prominent. How much should you reveal, and when? The other dialectics become more of an issue as the relationship progresses. How do you retain your freedom and identity, and yet be close? How do you maintain excitement, and yet retain the safety of predictability? The negotiation of these ongoing dialectics is key to survival of the relationship. Imagine, for instance, a case in which one partner is feeling a stronger pull toward connection, and the other toward autonomy. This may spell doom for the relationship, or the partners may agree to changes that make the relationship workable. Research supports the relational dialectics view of relationships (Baxter, 1990; Braithwaite & Baxter, 1995; Canary & Stafford, 1994; Montgomery, 1993).

Concept Review

- **Group development** is about how groups develop over time as members interact, learn about one another, and structure relationships and roles within the group.
- **Sequential stage theories** suggest that group development proceeds through a fixed series of stages. Certain developmental tasks must be accomplished in order to move from one stage to the next. Groups can be stuck in a stage, but ideally, groups develop toward maturity.

The Basic Group Development Model (Tuckman)

- The best-known model of group development is Tuckman's model, which identifies five stages of group development: forming (orientation), storming (conflict), norming (structure), performing (work), and adjourning (dissolution).
- **Forming** is a stage of "hesitant participation" as members figure out what is acceptable behavior in the group and rely on the group leader for structure and guidance.
- **Storming** is a phase of conflict within the group. Members disagree about such things as leadership and how to approach the task. Contrary to the basic model, storming does not always occur; when it does, it may be dramatic or subtle, depending partly on culture.

- In the **norming** stage, structure, roles, and group cohesion emerge. **Group cohesion** is a multidimensional concept that includes attraction to the group, a sense of unity, and commitment to the group.
- In the **performing** stage, the group's energies are focused on successful task completion. Many factors influence group performance, including leadership, resources, coordination and communication, and member skills.
- The **adjourning** stage is characterized by members' disengagement from the group as they begin to cope with its termination. The adjourning stage can provide for personal and professional growth if time is taken to reflect and review the group's experiences.

The Integrative Model of Group Development (Wheelan)

- Wheelan's model consolidates group development research and concludes that although development varies with the type of group, most models can be integrated into five stages.
- In Stage 1, **dependency and inclusion,** new members worry about the group's rules and whether they will be accepted. They rely on a leader for protection and structure.
- Stage 2, **counterdependency and fight,** is characterized by conflict between a single member and the leader, or among members and leaders.
- The focus of Stage 3, **trust and structure,** is on the open negotiation of group goals and structure—what the group is going to do, and how they are going to do it.
- In Stage 4, **work and productivity,** the group works to create a product. Good communication, awareness of time, and the availability of resources are essential.
- Stage 5, **termination,** encompasses the multiple endings associated with every group. Impending termination may result in regression to earlier stages, and conflict and negativity may occur.

Membership Change and Group Development

- Changes in the relationship between a group and its members are called **group socialization.** Levine and Moreland offer a five-stage theory that describes the development of the relationship between a new group member and the group. At the beginning, in the **investigation phase,** the group and potential member check each other out, and the role transition of entry occurs if they meet each other's entrance criteria. In the **socialization phase,** the group and the new member attempt to change one another to better fit their needs. The **maintenance phase** occurs as the person and the group agree on the member's role in the group. The **resocialization phase** occurs when the member seeks accommodations in the group and the group seeks to assimilate the member. If resolution takes place, then the role transition of convergence occurs and the person regains full membership. Group membership ends with a **remembrance phase** in which both the person and the group evaluate their experience.

■ Arrow and McGrath's model examines factors affecting the impact on the group of membership change. They note that groups with a relatively fixed and stable membership are more affected by membership changes and that the reason for member change affects the impact of the change on the group. Other important factors affecting the impact of member change are the frequency and predictability of membership change, the size of the change relative to the group's size, and the centrality of the departing members to the group.

Group Development in Specialized Groups

■ **Worchel's developmental approach** describes the development of groups that "spin off" from other groups because some members' needs are not being met. In Stage 1, the **period of discontent,** discontented members express their frustrations with the group. In Stage 2, **precipitating event,** discontented members are unified by some event that symbolizes their concerns. The new group begins in Stage 3, **group identification,** when the group starts to distinguish itself from the parent group. In Stage 4, **group productivity,** members focus on group goals and tasks and how these will be accomplished. In Stage 5, **individuation,** group members shift from a focus on the group to the satisfaction of their own needs in the group. In Stage 6, **decay,** the group begins to disintegrate as members begin to question the value of the group, power struggles occur, and leaders are challenged. The cycle repeats.

■ Gersick's **punctuated equilibrium model** focuses on the development of small, short-term task groups with specific deadlines for task completion. Gersick's study of eight teams found that the groups exhibited **punctuated equilibrium,** alternating between periods of inertia and periods of creativity and change. She also found that at the halfway point, the group underwent a major transition, and then made dramatic progress toward task completion.

■ **Corey and Corey's therapy group development model** proposes four group stages. During the **initial stage,** members are anxious about revealing themselves. In the **transition stage,** members learn the importance of saying what they think and feel about the group and how to confront others in a caring way. Defensiveness and resistance are common in this stage. In the **working stage,** members are willing to initiate work on their issues, to have meaningful interactions with other group members, and to work through conflicts with one another. The final stage is **termination,** in which participants discuss what they have learned in the group and what they will do with that learning.

■ **Social penetration theory** is a theory of dyadic relationship development that suggests that relationships develop as people gradually engage in reciprocal self-disclosure. In the **orientation stage,** people exchange superficial information about themselves. The areas about which information is exchanged are expanded in the next stage, the **exploratory affective stage,** but the information is still not very personal. In the **affective stage,** close friendships develop. People talk about many different aspects of themselves and offer praise and criticism to each other. Some intimate details are exchanged, but some barriers remain. Few relationships reach the final **stable exchange stage,** in which both people share very private feelings and personal possessions.

- Current thinking on the development of dyadic relationships is that they change constantly in response to powerful dialectics (opposing yet related forces). This is called **relational dialectics.** Three relationship dialectics are **openness/closedness,** referring to the tension between revealing ourselves and maintaining our privacy; **novelty/predictability,** representing our desire for excitement and our competing desire for the comfort of the familiar; and **autonomy/connection,** the tension between our desire to be independent and our desire to be emotionally connected to another. The negotiation of these dialectics is key to survival of the relationship.

Skill Review

Promote Movement Through the Basic Group Development Stages

- Structured leadership and "icebreaker" activities may be used to stimulate interaction among new group members and foster movement through the forming stage.
- To promote constructive conflict, group leaders or coordinators should confront and problem solve, reason and negotiate, and encourage solutions that respect members' autonomy and individuality.
- Group cohesion may be promoted by physical proximity, assembling a group of like members or creating similarity through shared experience, emphasizing goals that members have in common, and separating the group from other units and giving it unique characteristics such as a name.
- Making members feel included (satisfying their belongingness needs) and showing the group's commitment to them by structuring the group to meet members' needs enhance commitment to the group. Giving members a chance to make sacrifices for the group also fosters commitment.
- To facilitate the adjourning stage, groups should take time to review group accomplishments or processes and share what other group members have meant to them. In functional groups, at each ending point, the group evaluates its work together and members express feelings about each other and the group.

Improve Group Socialization

- A group and a potential member should be clear and honest about their expectations of one another and what they have to offer. If they are not, a new member and a group may not be able to work out differences, commitment to one another may wane, and the relationship may even end.

Be Aware of Member Change

- Group leaders should be sensitive to the fact that member change can have a profound effect on the group, depending on when and why it occurs and how many members are lost or gained. In cases where member changes strongly impact the group, it is a good idea to talk openly as a group about how the group is affected.

Deal With Discontented Members

- Groups should seriously address the concerns of discontented members. Otherwise, those members may leave and, in some cases, form their own group.

Better Dyadic Relationships

- To increase the closeness of a relationship, gradually self-disclose more about yourself if the other person reciprocates your self-disclosures.
- Be aware of relational dialectics, and understand that the negotiation of these is important to relationship survival.

 ## Study Questions

1. What is group development?
2. What assumptions are common to sequential theories of group development?
3. What is the best-known theory of group development?
4. What features are typical of each of Tuckman's stages? What factors might influence them? How can movement through each stage be facilitated?
5. What is Wheelan's integrative model of group development, and how can it be used to promote group effectiveness?
6. What is group socialization? What are the three psychological processes used to analyze group socialization? What are the five phases of group socialization?
7. According to Arrow and McGrath, what factors determine how membership change will affect the group?

8. What are the focus and the key stages of Worchel's developmental approach to group development? How is it a cyclical theory of group development?
9. What are the main features of Gersick's punctuated equilibrium model?
10. Corey and Corey's model of development in therapy groups has four stages. What distinguishes each of these stages?
11. What is social penetration theory, and how does it describe dyadic relationship development? What guidelines were given in the chapter regarding appropriate self-disclosure?
12. What are relational dialectics?

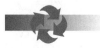

Group Activities

Activity 1: Practice Icebreakers

In a group of five or six, each member is to lead the group through an icebreaker (give members at least five minutes to create or remember one). After all the icebreakers have been completed, answer the following questions: Do you believe icebreakers are useful in facilitating the forming stage? Are certain types of icebreakers more helpful than other types, and if so, which ones? Are icebreakers more or less useful depending on the group?

Activity 2: Create a Plan to Promote Cohesion

Get into a small group of students with similar career goals. Next, pretend that your group has been charged with the task of promoting cohesiveness for one of the following new groups (choose according to your career goals): (1) a sports team, (2) a children's camp, (3) a student project group, (4) a work team, (5) a therapy group. Use the guidelines provided in the chapter to create a specific plan.

Activity 3: Analyze Group Development Case Studies

With your small group, read the following cases and decide which group development theory described in the chapter best applies. Identify key steps of the theory as illustrated in the case. Next, discuss with your group and arrive at a consensus. Did your group go through the sequential model as it discussed the cases?

   CASE 1   For as long as I can remember, music has been a big part of my life; I can't live without playing it, and listening to it. I recently left a band I had played with for five years and it was a struggle. I wanted to play guitar in a band again and lo and behold, an opportunity presented itself to me.
   I went to a bar to hear a friend's band play and ending up watching the next band as well. It was love at first sight. They were amazing. In between sets they

interacted with the audience and it was clear they were looking for a new guitarist. We talked a little and we found we had similar musical interests. After the show, we had a long conversation and they gave me a CD of their songs. I was to learn five songs to audition with at their next rehearsal. For two months, I waited until they finally agreed to let me rehearse with them. I liked many of their songs but I had my own ideas too. They liked some of my ideas but sometimes they liked their ideas better, so we played a bit of tug-of-war with some of the music. I wanted to be in a band where I had input and they wanted a member who didn't have to get everything he or she wanted.

I went to every practice for two months, added my input, but wasn't really considered a member until I actually performed with them at a party. It took a while for me to feel comfortable saying it was my band, but now I would say I am an equal member. We did have problems with another member though, due to his lack of commitment and practice. We decided that if he didn't start to pull his own weight and work harder, we would have to ask him to leave the band. After a long winter vacation, we did manage to work things out with him. Now everyone is working harder than ever to write new songs, practice as much as possible, and share time working on different band projects.

CASE 2   A couple of months ago, I entered a training group for the restaurant where I now work. The group consisted of two trainers, me, and my fellow trainees Josie, Jim, Andrea, Will, and Lisa. On our first day, we met with the restaurant manager who showed us videos and handed out literature about sexual harassment, showed us videos, and had us fill out forms. When there was a free minute we trainees exchanged information about our previous jobs and our past restaurant experience. On the second day, we met with Lenny, a "certified trainer." He seemed nice enough as he taught us about restaurant policies and gave us a tour of the restaurant. It was on this day that a leader in our group emerged. Jim was a thirty-five-year-old talkative Christian man. He was very warm and friendly and asked a lot of intelligent questions. Will, who had just graduated high school, emerged as the group "clown." The next day we met Michelle, another certified trainer. She was the sweetest person.

The next day Lenny was back, and the trainee group argued about who was the better trainer, Lenny or Michelle. Some of us thought that Lenny was too strict and cold and that we should stand up to him, while others thought Michelle was too nice for our own good. We also had some conflict over Jim. He seemed to like drinking wine too much. When we had food pairing activities (what type of wine went with what type of food), he would take more than his share of both. This bothered some of us more than others.

On our fifth day, we realized that we would soon be on our own waiting on tables. We had a sense of togetherness and promised each other we would help each other out. Despite our minor annoyances with one another, we realized that things would be worse if we didn't support one another. Our sixth and seventh days were spent with other servers. We followed them around and watched what they did. On the last day of training, we wished each other good luck since we would no longer be in training. It was a little scary leaving the comfort of the group. We knew eventually that training would end and we'd have to face demanding guests, botched orders, spilled drinks, and bad tips. However, it was still difficult. Today, months later, I still feel a sense of relief when I come to work and find that I have the same station with someone from my training group.

InfoTrac College Edition Search Terms

To do research for your papers and assignments, use InfoTrac that's provided free with new copies of this book. Go to http://infotrac.thomsonlearning.com and enter the following search terms:

- Icebreakers
- Group Cohesion
- Self-disclosure

Chapter **7** **Understanding and Managing Conflict**

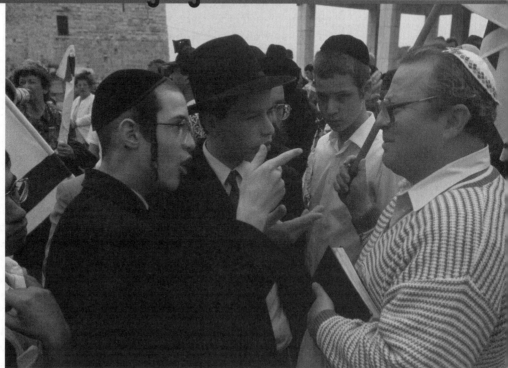

© Annie Griffiths Belt/CORBIS

Where there are groups, there are conflicts. Conflicts arise because group members are individuals with different opinions and goals; because members have trouble with people who differ from themselves; and because in some situations, what benefits one member or one group does not benefit another member or group. One of the themes of this chapter is that although conflict is a fact of group life, destructive conflict does not have to be. Take a look at the examples that follow. These examples show that conflicts in groups can be a good thing or a bad thing, depending on how they are handled. In some of these cases, the conflict was dealt with constructively and led to a good outcome; in other cases, it was not, and the group suffered.

- At a staff meeting, colleagues disagree about how to implement a policy change handed down from upper management. Although the discussion is heated, it does bring out members' chief concerns and allows the group to create a plan that satisfies the major issues of all members. Afterwards, members feel even more committed to the group, confident in the knowledge that they can disagree and work things out.

- A family hasn't gotten together for three years because two members are not speaking to each other since one missed the other's wedding. Now some members are taking sides, and others are so disgusted they are distancing themselves from the group.

- On a project team, one member thinks critical comments made by another member are directed at her culture and becomes defensive. The group ignores the situation, hoping it will go away. Unfortunately, productivity suffers because the two conflicting members refuse to talk to each other, making completion of the group's work difficult.

- A once friendly roommate group fragments into two groups—one that is party loving and noisy, and another that is studious and quiet. Because they were once all friends who got along well, one member decides that she'll get both groups together in a last-ditch effort to solve the problems. When they finally sit down to talk, they realize that each side has misunderstood the actions of the other, and everyone cooperates to create a plan they can all live with.

- The night shift deliberately sabotages the day shift because they believe that the day shift convinced management to give the night shift smaller raises. The day shift retaliates, and productivity declines. Management convenes the two groups to mediate the conflict. The night shift finds that management made the decision to give the day shift more because they believed that the day shift had additional duties to justify it. Once the day shift learns what the night shift group thought, they understand why the night shift acted the way they did. The day shift takes the night shift's side, pointing out to management that the night shift has duties the day shift doesn't, so they should all get paid the same. Management agrees.

This chapter focuses on conflict and its resolution. It is one thing to say that conflict has the potential to be constructive rather than destructive; it is yet another thing to realize this potential. After reading this chapter, you will be able to identify the seeds of destructive conflict and know how to prevent such seeds from taking root. You will also have some tools to resolve conflicts before they destroy groups or group members.

Destructive Conflicts

Destructive conflicts
Conflicts that damage the group and relationships between members or groups.

Destructive conflicts are those conflicts that damage the group and relationships between members or groups. Destructive conflicts include conflicts that spiral out of control and in which people say extreme things, become entrenched in their positions, and are more interested in winning than coming to a mutually agreeable solution. Conflicts that are not dealt with but prevent the group from realizing its full potential or quietly lead to its demise are also considered destructive conflicts. Destructive intergroup conflicts can lead to aggression between groups and to the denial of rights or resources to the less powerful group. It is a fear of destructive conflicts that makes so many people hesitant to face the differences they have with other group members.

Conflict Spiraling

One of the most important things to understand about the dynamics of conflict is that destructive conflicts arise out of a series of negative reciprocal interactions. One party does something that is perceived as aggressive by a second party, who then retaliates. The first party believes that this retaliation is excessive or unjust and counter-retaliates. The second party is angered by this counter-retaliation, believing that its own retaliation was only to even the score, which leads to counter-counter-retaliation, and so on. Understanding this conflict spiraling dynamic is important because preventing and breaking destructive cycles often depends on *not* reciprocating others' aggressive acts. This is no easy feat, because it goes against our natural tendency to return any ill will and to reciprocate (return in kind) negative actions or perceptions.

Conflict spiraling

The escalation of conflict in a progressive pattern of attack and counterattack.

The term **conflict spiraling** refers to the escalation of conflict in a progressive pattern of attack and counterattack (Deutsch, 1973). In destructive conflicts, the parties get away from problem solving and spend their time reacting to the previous "enemy attack," with each round getting progressively nastier. The conflicting parties mirror each other's negative actions (Fisher & Brown, 1988). If one is angry, the other is angry; if one does not listen, the other will not listen; if one is deceptive, the other will be deceptive; and so on. This "eye for an eye" approach means that conflict can get destructive quickly.

The famous conflict theorist Morton Deutsch (1994) once likened spiraling conflicts to malignant tumors, growing out of control and enmeshing the participants in a web of hostile interactions and defensive maneuvers that continuously worsen their situations, making them feel less secure, more vulnerable, and more burdened. Both parties end up feeling "wronged" by the other's seemingly deliberate effort to make them look bad and misunderstand them. This erodes trust between the two parties, and they both seek retaliation for the other's negative actions. The relationship disintegrates. The resulting suspicious, hostile attitude increases sensitivity to differences and threats while minimizing awareness of similarities (Deutsch, 1994). Communication becomes unreliable and impoverished, and contact and communication are often broken off. Deutsch (2000) terms this **autistic hostility** and notes that it perpetuates hostility because one has no opportunity to learn that it may be based on misunderstanding or misjudgment, nor to learn if the other has changed for the better.

Autistic hostility

When conflicting parties break off contact, making conflict resolution difficult because there is no opportunity to correct misperceptions.

Perceptual Distortion

Perceptual distortion

The exaggerated misinterpretation and attribution of hostile intentions to an opponent's actions.

Another feature of the destructive conflict is **perceptual distortion.** Indeed, the exaggerated misinterpretation and attribution of hostile intentions to an opponent's actions fuel conflict escalation. As the conflict develops, each side has a negative, "enemy" stereotype of the other that leads to biased processing of one's own and others' actions. Each side views its own negative actions as justified in reaction to the situation, while seeing the other's negative actions as evidence of an evil nature bent on terrorizing, aggressing, or dominating (Bettencourt, 1990; Burn & Oskamp, 1989). This is known as the **ultimate attribution error** (Pettigrew, 1979).

Ultimate attribution error

When each side in a conflict views its own negative actions as justified by the situation, while seeing the other's negative actions as evidence of an evil nature.

Likewise, each side fails to appreciate that its adversary's aggression is a response to its own behavior (which is perceived as threatening). Instead, the aggressive behavior is seen as evidence of the other's hostile intentions and power motivations (Kemmelmeier & Winter, 2000). Each side tends to perceive the other in a similar, negative way, a tendency called the **mirror image** (Bronfenbrenner, 1961; White, 1984). Self-fulfilling prophecies often arise as attributions of hostile intentions to the other side trigger defensive and hostile behavior toward them. When the other responds aggressively to these behaviors, it is taken as evidence that the negative assumptions about the other were correct.

Mirror image

The tendency for the two sides in a conflict to perceive each other in a similar, negative way.

By the time a conflict has escalated to the point of autistic hostility and perceptual distortion, both sides have generally done some pretty despicable things. These become new sources of conflict, as each side is angry about the actions taken by the other side during the course of the conflict. As Deutsch (1994) notes, destructive conflicts take on lives of their own, continuing even though the issues that initially gave rise to them have long been forgotten or become irrelevant. The term **metaconflict** is sometimes used to refer to a situation in which new issues produced by the conflict overshadow the issues that initially triggered the conflict (McEwen & Milburn, 1993).

Metaconflict

A situation in which new issues produced by the conflict overshadow the issues that initially triggered it.

Competitive Goal Structure

Competitive goal structure

A conflict context where it is believed that the goals of the two parties are divergent and cannot be reconciled.

One major source of conflict is competition for scarce resources or rewards. When resources or rewards are limited, and attaining them means that some "win" and others "lose," conflict is likely as competition occurs. Siblings or roommates may fight over who gets the best room. Coworkers may argue about who gets to take time off at the holidays. Departments may come into conflict over resources. Groups may fight over territory. Underlying destructive conflict is a **competitive goal structure** in which it is assumed that one party will win, and one will lose. The perception is that the goals of the two parties are divergent and cannot be reconciled. This is often called a **zero-sum conflict** because the conflicting parties perceive that anything gained by one side must be lost by the other. They see the interests of the two sides as mutually exclusive; to win,

Zero-sum conflict

A win-lose conflict in which it is believed that anything gained by one side must be lost by the other.

BOX 7-1 / A CASE OF DESTRUCTIVE CONFLICT

A conflict at a condominium complex in Huntington, California, began when some neighbors complained to the condo association board that another neighbor, John Rogers, was taking too many parking spaces (Allison, 2002). Rogers complained that he was being unfairly targeted and accused other neighbors of parking illegally also. The board responded by ordering those cars in violation to be towed. A few days later, Rogers found that his tires were slashed. Rogers responded with a videotaping campaign to document offenses, and other neighbors responded by videotaping him. The conflict has become especially heated between Rogers and neighbor Michael Richardson, who take turns shouting at each other through security gates and shining powerful flashlights through each other's windows at night. Both now have restraining orders against the other and have filed legal charges of harassment. Meanwhile, the other neighbors have taken sides and constantly videotape one another in the commons areas. The police have been called more than 200 times and have made more than 125 visits to the complex. Police lieutenant J. B. Hume says, "Basically you have a group of people not getting along, and they're doing everything they can to irritate each other. . . . What gets me is that they don't see themselves as being part of it. It takes two to tango. If you want to call them victims, both of them have been victimized by the other. We are still making attempts to mediate and improve things. . . . It could go from name-calling to actual violence."

Apply It! ••• **Analyze a Past Destructive Conflict**

Describe a conflict you were part of, using the concepts described above.

---

the other must lose. Advantage for one's own side is sought through coercion, misinformation, and obstructing the fulfillment of the other's wants (Deutsch, 2000a). **Box 7-1** presents a case of destructive conflict.

Constructive Conflict

Constructive conflict

A conflict that is primarily cooperative and oriented toward joint problem solving and the maintenance of a working relationship.

Remember that conflict is an inevitable part of human relations and that although conflict can be destructive, it can also be constructive if skillfully managed. **Constructive conflict** is primarily cooperative; it is oriented toward joint problem solving and the maintenance of a working relationship (Johnson, Johnson, & Tjosvold, 2000; Wilmot & Hocker, 1998). In constructive conflicts, participants interact with the intent of learning instead of the intent to protect themselves or dominate the other.

Benefits of Constructive Conflict

Donohue and Kolt (1992) point out that conflicts can motivate positive change by increasing awareness and leading to a deeper understanding of others and ourselves. Conflict can deepen, enrich, and save relationships. As the writer James Baldwin once said, "Not everything that is faced can be changed, but nothing can be changed until it is faced." Johnson (2000) argues that conflict can be beneficial because it focuses attention on problems that need to be solved, clarifies how we need to change, illuminates our values and what matters to us, and helps us understand other people and their values. Chapter 5, Communication in Groups, emphasized the importance of assertiveness and constructive confrontation. These behaviors increase the likelihood that facing an issue with another group member will in fact lead to needed change.

Chapter 6, Group Development, pointed out that conflict is a part of the development of most groups. Groups "storm" in order to decide what to do and how to do it. As Wheelan (1994) noted, ideally conflict is the way that the group arrives at a unified direction from divergent points of view. It is also a way for members to establish trust. It lets them know that they will be accepted despite differences, and permits greater intimacy and collaboration. Groups are strengthened when members disagree in a climate of friendship and support and cooperate to reach agreement. In a successful group, conflict increases trust and cohesion, and consensus about group goals and structure.

Conflict may also enhance a group's decision making because it leads to a more complete consideration of the issue. A group that fears internal conflict may adopt the first plausible suggestion in order to reduce debate among its members and may therefore make an inferior decision (Rubin, Pruitt, & Kim, 1994). Likewise, conflict often plays an important role in achieving justice for exploited groups and individuals (Rubin et al., 1994). As Deutsch (1994) once said, the issue is not how to eliminate or prevent conflict, but how we can promote the conditions that lead to lively controversy rather than deadly quarrel.

Cooperative Goal Structure

Cooperative goal structure

A context in which conflicting parties believe that they can work together to satisfy both parties' goals.

In contrast to destructive conflicts, which are characterized by a competitive goal structure, constructive conflicts are characterized by a **cooperative goal structure.** The conflicting parties are open to working together as a team to engage in mutual problem solving. Instead of asking "How can I/we get what I/we want at the expense of the other?" the question becomes "How can we all work together to create a solution that satisfies both sides' major concerns and needs?" In a competitive context, people refuse to seriously consider their opponent's viewpoints, making conflict resolution difficult and conflict escalation likely. In a cooperative context, constructive conflict is more likely because both sides make a sincere effort to listen to and understand the other's position. This enables them to come

---

Apply It! ••• **Evaluate Your Constructive Controversy Skills**

Box 7-2 enables you to assess your use of constructive controversy and identify areas in need of improvement.

---

up with solutions that satisfy the fundamental needs of both sides. Simply put, in destructive conflict the parties work against each other, whereas in constructive conflict they work together to solve a problem or come to an understanding.

Constructive Controversy

Constructive controversy

When parties seek a collaborative agreement in a respectful climate.

Constructive conflict embodies the features of **constructive controversy.** Constructive controversy occurs when there are differences between ideas, information, conclusions, theories, or opinions and agreement is sought (Johnson et al., 2000). Constructive controversy requires a cooperative goal structure and collaborative

---

BOX 7-2 / DO YOU DISPLAY BEHAVIORS CONSISTENT WITH CONSTRUCTIVE CONTROVERSY?

Instructions: Think about the three most recent disagreements you have had with others, describing them briefly on a separate piece of paper. Then, place a T (true) or F (false) next to the statements below.

_____ 1. I challenged and refuted the ideas of the other participants, while confirming their competence and value as individuals.

_____ 2. I separated my personal worth from criticism of my ideas.

_____ 3. I focused on coming to the best decision possible, not on winning.

_____ 4. I listened to everyone's ideas, even when I didn't agree.

_____ 5. I restated what someone said if it was not clear.

_____ 6. I tried to see the issue from the opposing perspective in order to really understand it.

_____ 7. I changed my mind when the evidence clearly indicated that I should.

_____ 8. I rationally sought the best possible answer given the available data.

_____ 9. First, I brought out all the ideas and facts supporting both sides, then I clarified how the positions differed, then I identified points of agreement.

_____ 10. I acted toward my opponents as I wanted them to act toward me.

Look back at your answers. What do you need to work on in order to become better at constructive controversy?

Source: Adapted from Johnson, Johnson, & Tjosvold, 2000

Differentiation

A part of constructive controversy in which parties illuminate the differences in their positions.

Integration

A part of constructive controversy in which the parties work to combine their positions into a new position.

conflict management skills. These skills include the ability to disagree with each other's ideas while confirming one another's personal competence. The focus is on the problem, not on personalities, and participants behave respectfully toward one another despite their differences. The ability to bring out differences (**differentiation**) while working toward combining the positions into a new, creative position (**integration**) is another important condition for constructive controversy. Reliance on rational argument is also central to constructive controversy. Participants must keep an open mind, changing their conclusions and positions when others are persuasive in their presentation of rationale, proof, and logical reasoning.

Conflict Resolution

The dynamics of destructive conflicts are such that perpetuation rather than resolution seems more likely. However, perceptions can change, and destructive competitive orientations can be turned to cooperative ones. Practitioners of conflict resolution work at many different levels, ranging from the interpersonal to the international, and share common insights and approaches to practice (Kelman, 1997).

Common Features of Conflict Resolution Programs

Most conflict resolution models are built on getting participants to recognize different perspectives, become aware of their biases, improve communication, and come up with integrative solutions that reconcile the interests of the parties. Conflict resolution programs require that participants be committed to fair solutions based on objective criteria instead of solutions based on bribery, threats, manipulation, or refusal to budge (Fisher, Ury, & Patton, 1991).

Many conflict resolution programs and techniques emphasize the development of communication skills to reduce the likelihood of conflict escalation and to increase cooperation (see, for example, Raider, Coleman, & Gerson, 2000). Conflict management skills also involve perspective-taking behaviors, such as paraphrasing the others' communications to ensure understanding and considering others when phrasing messages so that they are easily understood.

Another common feature of conflict resolution programs is an emphasis on clarifying the differences between the two parties, after which agreement is sought. For instance, in the ARIA (Antagonism, Resonance, Invention, Action) conflict resolution model described by Rothman (1997), the *antagonism* stage is where differences are identified; the *resonance* stage is where the parties work to understand what each side cares most about in the conflict and why it matters so much (each sides' true issues); *invention* is where the parties generate alternatives; and the *action* stage is where parties create a plan for action. The resonance stage is especially critical.

Once we understand what the real issues are, finding integrative solutions that satisfy the interests of both parties is not as difficult. We now have empathy for the other side, and this makes it possible to work cooperatively toward a solution. Rothman (1997) calls this mutual understanding **analytic empathy,** while White (1984) called it **realistic empathy.**

Analytic empathy (realistic empathy)
When parties understand what each side cares most about in the conflict and why it matters so much (each sides' true issues), making integration possible.

Because the escalation of destructive conflict erodes trust and makes conflict resolution difficult, **trust building** is another element recommended by conflict resolution researchers. Research indicates there are two basic ways to create trust in a conflict situation (Lewicki & Wiethoff, 2000). One is to act consistently and reliably, meet deadlines and commitments, and to do so over time. For instance, to rebuild trust, participants may undertake a series of conciliatory actions, giving the other time to see that the actions are not a "trick" and to respond in kind (Osgood, 1962; Rubin et al., 1994). A second way to build trust is to identify common goals, values, purposes, or identities that may form the basis for a cooperative relationship. Because rebuilding trust can take a long time, it may be necessary to put in place strategies to manage distrust in the meantime (Lewicki & Wiethoff, 2000). Each party responsible for a trust violation or act of distrust should apologize, explain, and express regret for any harm done. Both parties should also restate and renegotiate the expectations for future conduct and commit to those behaviors (and, of course, stick to those commitments). Last, the parties should agree on procedures for monitoring and verifying compliance with new commitments.

Trust building
Efforts to rebuild trust after it has been eroded by conflict.

Negotiation

Negotiation
When conflicting parties use an exchange of offers and ideas to come to a settlement.

Negotiation occurs when two or more parties to the conflict use an exchange of offers and ideas to come to a settlement. In all cultures, there are three broad strategies for reaching agreement in negotiation (Carnevale & Leung, 2001). One is *concession making,* where one reduces one's goals, demands, or offers ("Okay, we'll settle for a 4 percent raise instead of the 7 percent we were asking for."). A second one is *contending,* where one tries to get the other to concede by using threats, harassment, or absolute refusal to move from a particular position ("We won't accept less than 7 percent, and we are prepared to strike."). Contending is risky because it is often perceived as an aggressive move that is reciprocated by the other side, leading to conflict spiraling rather than resolution, but sometimes it works (Pruitt & Carnevale, 1993). A third strategy is *problem solving,* where an effort is made to satisfy both parties' goals ("It appears that we would both be satisfied with a deal in which my group took a lower raise but received stock options equivalent to an additional 3 percent."). These three different strategies are often seen during contract talks between unions and management. For instance, in 2002, the Major League Baseball Players Association refused to accept the owners' demands for increased revenue sharing and a luxury tax, and threatened to strike. Eventually, both sides were motivated to problem-solve to avoid a costly strike. Each made some concessions—the owners agreed to reduce their demands, and the union agreed to some increases in revenue sharing.

Carnevale and Leung (2001) note several things that are true of negotiation regardless of culture. One is that choice of strategy depends on the relationship. If a positive relationship is important, then contending is the least desirable option. A second cross-cultural similarity is that negotiation often follows a period of struggle. In other words, people first fight and then negotiate, once they realize the other side will not give in or the costs of the struggle are too great. For instance, in September of 2002, on the final night of the legislative session, the California legislature finally passed a new state budget after the longest Democrat–Republican standoff in California legislative history. For months, neither side would budge, but as the stalemate dragged on, both sides faced increasing pressure from constituents dependent on state programs, vendors who sell to the state, and state workers who were in danger of not getting paid. The state's controller was about to borrow billions of dollars to cover California's basic operating expenses. Both sides made significant concessions in order to get the budget passed.

In the research literature on negotiation, you will find two main models: the concession-convergence model and the mutual gains approach. In the **concession-convergence** or **distributive bargaining model,** each side stakes out a tough and extreme position and takes "baby steps" toward some point of convergence (Rubin et al., 1994; Walton & McKersie, 1965). For instance, in union and management negotiations, each side commonly makes a series of offers, counteroffers, and concessions, until an agreement is reached. In this case, negotiation is a game in which both sides misrepresent what they expect to get and what they are willing to give up, and only gradually does it become clear what each side's bottom line is (Rubin et al., 1994).

As in constructive controversy and the ARIA models, in the **mutual gains** or **integrative bargaining approach** (Fisher et al., 1991; Rubin et al., 1994), the two sides share what they want and why they want it, with the goal of coming up with a solution that satisfies the major issues of both parties. The idea is that too often in negotiation, we focus too much on the positions of the parties (which appear mutually incompatible) and not enough on *why* they hold these positions (their underlying motivations or interests). The following story is often used to illustrate. Imagine two sisters arguing over an orange. One argues that she should get 80 percent and the other responds that no, she wants 75 percent and the other can have 25 percent. Eventually, they decide to split it 50-50. The one takes her half, throws away the peel, and eats the fruit. The other throws away the fruit and uses the peel to bake a cake. Had they talked about why each wanted the orange, both would have gotten everything that they wanted. **Box 7-3** provides an example of the steps you could follow to use a version of the mutual gains model in negotiation.

The concession-convergence and mutual gains models differ in some important ways (Rubin et al., 1994). Threat has a place in the concession-convergence approach, as when one side threatens to walk away from negoti-

Concession-convergence model (distributive bargaining)
Negotiation model in which each side stakes out a tough position and "baby steps" are made toward agreement.

Mutual gains approach (integrative bargaining)
Negotiation model in which both sides share what they want and why they want it, with the goal of coming up with a solution that satisfies the major issues of both parties.

BOX 7-3 / A MUTUAL GAINS APPROACH TO NEGOTIATION

1. To build a relationship in which you can work cooperatively, talk with the other to build rapport and establish common ground.

2. In a nonattacking way, take turns identifying the positions that frame the conflict and clarifying the needs and issues that drive them. Each listens carefully, probes for additional information, and paraphrases the other's position to make sure that it is understood.

3. Clarify everyone's underlying interests or issues. If more than one emerges, a mini-negotiation occurs in order to prioritize them.

4. In a collaborative, respectful climate, brainstorm with the other to come up with a list of possible solutions to the problems.

5. Review the list to identify those alternatives that are feasible and optimize the satisfaction of each party's needs and concerns. Find external standards of legitimacy to evaluate and improve options.

Source: Derived from Bodine & Crawford, 1998, and Raider, Coleman, & Gerson, 2000

Third-party intervention

When an individual or group distinguishable from the conflicting parties interposes itself in an effort to move them toward agreement.

ations if they do not get what they want, but makes little sense in the mutual gains model. Open communication is key to the mutual gains approach, but secrecy regarding what one will settle for is key to the concession-convergence approach. Also, the mutual gains approach is time-consuming and may not be an option if social norms are such that concession-convergence negotiation is expected. For instance, union leadership is often expected and pressured by their membership to take tough and extreme positions, and CEOs typically require the same of their negotiators.

Mediation

Mediation

A type of third-party intervention in which advisory recommendations are made but do not have to be heeded by the disputants.

Arbitration

A type of third-party intervention in which the third party's recommendations for settlement are binding.

Third-party intervention occurs when an individual or group distinguishable from the conflicting parties imposes itself in an effort to move them toward agreement (Rubin et al., 1994). Such intervention can assume a number of different forms, including **mediation** (where advisory recommendations are made but do not have to be heeded by the disputants) and **arbitration** (where the third party's recommendations for settlement are binding). The focus here is on mediation. Mediators help negotiations along when the parties are stalemated, or stuck. In the United States, mediators are used to solve disputes between neighbors, employees, divorced parents, and to reach legal agreements. Mediators may be professionals, such as therapists or trained mediators, but they may also be concerned group members or leaders.

Mediation is usually a three-stage process (Pruitt et al., 1989). In Stage 1, *setting the stage,* the mediator shares the mediation ground rules with the disputants and gathers information about the dispute. In Stage 2, *problem solving,* the goal is to generate alternatives. In Stage 3, *achieving a workable agreement,* the parties are encouraged to reach agreement. Skilled mediators seek win-win, integrative solutions where both parties are satisfied with the outcome. Toward this end, they structure the situation so that it is conducive to cooperation and mutual problem solving. If hostilities are high, they may first meet with the parties separately in private caucuses. Pruitt and Carnevale (1993) suggest that in order to generate creative win-win solutions, mediators gather as much information as possible from both parties and then answer the following questions: "How can both parties get what they demand? Is there a resource shortage? Can the resource be expanded? Are some of the issues that are of high priority to one party of low priority to the other so that some concessions are possible? What are the risks and costs associated with the proposals being made? Can those risks and costs be mitigated so that the agreement is acceptable? What goals and values are served by the parties' proposals? Can they be served in some other way?"

The following mediation guidelines, synthesized from Rubin et al. (1994) may be helpful when you find yourself in a mediator role.

1. Initiate direct contact between disputants only if hostility is low and common ground is high. When hostility is high, direct contact may escalate the conflict. Therefore, it is advisable to "caucus" with the two parties separately to identify underlying interests and present the other side's position in a sympathetic way.
2. Teach the disputants constructive communication skills and negotiation concepts so that direct communication and resolution become possible.
3. Situate the negotiations at a neutral site to prevent one side from gaining a tactical advantage, and to enhance mediator control.
4. Promote trust between the parties by emphasizing overlapping interests and by encouraging them to make small but irrevocable concessions to show they are committed to a conciliatory process.
5. To cool off parties' emotions, listen carefully and sympathetically to participants' expressions of emotions, such as anger and resentment, in private caucuses with each side.
6. Use the parties' underlying interests to come up with integrative solutions.
7. Emphasize superordinate goals (common objectives) to promote cooperation.
8. Frame agreements in such a way that each side can make concessions without appearing weak or threatening its image.
9. To create a sense that agreement is possible, arrange the issues so that participants can work on easier issues first.
10. After significant progress has been made toward an integrative solution, impose a deadline by which a final agreement should be reached. Do not impose a deadline too early because time pressure makes joint problem solving less likely.

| *Apply It!* ••• | **Analyze Your Role as Mediator** |

The mediator role is a common socioemotional role in groups. How often do you assume this role in groups? Do you occupy this role in some groups, but not in others? To what extent do you use the techniques described above in your efforts to mediate a conflict between group members or between groups? What personal qualities do you think are possessed by an effective mediator?

Conflict Resolution Styles

Group members are individuals, often showing individual differences in their styles of dealing with conflict. These differences result from personality, culture, and sometimes gender. It is often useful to consider these differences so that our conflict resolution efforts will be more effective.

Individual Differences in Conflict Resolution Style

Dual-concern model
Suggests five conflict resolution styles that vary depending on how concerned the person is with his or her own outcomes as compared with the other party's outcomes.

The **dual-concern model** of conflict style postulates five styles that vary depending on how concerned the person is with his or her own outcomes as compared with the other party's outcomes (Gabrielidis, Stephan, Ybarra, Dos Santas Peason, & Villareal, 1997; Pruitt & Carnevale, 1993; Rahim, 1983; Rubin et al., 1994). *Accommodators* are people high in concern for others and low in concern for self; they sacrifice their own goals for the sake of others. *Avoiders* are low in concern for self and others; they are willing to let conflicts go unresolved or let others take care of them. *Compromisers* show intermediate levels of concern for self and others; therefore, they are willing to make some concessions if the other does so as well. *Collaborators* are high in concern for self and other; they seek to integrate the needs of both parties into a solution that will maximize the interests of both. *Competitors* are those with a high concern for self and low concern for others; consequently, they attempt to maximize their own outcomes with little regard for the costs to others.

Johnson (1994) has proposed a similar typology of conflict strategies, noting that the advantages and disadvantages of each depend on whether the goal is to achieve your goals, maintain a good relationship, or both. *Turtles* give up their goals and the relationship by avoiding the person and the issue. If the goal and the relationship are not important, then withdrawing may be a good strategy, but most of the time withdrawal creates resentment and hostility and interferes with conflict resolution. *Sharks* are "forcers" who achieve their goals at all costs with little concern for the relationship. If the goal is very important and the relationship is not, this style may be appropriate. However, because this strategy creates resentment and a desire for revenge, it is not advisable in long-term relationships.

Teddy bears are "smoothers" who will give up their goals to maintain the relationship. When the goal is unimportant to the teddy bear and the relationship is important, smoothing is okay. But it should not be one-sided, and is not a good idea if the goal is important. The *Fox* is a compromiser, willing to give up part of his or her goals and part of the relationship to reach an agreement. When the goal and relationship are of moderate importance, compromising may be appropriate, but generally problem solving is better. The *Owl* is a problem solver who negotiates to find a solution that meets both parties' needs and keeps the relationship positive. When both the goal and the relationship are important, problem solving and negotiation are the best routes.

Culture and Conflict Resolution Style

Intercultural conflict
Conflict involving parties from different cultures.

Conflict researchers realize that culture may play a role in how the conflict game is played, as well as in the success of efforts to manage **intercultural conflict** (conflict involving parties from different cultures). Different cultures do have different norms regarding acceptable conflict behavior (Mayer, 2000). For instance, some favor a direct and rational approach, and others a more indirect and intuitive style. In some cultures, it is acceptable to express strong feelings; in others, it is not. In some cultures, the message is communicated in *what* is said (low-context communication); in other cultures, the message is in *how* it is said or what is *not* said (high-context communication). People learn the values, norms, and rules of appropriate or inappropriate conflict conduct, and effective or ineffective conflict behavior, within the primary socialization process of their culture (Ting-Toomey, 1994).

Much of the research on culture and conflict has involved comparisons of the conflict resolution styles of individuals from individualistic cultures and collectivist cultures using measures of the conflict styles described by the dual-concern model. Examples include Gabrielidis et al. (1997); Leung, Au, Fernandez-Dol, and Iwawaki (1992); Ohbuchi, Fukushima, and Tedeschi (1999); Ohbuchi and Takahashi (1994); Trubisky, Ting-Toomey, and Lin (1991); and Wilson, Cai, Campbell, Donohue, and Drake (1995). Individualistic cultures are those that emphasize the individual's own self-interest, independence, and autonomy. Collectivist cultures place more emphasis on conformity to group norms and stress concern for the group (family, community, workgroup). In general, studies find that individuals from collectivist cultures are less confrontational, are more likely to avoid conflict out of a concern for others, and are more likely to seek solutions that integrate the needs of both parties. In contrast, individuals in individualistic cultures are more direct and competitive in their conflict resolution strategies. For example, in one study, Brazilians and Mexicans showed a greater preference for styles high in concern for others (collaboration and accommodation) compared to Americans (Carnevale & Leung, 2001).

Although some broad generalizations can be made about culture and conflict style, several caveats are in order. First, a number of studies indicate that not all collectivist cultures approach conflict in the same way, nor do all individualistic cultures (Gabrielidis et al., 1997; Gire & Carment, 1992). For instance, in one study, Canadians (an individualistic culture) preferred harmony-enhancing conflict resolution styles, and Nigerians (a collectivist culture) favored harmony-enhancing and competitive styles equally (Gire & Carment, 1992). Second, as Mayer (2000) reminds us, no culture is characterized by one specific conflict style that all its members exhibit. For instance, Diamant (2000) found regional, class, and gender variation in the way conflict is manifested and resolved in China. Although a culture may reinforce one style more than others, there is still likely to be great variation (Mayer, 2000).

Researchers studying conflict styles in different cultures have often assumed that such information will be helpful in conflict situations where the disputants are from different cultures. However, further research is needed to tell us whether intercultural conflict resolution style preferences are mirrored in intercultural encounters and have implications for conflicts among people from different cultures (Gabrielidis et al., 1997). What we do know is that cultural misunderstandings can contribute to the escalation of conflicts and interfere with their resolution. For instance, Kimmel (1994) identified a number of mistakes the United States made when dealing with Iraq's invasion of Kuwait in 1991, mistakes that could have been avoided had the U.S. government been more culturally aware. Chapter 5, Communication in Groups, provided some recommendations for improving intercultural communication that may be helpful in reducing conflicts that result from misunderstanding. Chapter 8, Member Diversity and Group Dynamics, also emphasizes multicultural skills to promote constructive conflict in intercultural interactions.

Gender and Conflict Resolution Style

Most people expect women and men to have different styles of handling conflict. Females are presumed to favor cooperative or compromising strategies, and males to favor competitive and forceful ones. These differences are expected because females are socialized to value relationships and seek harmony, and males are socialized to be competitive and value victory (Ruble & Scheer, 1994). Regardless of the apparent logic of this position, research support for it is mixed. Some studies do find support for such gender differences in conflict style (Gottman, 1994; Rahim, 1983; Todd-Mancillas & Rossi, 1985). For instance, Gottman (1994) reports that in marital relationships, 85 percent of stonewallers are men, men are more defensive, women complain and criticize their spouses more, and wives more often confront marital problems. However, many studies do not find gender differences, find differences in the opposite direction, or find mixed support (Chusmir & Mills, 1989; Conrad, 1991; Duane, 1989;

Apply It! ••• Examine Conflict Resolution Styles

Look at the five basic styles of conflict resolution, and decide which style best characterizes you and several other people you know quite well, such as your romantic partner, family members, and friends. Did you find a variety of styles among those sharing a common culture? Have conflicts been difficult because of style differences? Do you think it is helpful to know someone's style in order to more productively handle a conflict with him or her?

Sorenson, Hawkins, & Sorenson, 1995). A study by Ruble and Scheer (1994) is fairly typical in its lack of clear-cut gender differences. In that study, no gender differences in style were found in conflicts away from work; no differences were found for accommodating, avoiding, or collaborating styles in work or task-oriented settings; but small gender differences were found for competing and compromising in work- or task-oriented settings (women competed less and compromised more).

Some researchers argue that when gender differences are found, these differences are more a function of power and status than they are of gender. In other words, women are more likely to be found in positions of low status and power, and people in these positions must rely on more accommodating and compromising conflict styles. People high in power and status (traditionally men) can rely on more competitive and coercive strategies. In support of this position, research finds that men and women in power positions handle conflict very similarly (Chusmir & Mills, 1989). As Sorenson et al. (1995) concluded, for the most part, gender does not appear to affect conflict style preference in any substantial way. To put it another way, the differences found are too small to reliably predict the behavior of individuals (Ruble & Scheer, 1994).

Interpersonal Conflict

Interpersonal conflict
Conflict between two group members.

Interpersonal conflict, or conflict between two group members, can interfere with the group's cohesiveness and the ability of individuals to work cooperatively. Such conflicts may also dominate the group's attention, taking energy away from the group's work. In some cases, these conflicts cause members to leave the group.

Dynamics of Destructive Interpersonal Conflicts

As discussed in Chapter 5 on communication, group members will disagree with one another and will have complaints about one another, but how they go about expressing these makes a big difference in the climate of the group.

If a member feels criticized by another—that is, their personality or character is under attack—they will respond defensively and counterattack. Contempt—cruel criticism calculated to insult and psychologically hurt another—also triggers defensiveness and conflict spiraling (Gottman, 1994). Common signs are insults and name-calling, hostile humor, mockery (making fun of someone's words or actions or using sarcasm), negative body language, and facial expressions such as sneering, rolling of eyes, and curling of the upper lip.

When people feel defensive, they engage in behaviors that escalate the conflict. For instance, they often try to make the other person look bad by twisting things in such a way that it is the other's fault or problem. The conflict quickly gets off track and instead of being focused on the issue, ends up focused on making and responding to personal attacks. According to Gottman (1994), other typical defensive maneuvers are *denial of responsibility,* in which the person simply refuses to take any blame; *making excuses,* in which external forces beyond one's control are blamed; and *cross-complaining,* in which a complaint is met with an immediate counter-complaint while ignoring the initial issue. See Chapter 5 for strategies for making complaints about others without evoking defensiveness.

Stonewalling

When one party refuses to talk about a conflict.

Conflicts are also escalated when one member expresses a problem and others refuse to talk about it. Gottman (1994) calls this **stonewalling.** Stonewallers act a like a stone wall when someone tries to talk to them about a conflict. Some do not react at all, some offer monosyllabic mutterings, some change the subject, and some literally leave. This kind of withdrawal often intensifies the complainant's behavior as they become more upset and try to get engage the stonewaller. Gottman's research suggests that, contrary to their uncaring appearance, stonewallers are actually quite upset—so much so that they have trouble articulating their thoughts and react defensively by shutting down.

The origins of stonewalling vary. For instance, some people appear to avoid conflict because of repeated experiences (usually during childhood) with highly emotional and abusive individuals where the safest strategy was to say nothing. Some stonewallers report that they are not very good at arguing spontaneously and stonewall when faced with an emotionally articulate counterpart who has little trouble finding words in an emotionally charged situation. Conversely, some stonewallers come from families that handled problems rationally and calmly, and consequently, they do not know how to cope with emotionally charged individuals. For others, it is a power play or a defensive maneuver. Refusing to talk about a conflict can put you in the more powerful position or protect you from dealing with painful information. Stonewallers often find that others will give up trying to talk to them about anything of real importance, thus saving them the anxiety that such discussions bring. Unfortunately, though, this dooms many of their relationships to the superficial level.

Reducing Destructive Interpersonal Conflict

Integrative bargaining often works to resolve interpersonal conflicts. The constructive confrontation guidelines provided in Chapter 5 embody many of the elements of constructive controversy and integrative bargaining. **Box 7-4** presents Johnson's (1994) Six-Step Model for Negotiating Mutual Beneficial Agreements, another blueprint for using integrative bargaining to resolve interpersonal conflicts.

Many of the suggestions for reducing destructive interpersonal conflict follow logically from the discussion of the contributors to destructive conflict. For instance, to avoid triggering defensive reactions, you should avoid personality and character attacks and should instead focus your complaints on specific behaviors. Likewise, you should avoid responding defensively to others' complaints about you and, instead, engage in an honest and respectful dialogue about the complaint. When dealing with a stonewaller, it is especially important to present your case calmly and rationally and to give the stonewaller time to think about it. If you are a stonewaller because others' intense emotions cause you to freeze up in a conflict, you may want to learn to say something like "I appreciate your concerns, and I need to think about them before I can respond." Then set up a reasonable time when you will be ready to talk about it.

If you find yourself in a destructive, escalating conflict, there are things you can do to de-escalate it (Donohue & Kolt, 1992). For instance, you can apologize for your extreme statements ("Look, that was unfair, I shouldn't have said that. What I should have said was . . ."). You can restate the other's position to show you are going to listen from now on ("Am I getting this right, is your point that . . ."). You can suggest that you summarize the other person's position as you

---

BOX 7-4 / JOHNSON'S SIX-STEP MODEL FOR NEGOTIATING MUTUAL BENEFICIAL AGREEMENTS

Person One	Person Two
I want . . .	I want . . .
I feel . . .	I feel . . .
My reasons are . . .	My reasons are . . .
My understanding of your wants, etc., is . . .	My understanding of your wants, etc., is . . .
Three plans to solve this problem are . . .	Three plans to solve this problem are . . .
We choose a plan and agree.	We choose a plan and agree.

Source: Based on Johnson, 1994

Apply It! ••• **Identify Your Stonewalling Tendencies**

Are you a stonewaller? If so, what do you think accounts for your stonewalling? How does your behavior affect conflict resolution? In what way are you motivated to change your behavior? In what way are you motivated to remain the same? If you are not a stonewaller, what was your reaction to the discussion of stonewalling? Have you had difficulties dealing with stonewallers? Are you motivated to change your approach?

---

understand it, and they summarize yours (this tends to get things back on track and lead to greater understanding of the positions). You can also admit that you are getting off topic and express a desire to get back on topic. Sometimes it is a good idea to call a "time-out" ("I am too emotional right now to rationally solve this problem with you; let's meet back here in twenty minutes.").

Intragroup Conflict

Intragroup conflict
Conflict within a group involving more than two members.

Conflict within groups, also known as **intragroup conflict,** is common but has not received much research attention. This may be because conflict within groups is messy and difficult to study scientifically. It may also be due to the assumption that intragroup conflict can be subsumed under the categories of interpersonal conflict or conflict between subgroups. And indeed, there is some truth to the idea that some intragroup conflict can be reduced to these other two types of conflict. After all, conflict in a group may be merely conflict between two members (interpersonal conflict) or between coalitions or subgroups within the larger group (intergroup conflict). But it is also true that intragroup conflicts have some unique dynamics of their own.

Dynamics of Destructive Intragroup Conflicts

Interpersonal conflicts sometimes widen into intragroup conflicts that embroil the whole group as the initial conflicting members attempt to get others on their side. Intragroup conflicts also occur when group members disagree on issues facing the group. There are many sources of intragroup conflict. Group members get on one another's nerves, disagree about what to do and how to do it, and have value, belief, or goal differences over which they struggle. Much of this conflict is relatively short-lived and is managed through good leadership, the adoption of the norms of constructive controversy, and the use of cooperative group decision-making and problem-solving strategies. However, some intragroup conflicts are destructive, producing interpersonal hostility, impaired performance, and in extreme cases, dissolution of the group (Levine & Moreland, 1995).

Like other types of conflict, intragroup conflicts can spiral out of control and exhibit common features of destructive conflict such as autistic hostility, perceptual distortion, and self-fulfilling prophecy. This is most likely when the group has difficulty managing conflict because it has not developed norms of constructive controversy. In some cases, disagreements escalate into shouting matches in which people engage in the standard series of destructive conflict behaviors. Group members are then angry and distrustful of one another, and the integrity of the group is compromised. In other cases, members feel that it is a violation of the group's norms to have conflicts. Ironically, their attempts to avoid open confrontation of differences lead to conflict escalation or, at the very least, prevent the group from realizing the benefits of constructive conflict.

Intragroup conflict may arise out of an interpersonal conflict between two members. Research indicates that when individuals have a conflict with a fellow group member, they often engage in informal discussions with other group members about the conflict (see Volkema & Bergmann, 1997). Although these conversations may help to resolve a conflict, in some cases they fuel or even spread the dispute. In talking with other group members, the conflicting individuals may intend to gain some insight into the conflict, but they may also intend to draw other members into the conflict to side with them.

It is common for conflicting members to avoid one another and to rely on other group members to provide them with information about what the opponent is thinking and saying about them (a good example of autistic hostility). Because the conflicting members are upset and want others to be on their side, they are prone to exaggeration and drama. Unfortunately, these extreme characterizations may be conveyed to the other person via other members. This person then becomes angered by what is seen as an unfair attack and as a deliberate attempt by the opponent to make him/her look bad in front of others. Of course, this escalates the conflict.

At this point, the conflict occupies the thoughts of many group members. Members talk among themselves as they attempt to figure out whom to side with. Members do not talk as a group about the conflict and how to resolve it. Disagreement among group members about who is right leads members to side with one or the other of the conflicting parties. What was once a conflict between two group members may become a larger and more complex group conflict, with most members enmeshed in one way or the other, and others distancing themselves from the group. A once-cohesive group becomes two (or more) conflicting groups that may have trouble cooperating to get a job done and may become increasingly aggressive toward one another.

In the destructive intragroup conflict, many interpersonal relationships in the group are damaged. The conflicting members may no longer trust or respect those who did not clearly take their side. Members may distrust and disrespect those who behaved badly during the course of the conflict. Members may no longer trust conflicting members because they wonder if these individuals might do "this" to them. The integrity of the group is severely compromised. Some members may leave. Outside intervention, such as by a supervisor, mediator, or counselor, may be sought or imposed.

Reducing Destructive Intragroup Conflict

Superordinate goal

A goal desired by both parties to a conflict.

Because destructive intragroup conflict frequently arises because the group has not developed norms of constructive controversy, one solution is to introduce these norms when controversy arises. Generally, the idea is to bring the group's attention back to the main issues and keep them on the track of solution generation. Specifically, the idea is to emphasize a cooperative goal structure. One way to do this is to emphasize **superordinate goals**—goals that group members value and must cooperate to achieve: "We have some differences of opinion here, but I think we'd all agree that our priority is to meet this deadline and that we can't do it without cooperating." Also, when members begin to engage in personal attacks, they can be gently reminded to focus on the problem and its solution: "Things are getting a little heated here. I understand that we're all upset, but let's stay focused on solving the problem." Reframing member statements so that the issues underlying them can be more easily understood may help other members to take the perspective of others and keep the group focused on integrative solutions. For instance, a concern may be reworded so that that person's essential interest is still expressed but the more "toxic" elements have been removed. Or the essential needs or concerns of all the parties may be incorporated into a statement of the issue as a mutual problem to be solved (Mayer, 2000). Once the main issues are obvious, the group can be asked to brainstorm integrative solutions that address them.

Remember that intragroup conflicts sometimes originate in an interpersonal conflict between two group members who enmesh and entangle others through third-party discussions. Prevent the conflict from embroiling the whole group by resisting gossiping, and consider giving a neutral response if others try to gossip to you. If such conflicts threaten the integrity of the group, you may wish to mediate, especially if you are in a leadership position. However, proceed carefully. As Rubin et al. (1994, p. 198) once said, "Third party intervention is like a strong medicine that may have undesirable side effects, and that should therefore be employed with caution and some reluctance. The best, most effective third parties become involved only when needed and are so successful at helping the principals find a settlement and develop a good working relationship with each other that their intervention is no longer necessary."

Triangulation

When a group member attempts to mediate a conflict and inadvertently maintains or worsens the conflict, or is hurt in the process.

Triangulation is one particular danger to the unskilled mediator. In clinical and counseling psychology and clinical social work, the term *triangulation* is used to refer to perils of a third person's becoming the go-between in a conflict between two other people. First, there is the peril to the conflicting individuals. Your involvement may make it easier for the conflicting individuals *not* to deal with one another and their conflict. Also, keep in mind that the disputants may become dependent on you whenever they are in conflict. If these individuals are to carry on a sustainable relationship, they probably need to learn how to manage their own conflicts.

The second danger of a third party's acting as a go-between is the potential harm to the third party. Counselors frequently caution clients to avoid becoming "triangulated." They try to point out to clients that getting in the middle of the conflict may harm them and not be very helpful anyway. Trying to solve a conflict between two people is an extraordinary responsibility to take on or have put on you. Sometimes the conflicting individuals are not interested in resolving the conflict and perpetuate it through you. They may also demand your loyalty to them and their point of view, and will pressure you to agree with them and reject the other. This puts you smack in the middle of a "loyalty conflict," as you struggle to support them both without having either get angry with you. Divorced parents often put their children in this situation, with devastating consequences to their mental health. This is not to say that you cannot mediate a conflict in your group. In fact, if you introduce norms of constructive controversy and follow the guidelines given in the mediation section, you may be successful.

Sometimes it is appropriate to call in a professional counselor or mediator. Many larger organizations have trained mediators as part of their employee assistance programs. Skilled mediators help each party to become aware of interests, feelings, and needs and to recognize the other side. They are good listeners, are able to maintain an objective stance, are good communicators, and are assertive (establish and maintain ground rules that protect parties during the mediation). They help the parties come up with an agreement that honors, or at least does not violate, the essential interests of the parties. The mediation may occur in separate meetings, joint meetings, or both.

Last, if you have a conflict with another group member, be mature and resist the temptation to drag other group members into it. Do not attempt to carry out your conflict through other people. It is unfair to ask others to fight your battles for you or to take sides, as this may put them in a "loyalty conflict"—wanting to support you, but wanting to support your opponent as well. Also, if you realize that you are escalating and widening the conflict by drawing others into it, and that you are trying to destroy another person's reputation with other group members, by all means snap out of it and try to resolve the conflict constructively. If the relationship with the other person has gotten so impoverished that it is not possible to talk with each other directly, ask for mediation.

Apply It! ••• **Analyze Your Experience With Destructive Intragroup Conflict**

Have you witnessed a destructive intragroup conflict in your family, friendship group, roommate group, or workplace? How did the conflict develop? How did the group handle it? What was the ultimate effect on the group?

Intergroup Conflict

Intergroup conflict
Conflict between groups.

Conflict between groups, or **intergroup conflict,** can be a source of intragroup cohesiveness as members unite against a common enemy. Intergroup conflict can range from the local to the global. Conflict may be between nations or groups within nations, or between local gangs, high schools, opposing sports team spectators, or other groups within a school, workplace, or community.

Like other types of group conflict, intergroup conflict can have good or bad consequences. On the plus side, conflict between groups may result in justice for traditionally discriminated-against groups and may promote changes in outdated policies or laws. Also, competition between groups can sometimes stimulate productivity. On the negative side, conflict between groups also has the potential to spiral out of control. Rivalries between high schools or gangs may become violent. Unions and management may become deadlocked and unable to agree on a contract. Warring factions in the group may come to view themselves as separate and competing groups, and what was an intragroup conflict now becomes an intergroup conflict. The conflicting groups may then become more interested in sabotaging each other's work or reacting to real or perceived attacks than in cooperating to get a job done.

Dynamics of Destructive Intergroup Conflicts

Enemy imagery
Stereotypes of the opposing party that suggest they are hostile or evil.

Many of the dynamics of conflict discussed at the beginning of the chapter are relevant to intergroup conflicts. For instance, stereotypes of the opposing group (the outgroup) are promoted by ingroup members and by the leadership. **Enemy imagery** is common as the other side is seen as dishonest, unfriendly, selfish, inhumane, and warlike (Rubin et al., 1994), and mirror imagery is present in that each side perceives the other in a similar, negative way. The preservation of stereotyped views is enabled by physical segregation and lack of personal contact with outgroup members, as well as by the fact that it is socially rewarded by the ingroup and is a source of solidarity.

Perceptual distortion is also seen in the selective processing of ingroup and outgroup actions in ways that preserve positive views of the ingroup and negative ones of the outgroup. For instance, if the ingroup behaves aggressively toward the other group, it is viewed as a necessary offensive maneuver or as justified given the enemy's actions; that is, the action is justified by the situation. In contrast, the outgroup's similar actions are interpreted as evidence of their evil nature. Earlier in the chapter, this was referred to as the ultimate attribution error (Pettigrew, 1979).

A cycle of hostile interaction leading to the malignant spiraling of aggression is also typical of the destructive intergroup conflict. Once one group performs an act that is perceived as hostile, the other will usually retaliate and escalate the level of aggression slightly. Of course, this escalation is not lost on the first group, which then counterattacks at a slightly increased level of hostility. For instance, the escalation of the Palestinian–Israeli conflict in 2000–2002 followed a predictable spiraling sequence; many died in the conflict that ensued, and the fragile peace between the two groups was destroyed. Every time the Palestinians killed Israelis, the Israelis responded by killing Palestinians, who then avenged the death of their people by another attack on the Israelis, which had to be avenged by the Israelis, and so on.

One of the hallmarks of intergroup conflict is an "us versus them" identity. In members' minds, their group is distinct from the other group and possesses more desirable characteristics—whether honor, intelligence, talent, superior culture, or whatever. Thus, people are biased in favor of their own group (**ingroup bias**) and biased against the "enemy" group (**outgroup bias**). There is the assumption of ingroup superiority and outgroup inferiority. Groups frequently build solidarity and unite diverse members by emphasizing the ways in which their group is different from (and better than) other groups. The resulting animosity toward the other group(s) and their members tend(s) to produce counter-animosity, and a group conflict is born, complete with the perception of incompatible goals and interests, and competition to prove who is the superior, mightier group.

You probably remember that social identity theory suggests that one important function of groups is as a source of meaning, belonging, and identity. Unfortunately, groups may serve this function at the expense of other groups. People are very quick to separate themselves into distinctive groups and to develop group identities in contrast to other groups. Researchers have long noted how easy it is to get people to view themselves as part of a superior group, even on the flimsiest of criteria (Brewer, 1979; Tajfel, Billig, Bundy, & Flament, 1971; Turner, 1981). For instance, at my university, there is a week of orientation for first-year students called Week of Welcome (WOW). The students are randomly divided into small groups led by senior students. The groups readily adopt their own unique identities and create signs, clothing, and other items with markers of these identities. Frequent comparisons with other groups are made, and rivalries between the groups quickly emerge. Of course, identity differences between groups are often real and significant. As noted by Rothman (1997), identity-driven conflict often involves struggles over group survival, dignity, and recognition. This muddies the conflict resolution waters because the stakes are so high.

As noted before, social comparison processes are such that we frequently compare ourselves to others to decide whether what we are getting is fair, and the perception of deprivation may create conflict. This also occurs at the group level when intergroup comparisons are made. Conflict is likely when a group and its members become discontented with their group's place in the status hierarchy and perceive this status as illegitimate (Gurin, Miller, & Gurin, 1980). You may recall from Chapter 4 that this is called fraternal deprivation (Brewer & Miller,

Ingroup bias

When members selectively process their own group's actions in order to maintain a positive view of the group.

Outgroup bias

When members of one group selectively process the actions of another group to maintain a negative view of that group.

1996; Rubin et al. 1994) and it is associated with the perception of social injustice and a desire for social change (Brewer & Miller, 1996).

Fraternal deprivation is likely to lead to conflict when members identify themselves as members of an oppressed group and this becomes an important social identity and a source of collective self-esteem (self-esteem derived from group membership). Research supports the idea that disadvantaged group identities may motivate group activism (Dion, 1986; Smith & Tyler, 1997; Walker & Mann, 1987). Members of disadvantaged groups who believe their lower status is illegitimate turn "what is painful at the individual level" into a "source of pride at the group level—a badge of distinction rather than a mark of shame" (Brewer, 1991, p. 481). One way to look at it is that the group develops an "underdog" identity that is a source of pride. In this way, equality is seen as justified, group solidarity is built, and a positive social identity is restored. Imagine the group of unpopular high school students who embrace their "weirdness," or the workers on the assembly line who are proud of the grease beneath their fingernails and disdainful of the suits worn by management.

These group identities are paradoxical. On the one hand, collective struggle is fueled when ingroup identifications and enemy imagery form the basis of group solidarity, pride, and the indignation that so frequently motivates action. On the other hand, the struggles of the disadvantaged group may increase membership in the advantaged group and enhance the social identity of the traditionally dominant group, thus exaggerating ingroup/outgroup bias (Burn, 1996; Burn et al., 2000). When one group becomes aware that another group perceives them as an enemy, this stimulates their sense of group identity, as they feel unjustly vilified. This creates a backlash and increases their resistance to the equality struggle of the disadvantaged group.

Reducing Destructive Intergroup Conflict

Contact hypothesis

The assumption that bringing conflicting parties into contact will be enough to reduce conflict.

As noted earlier, conflict between groups is often aggravated by the tendency for the groups to physically segregate themselves from one another and to stop direct communication and interaction. This, we noted, contributes to autistic hostility and makes it easier for the groups to maintain extremely negative views of one another. You might think, then, that bringing the two groups into contact with one another to see that their extreme views are wrong would help to reduce the conflict. This notion is sometimes called the **contact hypothesis.** Unfortunately, simple contact often has the effect of escalating hostilities as the groups hurl insults or engage in aggression. This is not to say that there is not some merit to the idea, but the conditions of contact must be carefully structured to engender cooperation and change the groups' customary ways of interaction. This typically requires the intervention of a third party. This point is illustrated by the classic Robbers Cave study conducted by Sherif and his colleagues in 1954 (described in Sherif, Harvey, White, Hood, & Sherif, 1961).

The researchers brought twenty-two 11-year-old boys to a three-week camp in Robber's Cave, Oklahoma, where they were randomly assigned to two groups. To create intergroup hostility, the researchers first segregated them and had them engage in group-building activities. The groups were encouraged to choose a name; one group became the Rattlers, and the other the Eagles. Next, they had the two groups engage in a series of competitive sports events. It did not take long for intergroup hostility to arise, as evidenced by fistfights, name-calling, and raids on each other's cabins. Even when the groups were brought into contact under pleasant conditions involving no competition (such as a Fourth of July celebration), the groups fought. At this point, the researchers figured that if incompatible goals fostered conflict (the competitive activities), then perhaps compatible goals would reduce it. They created several situations in which the groups would have to cooperate in order to attain a superordinate, or mutually desirable, goal. These included a breakdown of the water tower that required the boys work together to disassemble it for repair. The cumulative effect of these cooperative events was that the boys were able to become friends. Notice that because groups in conflict are so antagonistic toward each other, they may need the help of a mediator to arrange superordinate goals or to help them identify mutually agreeable goals (Rubin et al., 1994).

The racial desegregation of American schools following the 1954 Supreme Court decision in *Brown* v. *Board of Education* is another good example of how mere contact is not enough to reduce intergroup hostilities. In general, research indicated that although desegregation increased the academic performance of minority children, it did not decrease racial tensions (Cook, 1985). After reviewing the research on school desegregation, Cook (1985) specified a number of conditions that must be present before contact will be successful in reducing intergroup conflict:

1. The situation must promote equal-status interactions between members of the groups.
2. The interaction must encourage behaviors that disconfirm the stereotypes the groups have of each other.
3. The situation should require that members of both groups cooperate to attain a mutually desirable goal.
4. The situation must promote personal acquaintance between members from the different groups.
5. The social norms in the situation must be supportive of reduced intergroup conflict.

Cooperative education
A set of techniques designed to reduce intergroup tensions in educational settings by engineering equal-status contact and superordinate goals.

Sherif et al. (1961) structured the situation at the Robber's Cave to provide superordinate goals and reduce intergroup conflict. Likewise, intergroup conflict resolution strategies essentially engineer the conditions identified by Cook (1985). For instance, a variety of educational techniques, generally known as **cooperative education,** seek to reduce intergroup hostilities and enable students from different groups to work cooperatively. Cooperative education techniques require coopera-

Have you seen conflict between groups at a school or in your community despite contact? To what extent did your school or community embody the conditions necessary before contact is successful in reducing intergroup conflict?

tion across racial lines, equal-status roles for students of different races, contacts across racial lines that permit personal acquaintance, and the communication of teacher support for interracial contact (Aronson & Bridgeman, 1979; Aronson & Gonzalez, 1988; Aronson & Patnoe, 1997; Slavin & Cooper, 1999).

Stalemate

The point at which it is clear that there is more to gain than lose from collaborating.

Because conflict with other groups boosts ingroup solidarity and group pride, groups are often unmotivated to end a conflict with another group until their losses are significant. The group must be at a point of **stalemate** where it is clear that it will not get what it wants through domination or coercion, it has few resources left to continue the struggle, and it has more to gain than lose from collaborating (Rubin, 1989). However, as Rubin points out, it is difficult to return to a cooperative relationship after a history of aggressive confrontation. "Residue" from the destructive conflict lingers. To get back on the path of cooperation and trust, one group has to make a unilateral collaborative overture, and persuade the other side that this overture is to be taken seriously (Rubin et al., 1994). For instance, an apology (a sincere "I'm sorry") can signal a willingness to move from a period of escalation to one of problem solving (Rubin et al., 1994). Osgood's (1962) GRIT strategy is a well-known example of a strategy for making a unilateral conciliatory initiative. **GRIT** stands for **Graduated and Reciprocated Initiatives in Tension-Reduction.** It calls for one party to announce in advance its intention to make a cooperative conciliatory gesture—for example, a cease-fire, or a release of prisoners. The first gesture should be relatively small so that if exploited by the other side, little is lost. The first side should then provide the other side with the opportunity to reciprocate with a similar gesture. A systematic program may then be initiated in which each side makes increasingly cooperative gestures.

GRIT (Graduated and Reciprocated Initiatives in Tension-Reduction)

A systematic conflict resolution program in which each side makes increasingly cooperative gestures.

Concept Review

Destructive Conflicts

- **Destructive conflicts** are those conflicts that damage the group and relationships between members or groups. Common features include **conflict spiraling** (an attack-counterattack sequence), **perceptual distortion** (the exaggerated misinterpretation and attribution of hostile intentions to an opponent's actions), and a **competitive goal structure** in which it is assumed that one party will win and the other will lose.

Constructive Conflict

- **Constructive conflict** is primarily cooperative. It is oriented toward joint problem solving and maintenance of a working relationship. Common features include a **cooperative goal structure** (where disputants engage in mutual problem solving) and conflict management skills.
- Constructive conflict can motivate positive change, help groups arrive at a unified direction from divergent views, promote the development of trust, enhance decision making, and result in more equitable resource distributions and justice.
- **Constructive controversy** is part of constructive conflict. Disputants cooperate to clarify differences respectfully and then reach an integrated position where both parties' major issues are satisfied. Reliance on rational argument is also central.

Conflict Resolution

- Most conflict resolution models are built on getting participants to recognize different perspectives and achieve **analytic empathy,** become aware of their biases, improve communication, and come up with integrative solutions that reconcile the interests of the parties. An emphasis on **trust building** is also common.
- **Negotiation** occurs when two or more disputants use the exchange of offers and ideas to reach settlement. There are two main negotiation models. **Distributive bargaining** (the **concession-convergence model**) occurs when both sides stake out tough and extreme positions and then take "baby steps" toward agreement. In **integrative bargaining** (the **mutual gains approach**), the two sides explain the motivations and interests underlying their positions, then seek creative solutions integrating these interests.
- **Third-party intervention** occurs when an individual or group distinguishable from the conflicting parties works to move them toward agreement. In **mediation,** advisory recommendations are made but do not have to be heeded by participants. In **arbitration,** the third party's recommendations are binding.
- Skilled mediators seek win-win, integrative solutions in which both parties are satisfied with the outcome. Mediation is usually a three-stage process. In Stage 1 (setting the stage), the mediator gathers information about the dispute and sets ground rules. In Stage 2 (problem solving), the goal is the generation of alternatives. In Stage 3 (achieving a workable agreement) the parties are encouraged to reach agreement.

Conflict Resolution Styles

- The **dual-concern model** postulates five conflict resolution styles that vary depending on how concerned the person is with his or her own outcomes as compared with the other party's outcomes. *Accommodators* sacrifice their own goals for others. *Avoiders* are willing to let conflicts go unresolved or let others take care of them. *Compromisers* are willing to make some concessions if the other does so as well. *Collaborators* seek to integrate the needs of both parties into a solution that will maximize the interests of both. *Competitors* attempt to maximize their own outcomes with little regard for the cost to others.

- Understanding how culture affects conflict is important in managing **inter-cultural conflicts.** In general, studies find that individuals from collectivist cultures are less confrontational, are more likely to avoid conflict out of a concern for others, and are more likely to seek solutions that integrate the needs of both parties. Individuals in individualistic cultures are more direct and competitive in their conflict resolution strategies. However, no culture is characterized by one specific conflict style that all its members exhibit.

- A common assumption is that females favor cooperative or compromising conflict resolution strategies and that males favor competitive and forceful ones. However, research findings yield mixed results, and the differences that are found are small (around 5%).

Interpersonal Conflict

- **Interpersonal conflict**—conflict between two group members—can interfere with group cohesiveness and productivity.

- Criticism and contempt trigger defensiveness and conflict spiraling in the interpersonal conflict. Conflicts are also escalated when one member **stonewalls,** as the complainant often becomes more upset and tries to engage the stonewaller.

Intragroup Conflict

- **Intragroup conflict**—conflict that involves three or more group members—is common and usually short-lived but can spiral out of control if group norms of constructive controversy have not developed. Intragroup conflicts may harm many member relationships.

- An interpersonal conflict between two members can become a larger, intragroup conflict as contenders take the conflict to other group members and try to get members to side with them.

- Interpersonal conflict may even turn into intergroup conflict as members take sides and factions develop.

Intergroup Conflict

- **Intergroup conflict** is a conflict between groups. Selective processing of ingroup and outgroup actions (perceptual distortion and ultimate attribution error) is typical and aggression spirals. Self-segregation contributes to autistic hostility.

- Social identities play a large role in intergroup conflict. The conflict is framed competitively in terms of "us" versus "them" (ingroup versus outgroup), and **ingroup/outgroup bias** (assumption of ingroup superiority and outgroup inferiority) is typical. Being a member of a superior ingroup is a source of identity, and ingroup solidarity is built by emphasizing differences from other groups.

- The **contact hypothesis** is the idea that bringing groups into contact will reduce hostilities. However, the contact must be structured carefully to reduce conflict. For instance, **cooperative education** promotes cooperative relationships between diverse students by requiring cooperation across racial lines, equal-status roles, contact that permits personal acquaintance, and communication of teacher support for interracial contact.

- Before groups are motivated to cooperate, they must reach a **stalemate.** To get back on the path of cooperation, one group can make unilateral collaborative overtures and persuade the other side it is serious.

Skill Review

Use General Conflict Resolution Strategies

- Use integrative bargaining by building rapport and seeking common ground; taking turns identifying the positions that frame the conflict, and the issues and needs that drive them; clarifying everyone's underlying interests or issues; brainstorming to come up with solutions; and reviewing solutions to identify feasible ones that optimize the satisfaction of each side's issues/needs.

- Rebuild trust by acting consistently and reliably, taking a series of conciliatory actions, and identifying common goals and values as the basis for a cooperative relationship. Manage by apologizing, explaining, and expressing regret for harm done, stating and negotiating expectations for future conduct, committing to these, and following through.

Mediation Guidelines

- If hostility is high, caucus with the two parties separately. Cool things down by listening empathetically to each side's emotional expressions. Identify underlying interests, and present the other's side in a sympathetic way, before bringing them together at a neutral site.

- Teach disputants constructive communication skills and promote trust by emphasizing common ground and small conciliatory steps.

- Use parties' underlying interests to come up with integrative solutions, and emphasize superordinate goals to promote cooperation.

Reduce Destructive Interpersonal Conflict

- Avoid criticizing others or expressing contempt.
- When dealing with a stonewaller, present your case calmly and rationally and give the other person time to process it. If you are a stonewaller, ask for time to process the other's complaint.
- De-escalate conflicts by apologizing for unfair statements. Restate the other's position to prove you are listening.
- Use integrative bargaining and constructive confrontation to resolve conflicts.

Reduce Destructive Intragroup Conflict

- Introduce norms of constructive controversy when conflict arises. Incorporate essential concerns of the parties into a statement of a mutual problem to be solved, and then brainstorm integrative solutions.
- Mediate carefully if necessary. Avoid triangulation.
- If you have a conflict with another group member, resist the temptation to embroil other group members. Seek professional mediation if necessary.

Reduce Destructive Intergroup Conflict

- Structure contact between conflicting groups to promote equal-status interactions and cooperation toward superordinate goals.
- Use the Graduated Reciprocated Initiatives in Tension Reduction (GRIT) method. One party announces its intention to make a cooperative conciliatory gesture and provides the other side with an opportunity to reciprocate. A systematic program in which each side makes increasingly cooperative gestures is then initiated. *cease fire*

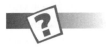 **Study Questions**

1. What are destructive conflicts? What are their common features and dynamics?
2. How does constructive conflict differ from destructive conflict?
3. What are the common elements of conflict resolution and management?
4. What are the two main approaches to negotiation?
5. What is third-party intervention? What mediation guidelines were given in the chapter?
6. What is the dual-concern conflict style model? What are the five styles described by the model? How do culture and gender affect conflict style?

7. What contributes to destructive interpersonal conflict? How can destructive interpersonal conflicts be reduced?
8. What are the dynamics common to the destructive intragroup conflict? What suggestions were given in the chapter for managing destructive intragroup conflicts?
9. What dynamics characterize the destructive intergroup conflict?
10. What role do social identities and fraternal deprivation play in intergroup conflict?
11. How must the conditions of contact between groups be structured in order to reduce intergroup hostilities?
12. How can unilateral conciliatory initiatives be used to get two conflicting groups to cooperate?

Group Activities

Activity 1: Analyze News Accounts of Conflict

Each group member brings a news story from a major newspaper about a group conflict and presents the case to the group, which then analyzes it using chapter concepts. Is there evidence of conflict spiraling, perceptual distortion, ingroup/outgroup bias, and a competitive orientation? Are oppositional social identities at work? Fraternal deprivation? Describe any conflict resolution efforts in the case, and discuss what would have to happen before the conflict can be resolved.

Activity 2: Role-Play a Mediation

This activity is done in a three-person group. Together, first review the guidelines on mediation. Next, look over the three scenarios provided, each involving two disputants and one mediator. Each role will be played by one member of your triad, making sure that each member acts as mediator for one of the scenarios. Work on the scenarios one at a time, beginning by deciding who will play each disputant role and who will play the mediator. Then take five minutes to familiarize yourself with the conflict and prepare to act out your role (you will improvise using the information provided). When everyone is ready, the mediator begins the "session." Following each scenario, briefly review the mediation guidelines and give the "mediator" feedback.

SCENARIO 1 J. is a supervisor who must mediate a conflict between two members of the same workgroup, C. C. and K. What was once a pleasant workgroup has become nasty as C. C. and K. constantly insult each other and try to get other members to side with them against the other.

C. C.'s side: "As far as I'm concerned, K. is new to this organization and should show me more respect. Many times, K. has corrected me in front of the rest of the workgroup and embarrassed me. To me, it feels like K. wants to knock me down to take my position in the group. I don't know how to respond other than to defend myself and reduce K.'s credibility in the group by trying to make K. look bad. I know that K. brings some good experience to the job, but I'm scared K. is trying to take over the group at my expense."

K.'s side: "C. C. should show me more respect because although I came on later, I do have a lot of experience. A few times, C. C. said things to the group that were just plain wrong, and I couldn't let them go just because C. C. had been on the crew a long time. C. C. couldn't handle it and is now intent on harming my reputation in the group and with supervisors. I have to defend myself. I appreciate that C. C. knows this system better than I do and that I can learn from C. C., but I've been doing this kind of work a long time and think C. C. can learn from me also."

SCENARIO 2 B. B. and J. J. are part of a four-person long-term friendship group, but their conflict threatens to destroy the group. One of the remaining members, D. D., attempts to mediate the conflict to save the group.

B. B.'s side: "Ever since I spoke honestly about J. J.'s new romantic partner X., J. J. won't even speak to me. Honestly, I don't see what I did wrong, and I am getting really mad that J. J. is making such a big deal out of this. I thought we had the kind of relationship where we could say what was on our minds. I just don't think X. is right for J. J., and I am convinced that J. J. is making a big mistake. J. J. also expressed some reservations, and all I did was agree and maybe add to what J. J. said. At this point, I feel like J. J. is choosing X. over me, and I am really hurt by it because we've been friends since high school. I guess our friendship isn't what I thought it was."

J. J.'s side: "B. B. said some really unkind things about X. and practically called me a total idiot for dating X. I was really insulted. I mean, after all this time, I find out that B. B. thinks that I am not smart enough to make my own decisions. Things are actually going really well with X., and a lot of the concerns I shared with B. B. turned out to be nonissues. I appreciate that B. B. wants to be honest, but it was a little rough, and I felt like I was being ordered to choose between B. B. and X. Frankly, if B. B. is going to act like that, I'll choose X., but I'd rather not have to choose at all."

SCENARIO 3 K. C. and J. C. are having a conflict that appears to be over scarce resources. They share a phone line that is used both for ordering supplies and making calls to clients and for the Internet. L. C., their coworker, is tired of hearing them complain about the other to her. L. C. is friends with both of them and would like to see them become friendly with each another again. L. C. decides to mediate.

K. C.'s side: "J. C. and I used to have a good relationship, but I was having some trouble getting to use the phone because it seemed like every time I wanted to make my calls, J. C. was on the Internet. So I decided to jump on the phone first thing in the morning to make my calls to be sure I'll get to make them. I can never predict when J. C. is going to be using the Internet, so it's risky to wait any longer. But when J. C. came in, saw me on the phone, and asked in a snotty voice when I'd be done, I felt kind of angry and said right back in a snotty voice that I didn't know. I mean, J. C. doesn't own the phone. I have a right to use it. Now when J. C. comes in, I get a look that makes me feel like I'd better watch my back! I'm not going to be intimidated, though, and I glare right back at J. C. At this point, it's getting kinda weird around here. I try to avoid J. C., but it's a small place, and the boss sometimes assigns us projects to work on together, so I don't know what's going to happen then. I wish they'd just put in another line, but I think J. C. and I would have to present a unified front to management, and I don't see that happening."

J. C.'s side: "Every day K. C. gets here before me and grabs the phone. I never know how long it will be before I can use it, and it makes it hard to plan my work for the day. One day, when I arrived after a nightmare commute on the freeway, I asked K. C. how long it was going to be before I could get on the Internet. K. C. gave me the rudest response, as if I had no right to even ask! From then on, I've just felt like if that's the way K. C. is going to be, well, I'll just be that way too. I have started staying logged onto the Internet a little more than I really need to, just to aggravate K. C. I know it sounds kind of immature, but I wouldn't act like this if K. C. weren't acting the same way."

Activity 3: Develop Recommendations for Different Conflict Styles

The chapter suggests that it can be helpful to understand the conflict styles of individual group members. This five-person group activity is intended to help with this. Members first individually review the conflict styles discussed in the chapter and decide which one best describes their own style. Next, each member writes down (1) advice to give to others that would be helpful when in a conflict with a member with this particular style and (2) how people with this style tend to respond to members with the other styles.

Next, group members take turns sharing what they wrote. The group then creates a set of written recommendations based on the discussion.

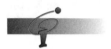

InfoTrac College Edition Search Terms

To do research for your papers and assignments, use InfoTrac that's provided free with new copies of this book. Go to http://infotrac.thomsonlearning.com and enter the following search terms:

- Destructive Conflict
- Constructive Conflict
- Interpersonal Conflict
- Intragroup Conflict
- Intergroup Conflict

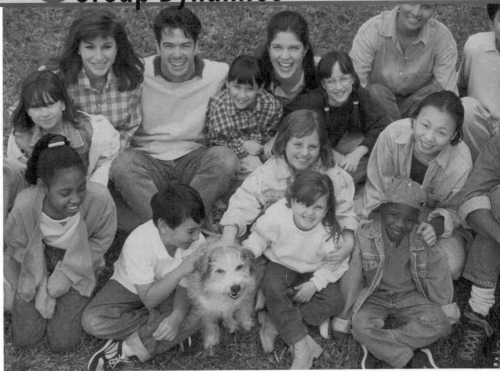

© Tom & Dee Ann McCarthy/CORBIS

Diversity is a popular word. Chances are that your college or university has programs and curriculum designed to enhance your appreciation of diverse cultures and people. This emphasis on diversity will follow you when you leave the university and enter the work world. There, diverse clients, patients, customers, and coworkers will require that you broaden your conception of what is normal and desirable. If you become a manager, you are likely to find yourself managing a workgroup of people varying in age, gender, ethnicity, culture, personality, religion, sexual orientation, physical ability, education, and skill level. Managers who are skilled at managing and working with people from different backgrounds are better able to serve clients and improve employee relations (Tung, 1997). Unfortunately, people who are different from us often make us feel uncomfortable, and this discomfort may interfere with fair treatment, cooperation, and growth. This means that instead of being a source of creativity and enrichment, diversity is frequently a source of miscommunication, conflict, and reduced productivity.

We must become better at working and socializing in diverse groups. One obvious reason is simply the reality of diversity. All contemporary societies are now culturally plural, made up of people who vary in ethnic origin, language, and religion (Berry, 1997). The 2000 United States census shows that the nation's diversity increased dramatically over the last decade and that there is nearly a 1 in 2 chance that two people selected at random will be racially or ethnically different (El Nasser & Overberg, 2001). Nearly 1 in 3 Americans is nonwhite, up from 1 in 4 in 1990, and virtually all areas of the country show rapid increases in the Latino and Asian populations (Cohn & Fears, 2001; Rosenblatt, 2001). The Hispanic population, at approximately 35.3 million, rose 58 percent over the last decade and now equals that of African Americans (Cohn & Fears, 2001). Each of these groups now comprises about 13 percent of the population, and Asian Americans comprise about 4 percent (Cohn & Fears, 2001). According to a 1998 study, 58 percent of Fortune 500 corporations have staff members specifically designated to work on diversity issues, and three out of every four have diversity programs (Terry-Azios, 1999).

Diversity is a reality, but it is also a human value. Our favorite groups are usually those whose members feel included, respected, known, and valued for who they are, despite their differences from other group members. Groups that value diversity and fully incorporate members from traditionally discriminated-against groups contribute to the realization of the values of social equality and justice.

Defining Diversity

In group dynamics, **diversity** refers to how similar (**member homogeneity**) or different (**member heterogeneity**) group members are from one another. There are many types of diversity and group members often bring into the group differing cultures (beliefs and behavioral patterns) based on these. Members may be diverse in demographic attributes, such as gender, age, country of origin, or ethnicity (**demographic diversity** or **social category diversity**); in personal attributes, such as personality and background (**personal diversity**); or in skills and abilities (**ability and skill diversity**) (Jackson, Stone, & Alvarez, 1993). **Informational diversity** refers to differences in knowledge bases and perspectives that members bring to the group (Jehn, Northcraft, & Neale, 1999). Harrison, Price, and Bell (1998) suggest two general categories of diversity: **surface-level diversity** (demographic and physical characteristics) and **deep-level diversity** (attitudes, beliefs, and values).

Diversity
How similar or different group members are from one another.

Member homogeneity
Similarity of group members.

Member heterogeneity
Differences among group members.

Demographic diversity (social category diversity)
Diversity based on attributes such as gender, age, country of origin, or ethnicity.

Personal diversity
Member differences in attributes such as personality and background.

Ability and skill diversity
Member differences in abilities and skills.

Informational diversity
Member differences in knowledge bases and perspectives.

Surface-level diversity
Member diversity arising out of demographic and physical characteristics.

Deep-level diversity
Member diversity arising out of attitudinal, belief, and value differences.

Laboratory studies on the effects of heterogeneity on groups date back to the early 1960s. For example, several researchers reported that heterogeneity decreased communication and increased communication errors (Barnlund & Harland, 1963; Triandis, 1960). Such research was relatively rare, though, and until recently, most group research was conducted with artificial groups comprised of demographically similar individuals. In the last several decades, however, it has become obvious that diversity in real-world groups has important effects on group processes such as conflict, communication, and cohesion. Heterogeneous groups do not always behave the same way that homogenous groups do, and although there are distinct benefits associated with diverse groups, there are also distinct challenges.

Our Discomfort With Diversity

If you are like most people, you are more comfortable in a group of people who look like you, are around the same age, and come from a similar background. Humans, it appears, come equipped with a number of tendencies that make diversity especially challenging to us. Indeed, people have a general discomfort with diversity that is driven by a natural inclination to categorize people as one of "us" or one of "them" and to prefer those who are similar to us. It is important to understand these dynamics, for they bring important information to bear on the challenges facing diverse groups. Understanding these forces is also important so that we can see our prejudices objectively. Once this awareness occurs, we become motivated to override prejudices and become more open to being in groups with people who are different from us. Our groups may then become more inclusive and are less apt to be dogged by tensions between members who are different.

The Similarity Attraction Paradigm

Similarity attraction paradigm

Tendency to be attracted to and to like people who are similar to us in interests, attitudes, values, and demographics.

The **similarity attraction paradigm** describes our tendency to be attracted to and to like people who are similar to us in interests, attitudes, and values, as well as on demographic variables such as age and ethnicity. Decades of research support the idea that we avoid associating with others who are obviously dissimilar, are indifferent to those who are low in similarity, and are drawn to those who are highly similar (Bersheid & Reis, 1998; Byrne, Clore & Smeaton, 1986). Rosenbaum (1986) suggests that it is not merely that we are attracted to those who are similar, but that we are downright repulsed by those who are dissimilar. Some research indicates that dissimilarity acts more strongly against attraction than similarity acts towards attraction (Singh & Tan, 1992).

There are two main reasons why we like people who are similar to us and dislike those who are not, both having to do with the relative rewards and costs *rewards + costs*

of interacting with similar or dissimilar others. First, similar others are easier to interact with, and this increases the rewards and reduces the costs of interaction. Similar others tend to use the same language and expressions, and it is easy for us to find things to talk about and do with them. We are also more comfortable because we are not as worried that miscommunication may occur and that what we say may be taken the "wrong way." In other words, **intergroup anxiety**—the worry and arousal that may occur when we interact with people who are not from our group—is lessened. Intergroup anxiety may result in avoidance or excessive politeness, either of which may interfere with group functioning (Stephan, 1994).

Second, interaction with similar others is rewarding because it provides consensual validation. Remember that social comparison theorists say that we frequently compare ourselves with others in order to assess our abilities and opinions. In short, similar others boost our confidence that our attitudes and behaviors are correct. Dissimilar others shake our sense of confidence that our way of thinking and doing things is right. Consequently, contact with dissimilar others is often very threatening. After all, we wonder, "How can we both be right?" Furthermore, we perceive the dissimilar other to be judging our behavior and attitudes as wrong or stupid, and this makes us defensive and rigid, and avoidant of the different other.

We also expect that dissimilar others will not like us, and we reciprocate by not liking them. A number of research studies indicate that one of the most crucial determinants of whether we like someone is whether we think the person likes us; this is called **reciprocal liking** (Bersheid & Walster, 1978; Condon & Crano, 1988; Kenny, 1994). Furthermore, if we think someone does not like us, then we are more likely to behave in less likable ways, such as being less warm and pleasant and more disagreeable; in this way, our behavior can contribute to a self-fulfilling prophecy (Curtis & Miller, 1986). Reciprocal liking is so important that it can override dissimilarity. In other words, if we believe that dissimilar others like us, then we will probably like them despite the fact that they disagree with us in some important ways (Gold, Ryckman, & Mosely, 1984).

Familiarity is another factor found by years of research to affect liking, and the appearances, communication styles, and cultures of diverse others are often strange and unfamiliar to us. Familiarity is largely the result of repeated exposure to something. In fact, more than 200 experiments have documented the **mere exposure effect:** the more often we are exposed to something, the more we like it (Zajonc, 1968; Bornstein, 1989). We like familiar things and people because they are predictable. Predictability increases our feelings of control and is therefore less stressful than unpredictability. We know what to expect from familiar others. We do not have to think hard about them, or about our behavior around them. People from groups with whom we have little familiarity make us feel uncomfortable. We do not know what to expect from them, we are distracted by our differences, and we feel less "natural." For instance, some people experience

---

Intergroup anxiety

The worry and arousal, and consequent avoidance or excessive politeness, that may occur when we interact with people who are not from our group.

Reciprocal liking

The idea that an important determinant of our liking of others is whether we think they like us.

Mere exposure effect

The more often we are exposed to something, the more we like it; explains why we like familiar things and people.

Cultural distance

The extent to which one culture differs from another.

intergroup anxiety when exposed to people from cultures very different from their own. The greater the **cultural distance**—that is, the more different the culture is from our own—the more likely intergroup anxiety is. Normally, we are able to react mindlessly and habitually to the behavior of others, but when dealing with people who behave in ways we do not understand, we feel a loss of control that may lead to feelings of incompetence, confusion, anxiety, depression, and helplessness (Triandis, 1994). Again, our discomfort often produces discomfort in them, and interactions between us become strained (self-fulfilling prophecy).

Our lack of familiarity with diverse others usually stems from the social segregation of different groups. We tend to have little contact with people outside our own group because we are more comfortable with similar others, because we seek consensual validation, and because cultural groups seek to socialize their children in the ways of the culture. In other words, **social distance** is often great between people from dissimilar groups, and ingroup norms often encourage this distance (Triandis, 1994). Even in so-called integrated schools, universities, and workplaces, when given the option, people tend to self-segregate into groups of similar people. Research suggests that we tend to use easily visible demographic characteristics such as age, gender, and ethnicity as indices of similarity (Tsui & O'Reilly, 1989).

Social distance

The extent to which members of one culture have contact with members of another culture.

The relationship between familiarity and social distance goes both ways. Lack of familiarity leads to increased social distance, and increased social distance results in lack of familiarity. Not only are we attracted to others based on similarity and familiarity, but we also tend to like and seek out food, media, and entertainment that are familiar to us based on our culture. This, of course, is what we like. However, these tendencies do mean that other ways of looking, communicating, eating, worshipping, and so on, remain unfamiliar and uncomfortable to us. This perpetuates a situation in which we avoid those who are different from ourselves.

Improving Group Effectiveness With the Similarity Attraction Paradigm

In the previous section, you learned about the role of similarity and familiarity in liking and the impact of this on our preference for homogeneous groups. You can use this information to enhance group effectiveness in the following ways:

1. Remind yourself of the rewards of interacting with diverse others. Although interacting with diverse others entails costs, such as discomfort and defensiveness, it offers distinct benefits as well. These include being exposed to new ways of thinking and doing things, and learning about how others live.

2. Remind yourself that you may have similarities with diverse others, regardless of apparent demographic and cultural differences. Do not let obvious differences prevent you from identifying similarities that can bring you together. Take

the time to look for things you share with seemingly different group members, and connect on that basis.

3. Make an effort to override the natural tendency to distance yourself from people who appear different from you. That only keeps them unfamiliar and interactions uncomfortable.

4. Avoid jumping to the conclusion that different others will not like you or will judge you. If you act distant and cool because of these assumptions, they will probably assume that you do not like them and are judging them. Remember that the reciprocity rule governs much of human relations—if you show an openness and warmth toward others, they will return it.

5. If you experience culture shock, hang in there. Once you become more familiar with diverse others and their differences, those feelings of discomfort will go away. *familiarize yourself*

The Social Categorization Approach

Social categorization approach

Emphasizes that we categorize members according to preexisting stereotypes, leading to biased perceptions and interactions.

The **social categorization approach** also suggests that member heterogeneity may create problems in groups. Our natural tendency to categorize people into "ingroup" and "outgroup" may interfere with our seeing diverse members as part of our ingroup. This approach emphasizes how our beliefs (stereotypes) about different demographic groups bias how we interact with members of those groups. Once we have negative beliefs about a group and its members, evidence that disproves our stereotypes is hard to come by. This is true for three reasons. First, we socially distance and avoid members of the outgroup, so that we do not have enough experiences with people from the outgroup to learn that we are wrong. Second, our prejudices influence our behavior toward members of the outgroup, so that we are likely to elicit behavior from them that confirms our stereotypes (we create a self-fulfilling prophecy). As you have already learned, our discomfort and suspicion trigger similar behavior from outgroup members, which we then interpret as evidence that we are right to be wary of them. Third, our natural information-processing tendencies mean that once we have a stereotype, it operates *schematically*. This means that we are more likely to notice, interpret, and remember things in ways that confirm what we already believe. The more prejudiced we are against a group, the more true this appears to be (Blascovich, Wyer, Swatt, & Kibler, 1997).

hard to find truth after biased judgement

Our natural information-processing strategies, particularly our tendency to categorize, influence how we perceive others. Think about it like this: The world is full of a potentially overwhelming number of people, situations, and things. To reduce the world's infinite variety into a cognitively manageable form, we categorize information. These categories are believed to exist in cognitive structures called **schemas.** These schemas influence how information from the environment is perceived, stored, and remembered. As you will see, schemas of people, also known as stereotypes, influence what we notice about others, how we inter-

Schemas

Cognitive structures that influence how information from the environment is perceived, stored, and remembered.

how we categorize/organize info. Any barely have to think

Stereotypes
Generalized beliefs about what members of an identifiable group are like that operate as schemas when perceiving members of those groups.

pret their behavior, and what we remember about them. **Stereotypes,** then, are generalized beliefs about what members of an identifiable group are like that operate as schemas when perceiving members of those groups. In other words, they influence perception and memory. *operate as schemas*

We often "process" people according to salient (noticeable) features that allow us to categorize them as belonging to some group. Gender, ethnicity, accent, weight, even haircut and clothing often "activate" schemas for these groups, putting us on alert for information consistent with our expectations. For instance, if you are not from the southern United States and a group member tells you in a thick southern accent that he was raised in Mississippi, this will probably influence what you notice and remember about him. Without this information, the same behaviors and qualities might go unnoticed or unremembered.

Research indicates that information consistent with our schemas is more likely to be noticed and remembered than is schema-inconsistent information (Cantor & Mischel, 1977; Hamilton, 1981; Howard & Rothbart, 1980; von Hippel, Sekaquaptewa, & Vargas, 1995). In one classic study, research participants watched a video of a woman's birthday party. Those told she was a waitress remembered her drinking beer and owning a television; those told she was a librarian remembered that she was wearing glasses and owned classical records (Cohen, 1981). In other words, "waitress" evoked a different schema than did "librarian," and participants' processing of the woman's party was guided by their schemas.

Snyder and Uranowitz's (1978) study provides another good research-based illustration, this one on the influence of stereotypes on memory. All research participants read an extensive story about "Betty K." Following the reading, one-third of the participants were told that Betty K. was a lesbian; one-third were told she was heterosexual; and one-third learned nothing about her sexual orientation. One week after reading the case history, they took a 36-item multiple-choice examination on the life of Betty K. The results: Those told that Betty K. was a lesbian were significantly more likely than the other subjects to choose answers consistent with lesbian stereotypes. In fact, they frequently went beyond the information given in the original story, choosing answers that were not in the story but that were consistent with lesbian stereotypes.

 The wonderful thing about schematic processing is that it is, as Markus and Zajonc (1985, p. 143) put it, "economical" because it reduces "an enormously complex social environment to a manageable number of meaningful categories. They fill in where there is too little information and allow the perceiver to go beyond the information given." Instead of taking a lot of time and thought to find out about somebody, you simply make assumptions based on what you believe you know about this type of person. By simplifying the way we form impressions of others, stereotypes free up cognitive resources for other activities (Macrae, Milne, & Bodenhausen, 1994). Of course, this simplification is the very shortcoming of schematic processing as well. As Fiske and Taylor (1984, p. 139) put it, "accumulated general knowledge about categories of people does not do justice to the unique qualities of any given individual." There is great diversity within any social category.

Just as Markus and Zajonc (1985) said, schemas allow us to go beyond the information given. Indeed, perceivers tend to overestimate the frequency of schema-consistent information (Hamilton & Rose, 1980; Martin, 1987; Schaller, 1991). Because our schemas draw our attention to instances that confirm our expectations, we may perceive a stronger relationship between two things than may actually exist. As I often tell my students, there are "walking, talking stereotypes" out there, people who exemplify almost any group stereotype you can think of. These people are more salient and memorable to us than those that do not fit the stereotype, although they are usually far from representative of their group. Slusher and Anderson (1987) even found that stereotype-based imaginings can lead to inflated associations of groups with their stereotypic traits. In other words, people sometimes have stereotypes that lead them to imagine people in an identifiable social group in ways that fit their stereotypes. But because the stereotype holder does not remember these imaginings as distinct from actual events, they are experienced as additional evidence that the stereotype is correct. Thus, stereotype holders have the impression that they have seen many instances of behavior that confirm the stereotype, although they may not be able to recall any specific instance.

Schemas, then, influence first what we perceive and then what we remember. Fiske and Taylor (1984) note that this is different from the way we normally think of perception. To most people, it appears that perception is a direct copy of the objective data. However, the schema concept is based on the idea that organized prior knowledge (that is, schemas) results in the active construction of social reality. Although the objective data do shape what you perceive, your existing beliefs and expectations shape how you view the data.

Although our categorization of people into groups is definitely a by-product of our natural tendency to categorize information, there is no doubt that these categorizations are strongly influenced by social factors. Social factors are one of the major determinants of the content of our stereotypes, and strongly influence how we categorize and process others. Because we tend to have relatively little experience with members of other groups, our stereotypes of other groups are frequently derived from what our groups tell us about other groups. A good example of this is heterosexuals' stereotypes of gays and lesbians. Most homosexuals are not very open about their sexual orientation because they believe they are likely to face prejudice and discrimination (called heterosexism). The content of heterosexuals' stereotypes of homosexuals is thus not derived primarily from experience, but from heterosexual culture and what other heterosexuals teach about lesbians and gays.

Fiske and Taylor (1984) point out that a schema's activation is based partly on how recently it has been activated and how frequently it is used. The more recently a schema has been activated, the more accessible it is to memory, and the more likely it is to be applied in another context. For instance, imagine that you have just heard a joke that puts down a certain ethnic group and shortly thereafter have an experience with a member of that group. The joke may have primed your stereotypes of this group, so that you are more likely to process this individual stereotypically than you might have otherwise. This is called the **priming effect.** A frequently used schema is, in a sense, permanently primed (Fiske & Taylor, 1984). Several studies indicate that when perceivers are primed to think briefly of a common group stereotype, this is enough to trigger subsequent processing based on the stereotype (Banaji, Hardin, & Rothman, 1993; Lepore & Brown, 1997).

Priming effect

The more recently a schema has been activated, the more accessible it is to memory, and the more likely it is to be applied in another context.

On the face of it, priming is a basic cognitive process. However, it is also a social one because your ingroup, and who it classifies as an outgroup, may influence how "primed" your stereotypes are and whether you even have a schema for a particular group. If another group is an outgroup to your group, your outgroup schema may be primed and ready to bias your perceptions. For instance, I teach at a university in California where there are so few Portuguese Americans and Puerto Ricans that they are not an outgroup to any other group. Most Californians, it seems, do not have schemas for these groups and do not process individuals from such groups schematically (unless they misclassify them as Mexican American, a group that some groups in California perceive as an outgroup). However, this would not be the case in New York, where Puerto Ricans are an outgroup to some other groups, or in Boston, where the Portuguese are a salient outgroup to some groups. Puerto Rican Americans and Portuguese Americans are much more likely to be processed according to stereotypes in those regions of the country.

Although we are generally hard-pressed to remember schema-inconsistent information (the cases that do not fit our stereotypes), there are times when we do. However, even if individuals remember the schema-inconsistent information, this does not mean that they will alter their stereotypes. When faced with a schema-contradictory instance, people often develop subcategories or subtypes that allow them to maintain the overall stereotype while acknowledging that it does not fit all members of the category (Taylor, 1981). Many times people respond to schema-disconfirming instances by developing an **exception-to-the-rule category** for individuals who do not fit. Most of us know a prejudiced person who has a friend from the group against which they are prejudiced. Such individuals usually insist that their friend is "different" from the others.

Exception-to-the-rule category

A schema created to accommodate what a person thinks is a rare case contradicting an otherwise "correct" stereotype.

All this is not to say that we are doomed to hold onto our stereotypes even in the face of disconfirming evidence. We can overcome our stereotypes and judge people as individuals rather than as stereotyped group members under certain conditions. For instance, individuals who are low in prejudice and high in motivation to suppress stereotypes may be able to keep stereotyped thoughts out of their minds (Monteith, Devine, & Zuwerink, 1993). However, in some cases, attempts to suppress a stereotype actually have the opposite effect of priming the stereotype, thereby increasing biased processing (Macrae, Bodenhausen, Milne,

& Jetten, 1994; Macrae, Bodenhausen, & Milne, 1998). This seems most likely if the person strongly believes the stereotype to begin with.

One of the most important factors in overcoming stereotypes is to obtain personal information about other group members. Research indicates that we will set aside our stereotypes and judge people on an individual basis when personal information is available to us (Hilton & Fein, 1989; Lord, Desforges, Fein, Fugh, & Lepper, 1994) and when we are highly motivated to form an accurate impression of someone (Hilton & Darley, 1991; Snyder, 1992). However, if we are busy, tired, drunk, or otherwise distracted, we are more likely to rely on the stereotypes that come automatically to mind and not notice personal information that might contradict our stereotypes (Gilbert & Hixon, 1991; Lambert, Khan, Lickel, & Fricke, 1997; Pratto & Bargh, 1991; von Hippel et al., 1995).

Improving Group Effectiveness With the Social Categorization Approach

In the previous section, you learned how our natural information-processing tendencies can lead to predictable errors in how we perceive others. These errors mean that we are inclined to notice, interpret, and remember things in ways that confirm our stereotypes unless we are motivated to override them and seek personal information about individuals. You can use this information to enhance your ability to work with diverse others.

1. Be aware of and question your stereotypes. Where did your ideas about different social categories come from? Do you really have good evidence that your stereotypes are accurate?

2. Work to form accurate impressions of individuals, especially if you must work with them in a group. Take the time to get to know people as individuals, because personal information overrides information from group stereotypes. Yes, demographic and cultural group memberships are part of who we are and do influence behavior. However, social category membership tells only a part of an individual's story.

3. Before concluding that a group member's behavior is evidence that your stereotype is correct, ask yourself: What stereotypes do I have that may influence the way I see this behavior? If a member more similar to me did the same thing, would I interpret it in the same way?

4. To override the tendency to notice and remember instances that confirm already-held stereotypes, challenge yourself to look for examples of individuals who do not fit your stereotypes. Get to know enough individuals from a social category that you can see the individual diversity within the category and the inaccuracy of your stereotypes.

5. When you are tired, distracted, or busy, be especially careful about jumping to conclusions about people based on their social category. It is at these times that we are especially likely to use our stereotypes as person-processing shortcuts.

when tired, distracted / busy

Apply It! ••• **Identify the Origins of Your Biases**

To what extent have you experienced segregated environments (residential, school, and work)? How has this influenced your comfort level and interaction with people from social categories other than your own? How have your prejudices (current or past) been influenced by what your family and peers taught you about different groups? How has this affected your interactions with people from those groups?

Group Process Challenges in Heterogeneous Groups

The similarity attraction and social categorization paradigms leave us with a somewhat pessimistic view of the effects of diversity on group processes and performance. When individuals in a group differ from one another, there is the potential for the creation of ingroups and outgroups within the group. This may prevent needed cooperation and contribute to conflict. Heterogeneity can also interfere with communication and lead to message distortion and errors in communication. Dissimilarity may result in group process and performance loss, including less positive attitudes toward the group and a higher likelihood of turnover from the group, particularly among those who are most different (Williams & O'Reilly, 1998).

Commitment and Cohesion

Members are expected to have less positive attitudes toward a diverse group because we are less inclined to like dissimilar group members and social categorization processes interfere with our sharing a common group identity. In other words, seeing other group members as part of a "them" interferes with the "us" that is part of group cohesion and commitment. Group members may perceive that they lack the shared experiences and identity necessary for cohesion (Knouse & Dansby, 1999). Diversity in a group may have a negative effect on member satisfaction because members do not feel socially integrated within the group and do not identify with it (Cady & Valentine, 1999). This may impede the motivation to work together as a group and may be especially problematic if the group's task requires cooperation between group members. Satisfaction and cohesion are also related to commitment to the group and leaving the group. Several studies indicate that group heterogeneity reduces satisfaction and commitment and increases turnover (Konrad, Winter, & Gutek, 1992; Riordan & Shore, 1997; Tsui, Egan, & O'Reilly, 1992).

A good example of this may be seen in the 2000 movie *Remember the Titans,* a slightly fictionalized account of a white high school football team in Alexandria, Virginia, forced to integrate in the early 1970s. Initially, the prejudiced white players refused to accept the black players as part of the team, and some even quit the team. At first, the white quarterback would not pass to the black wide receiver who was wide open. The white offensive linemen would not block for the black running backs, leaving them wide open to attack from the other side's defense. The group's performance was abysmal until the coach introduced activities designed to make diverse members get to know one another as individuals and appreciate one another's cultures. The shared experience of grueling training sessions and an emphasis on a team identity also brought the group of diverse players together into a winning team.

Conflict

The similarity attraction and social categorization paradigms both suggest that conflict will be less in homogeneous groups. To the extent that members are similar, there are likely to be fewer areas of disagreement. Coming from the same perspective, group members are more likely to agree about what to do and how to do it. Several studies indicate that such disagreements are more likely in heterogeneous groups (Jehn, Chadwick, & Thatcher, 1997; Jehn et al., 1999). Similarity eases communication, so that communication errors, misunderstandings, and intercultural conflicts may be less likely to occur. From a social categorization standpoint, conflict in the heterogeneous group is also more likely because categorizing individuals in the group into different groups can provoke hostility or animosity between members (Jehn et al., 1999) and can separate a group into rival groups. Stereotypes may lead to the biased processing of the behaviors of dissimilar group members, causing us to misperceive their acts as arrogant and hostile, and to respond accordingly.

Overcoming Group Process Challenges Related to Member Heterogeneity

Because members of diverse groups are often less attracted and committed to the group, resulting in lower satisfaction, poorer task performance, and increased absenteeism and turnover, a major issue is how to enhance cohesiveness in a diverse group (Linnehan & Konrad, 1999). Here are some suggestions to help group members note and accept differences, while also identifying similarities and superordinate goals.

1. To increase cohesion and reduce the stereotypes that may engender conflict, create opportunities for socializing, so that members have positive experiences in common and get to know one another as individuals. Consider playing games or organizing activities at such events that require positive, cooperative interaction between group members.

2. To integrate new or minority group members and to make sure that valuable input from them is not suppressed, make an extra effort to solicit the input of new and minority group members. Emphasize to the group what these members bring to the table, so that everyone will be reminded that these members belong.

3. Create a superordinate group identity by emphasizing shared goals and giving the group a name, logo, or common opponent. This will increase cohesion and unite diverse subgroups.

4. As a group, create a shared understanding of the group's issues, concerns, and tasks that incorporates the different views, perspectives, and experiences of all members.

Differences in perspectives can increase conflict because members are less likely to agree about what to do and how to do it, but remember that conflict can increase group performance if it is managed constructively (see Chapter 7).

1. All sides should listen to opposing positions with the goal of analytic empathy (understanding not just what people want but why). Once this occurs, they can work cooperatively to arrive at a final position that integrates everyone's interests.

2. Make time to talk about the group's process and performance. According to Watson, Kumar, & Michaelson (1993), initial group process problems of diverse groups can be solved. First, provide group members with an assessment of their group's process and performance. Then, encourage and provide time for group members to discuss how things are going and to decide on a plan of action for improving their problem solving.

- rate performance
- make plan together -

The Value-in-Diversity Hypothesis

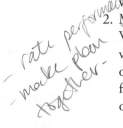

Value-in-diversity hypothesis

Posits that diversity in groups offers distinct benefits, such as greater creativity and better problem solving.

Not all theorists agree that member heterogeneity has largely negative effects on groups. For instance, Blau (1977) said that the "social experience of associating with persons with different backgrounds undoubtedly affects attitudes and conduct. It may well broaden people's horizons, promote tolerance, and stimulate intellectual endeavors" (p. 36). The **value-in-diversity hypothesis** posits that there are distinct benefits to diversity in groups (Cox, Lobel, & McLeod, 1991). In **Box 8-1,** you will find a student story about the benefits of diversity.

Enhanced Problem Solving

Information and decision-making theories predict that diversity can enhance group performance by increasing the range of knowledge, skills, and contacts that enhance problem solving (Williams & O'Reilly, 1998). For instance, one study of 92 workgroups found that although informational diversity (differences in educational background, training, and work experience) increased conflict, it also increased group performance (Jehn et al., 1999). Studies support the idea that diversity in gender, ethnicity, and nationality can increase the number of alternatives and perspectives that a group considers when making a decision (Kirchmeyer & Cohen, 1992; Watson et al., 1993). Of course, this potential may not be realized if minorities perceive that expressing different points of view will be ignored or punished (Granrose & Oskamp, 1997). Therefore, it is important

BOX 8-1 / STUDENT STORY

Kristin writes about how a superordinate identity at her church unites diverse members.

When I went to church last Sunday morning, the service started out with the youngest children reciting verses from the Bible. The middle-aged white pastor then hugged a young African American woman in the congregation, announcing that her daddy had just went to be with the Lord this week. We spent twenty minutes singing with our choir, a choir comprised of young, old, wealthy, poor, European Americans, African Americans, Asian Americans, and Latin Americans. The service ended when the oldest member of the church (102 years old!) prayed for us.

Our church did not push diversity when it was first established; it simply welcomed it. The idea was that anyone who had the common bond of the Christian faith could unite in a comfortable and relaxed atmosphere. All who came were treated equally, which triggered rapid growth. The only way to unite such diverse people is to start out with a unified goal and then to give each person a role in reaching that goal. The belief system of the church is that we are worshipping the same God and our goal is to give Him glory and spread His word. The church's philosophy is that each person must come to have their faith in the way that they are most comfortable. And so, the producers and actors that attend our church create plays and shows for the congregation, the musicians create music, teachers run our day care, architects designed our new church, and landscapers did our landscaping.

Diversity makes my church an interesting and exciting place to be. I never really know what to expect on Sunday, other than that I will learn something new each time that I go and will learn it in a new and unexpected way.

that groups establish norms and use problem-solving and decision-making strategies that support the expression of varied points of view.

Enhanced Creativity

Diversity can also enhance a group's creativity and innovativeness—the generation of new ideas. The creation of knowledge and the discovery of insight by groups depend on the presence of diverse viewpoints and perspectives about the task (Jackson, 1992; Jehn et al., 1999). Studies indicate that the insights and sensitivities brought by people of varying backgrounds (including gender, ethnicity, and functional knowledge) increase flexibility and promote high-quality innovations (Cady & Valentine, 2000; Damanpour, 1991; McLeod, Lobel, & Cox, 1996; Milliken & Martins, 1996; Rogelberg & Rumery, 1996; Watson et al., 1993). Some research suggests that although homogeneous groups may initially perform better than heterogeneous ones, over time, heterogeneous groups surpass homogeneous ones in terms of problem solving and innovativeness (Harrison et al., 1998; Knouse & Dansby, 1999; Watson et al., 1993). It appears that groups need some time to appreciate and make good use of diversity and to re-

---

Apply It! ••• **Comprise the Ideal Group for the Task**

A community organization receives a large grant from the state to educate citizens on how to reduce sexually transmitted diseases. The Euroamerican staff creates a number of educational materials and programs but discovers that their safe-sex program has had no effect on the sexual practices of teenagers, Latin Americans, and African Americans in their community. They realize that they may not understand these groups well enough to know how to serve them and have asked you to hire five new staff members to develop new materials and programs. What types of people would you hire, and why?

---

solve group process issues (Cady & Valentine, 2000; Watson et al., 1993). In other words, despite some negative effects of diversity on group process, ultimately, diversity may have positive effects on creativity and innovation.

Contextual Influences on Diversity and Groups

Researchers are still hard at work trying to solve the group diversity puzzle. It is confusing—after all, it is easy to see how diversity can exert positive or negative effects on groups. In 1998, Williams and O'Reilly reviewed forty years of diversity research on group process and performance and concluded that there are no consistent main effects of diversity because the influence of diversity on groups is affected (mediated) by a number of other factors, including type of task and type of diversity.

Task Type

The effects of diversity on a group's process and performance depend in part on the group's task. For instance, a meta-analysis by Bowers, Pharmer, and Salas (2000) found that on tasks high in difficulty, heterogeneous teams performed significantly better than homogeneous ones. Homogeneous groups may be more effective at performing tasks that rely on perceptual and motor skills (Jackson et al., 1993). Diversity is expected to have an especially positive impact when a group's task can benefit from multiple perspectives and diverse knowledge, and when disagreement arising from differing perspectives is well managed (Jehn et al., 1999; Williams & O'Reilly, 1998). Cognitive tasks such as generating ideas may especially benefit from diverse backgrounds (Pelled, Eisenhardt, & Xin, 1999).

Diverse groups appear to have performance advantages over homogeneous groups on creativity tasks requiring knowledge of different cultures (McLeod et al., 1996). Many companies are interested in increasing diversity because they believe that it has the potential to help them develop products, services, and market

Marketing argument (cultural rationale) for diversity

Suggests that diversity's value lies in its potential to increase profits or create better products or services.

campaigns that appeal to a larger market. This has been called the **marketing argument for diversity** (Cox & Blake, 1991) or the **cultural rationale for diversity** (Linnehan & Konrad, 1999). As Konrad and Linnehan describe it, the demographics of the U.S. labor force and customer base are changing, and because the economy is increasingly global rather than national, organizations must be able to deal effectively with cultural differences in order to enhance competitiveness. In the United States, most organizational leaders and decision makers have been males of Western European descent. Their unfamiliarity with other cultures may interfere with their ability to generate ideas that will resonate with diverse customer populations and with their adoption of effective management styles for use with diverse employees.

The example of Avon, a cosmetics company, shows how culturally and ethnically diverse groups may be especially effective in helping organizations reach a variety of markets. In the 1980s, Avon's sales were down. The task was to figure out how to turn things around. Avon was able to significantly increase its revenues by listening to one of its directors who grew up in a Latin American community. She used her knowledge of Latin American culture to expand Avon's client base. She had ideas for products that would appeal specifically to that market, and recommended a return to a door-to-door strategy using Spanish-speaking salespeople. Sales to Latin Americans now comprise a significant source of company revenue.

An experimental study conducted by McLeod, Lobel, and Cox (1996) also shows how heterogeneous groups may be more effective on creativity tasks involving knowledge of different cultures. They compared the performance of groups comprised only of Euroamericans with heterogeneous groups comprised of Euroamericans, Asian Americans, African Americans, and Latin Americans on a brainstorming task called the "tourist problem." The groups were asked to spend fifteen minutes generating as many ideas as possible to bring more tourists to the United States. Experts from the travel industry rated the groups' ideas on effectiveness and feasibility. Statistical analyses indicated that the ideas produced by the diverse groups were judged as significantly more effective and feasible than the ideas produced by the heterogeneous groups. ?

The nature of the task is also important. For some groups, interaction and coordination are critical for group performance; for others, this is less so. For instance, diversity appears to have more impact when a group is performing a nonroutine task in which members must interact and rely on one another (Pelled et al., 1999). In such cases, conflict between members is more likely than it is in situations where members perform routine tasks requiring relatively little interaction and negotiation. In general, the more the group's work requires interaction and cooperation—that is, the more interdependent members are—the more influence diversity seems to have (Jehn et al., 1999). Timmerman (2000) demonstrated this in a study comparing the effects of age and racial diversity on the performance of professional baseball and basketball teams. In contrast to basketball, baseball is a low-interdependence activity; a team's performance approximates the sum of the individual players' performances. Basketball, however, is a high-interdependence activity; members work physically close to one another and must interact, cooperate, and coordinate to win. Age and racial diversity were unrelated to team performance for baseball teams, but for basketball, greater diversity was associated with lower winning percentages.

Type of Diversity

Not every aspect of diversity has the same effect on group process and performance (Williams & O'Reilly, 1998). At the beginning of the chapter, you learned that there are a number of different types of diversity, and if you think about it, it makes sense that these would exert differing effects on group process and performance. This is a relatively new area of research; there is a lot we do not know, and many contradictory research findings. Overall, though, the research so far suggests that type of diversity does make a difference. More visible or salient characteristics, such as ethnicity, age, and gender, are expected to have a greater impact because they are "markers" of difference and are more likely to be used for social categorization (Williams & O'Reilly, 1998). However, other types of diversity may also affect group functioning. For instance, one study of 545 employees from three top firms in the household goods moving industry found that informational diversity (differences in knowledge and perspectives) enhanced performance, whereas value diversity (differences about what the group's goals or mission should be) reduced performance (Jehn et al., 1999).

In their review of forty years of research on the effects of diversity in groups on process and performance, Williams and O'Reilly (1998) examined separately the literature on tenure diversity (time of entry into the group), age diversity, background diversity (functional diversity), gender diversity, and racial and ethnic diversity. According to Williams and O'Reilly, there is strong evidence suggesting that tenure diversity is associated with less effective group process. Presumably, this is because individuals identify more with group members who enter the group at the same time; therefore, cohesion is greater and communication better when tenure diversity is less. Although tenure diversity can lead to increased performance by providing a wider variety of perspectives, process problems and the isolation and exclusion of newer members often prevent the realization of this potential. The research on background diversity indicates that although functional diversity (differences in education and specialization) increases conflict, it also improves performance. The effects of age diversity on group process and performance are not strong, but it appears that age diversity is associated with higher absenteeism and turnover.

Some research suggests that diversity based on racial and national differences appears to interfere with group process more than heterogeneity based on gender or personality (Watson et al., 1993). Like the research on age diversity, the research on ethnic diversity indicates that racial and ethnic minorities in a group may be less committed to the group, more likely to leave, and more likely to be absent (Tsui et al., 1992). Whites who are minorities in a group appear to experience more of these negative effects than nonwhites (Williams & O'Reilly, 1998). However, some studies find a positive relationship between ethnic diversity and creativity and the ability of the group to implement decisions (O'Reilly, Williams, & Barshade, 1997; Williams & O'Reilly, 1998). This may be more likely when group members identify strongly with the task and when group members committed to fairness consciously override their biases in an effort to work with diverse others (Gaertner & Dovidio, 1986; Mullen & Copper, 1994; Williams & O'Reilly, 1998).

The research on gender diversity suggests that the effects of diversity on a group may depend on the proportion of individuals in a group that possess a particular characteristic. Thus, the ratio of males to females in a group, known as gender composition, may influence the impact that gender diversity has on the group. As the proportions of males and females in a group diverge, conventional gender roles often become more salient, and members may be treated accordingly (Levine & Moreland, 1995). "Solo" or "token" members are individuals in the numerical minority who represent a relatively less powerful social category (Kanter, 1977). These minority members attract more attention from other group members (Lord & Saenz, 1985) and are more likely to be processed in stereotypical ways (Mullen, 1991). For instance, solo women may be treated as the "mother" of the group or the "cheerleader" (Levine & Moreland, 1995). As noted in the discussion of stereotype threat in Chapter 4, this visibility and awareness of others' stereotyped perceptions may create anxiety in minority members that may lower performance (Spencer, Steele, & Aronson, 1999; Steele & Aronson, 1995). Ironically, though, as tokens, there is extra pressure to match or exceed the performance of majority coworkers (Levine & Moreland, 1995).

Being a solo in a group is often a difficult experience (Kanter, 1977). Imagine for a moment being the only one of your gender in a ten-person group, versus being one of a minority of four. Would you feel less comfortable and less a part of the group when you were a minority of one? Several studies find that the fewer women in a group, the greater their perception of isolation and the lower their job satisfaction (Burke & McKeen, 1996; Konrad et al., 1992). Some studies indicate that being a gender minority is more difficult for women (Crocker & McGraw, 1984; Wharton & Baron, 1987), whereas others indicate that males, more than females, have difficulty as gender minorities in a group (Tsui et al., 1992). Other studies indicate that being a gender minority in a group reduces satisfaction and increases dropout for both men and women (Popielarz & McPherson, 1995). Research also indicates that both women and men experience more emotional conflicts as the proportion of group members of the other gender increases, and that this negatively affects group performance (Pelled, 1997).

Apply It! ••• **Analyze Your Experiences as a "Solo" Group Member**

Describe your experiences as a "solo" group member. How did being solo affect your level of comfort, your feelings of belonging, your level of contribution to the group, your assumption of a leadership role? How were your experiences affected by the way "majority" group members acted toward you? (Even if you are usually a majority group member, it is likely that you have had the experience of being a minority group member at some point. For instance, a white heterosexual male may find himself the solo male among a group of women. Or you may have been the only person at a family gathering who was not related to everyone else by bloodline.)

The Interaction Between Type of Diversity and Context

It is actually somewhat difficult to generalize about the effects of type of diversity on group process and performance because these effects can depend on the particular situation, or context. The context is an important determinant of what differences are salient (perceptually noticeable) and task-related. For instance, Williams and O'Reilly (1998) note that being an African American physician in a hospital with a diverse workforce may have very different effects on group process than being the only American female engineer in a group of male Japanese engineers.

As mentioned earlier with regard to gender diversity, it is also known that the relative proportions of members from different subgroups may make a difference. Rosabeth Moss Kanter (1977) was one of the first theorists to emphasize that when a group is comprised of a large majority group and a small minority group, majority group members may treat minority members in ways consistent with common stereotypes. She theorized that in response to this, minority members would experience social isolation and performance pressures. Some theorists suggest that once a subordinate minority reaches a certain size, the majority's prejudices are more likely to wane as a result of their greater experience with the minority. Also, minority members are more likely to be comfortable in the group because of increased support from other minority members, and more likely to assert themselves regarding perceived inequalities (Blau, 1977; Ely, 1994). Sometimes, however, when the size of the minority group within a larger group increases to a certain point, the minority and majority groups within the larger group may develop distinctive, salient ingroup identities and begin to compete for power and resources. Majority group members may feel threatened as the size of the minority group increases (Tsui et al., 1992; Tolbert, Simons, Andrews, & Rhee, 1995). All of this may interfere with the functioning of the larger group (Tolbert, Graham, & Andrews, 1999).

Finally, type of diversity and type of task may interact to determine the influence of diversity on a group. For instance, some types of diversity may be more relevant in some situations than in others, and factors such as job-relatedness, status differences, and cultural stereotypes may determine the strength of the effects of diversity (Moreland & Levine, 1995; Pelled, 1996). Jehn et al. (1999) offer the following examples. If the task of the group is to define a strategic financial direction for the organization and all group members have backgrounds in finance, then being female is not likely to make a difference in what that individual brings to the group and in the group's performance. However, if the group must select product features for a new model of automobile, the experience of being a woman may bring a different orientation to the group and add to the group's performance, even if that woman is an engineer just like other members. Even the influence of group proportions (the relative size of different subgroups) may depend on contextual variables such as culture and status. For instance, a study of groups comprised of Chinese and Caucasian males in Canada found that being a numerical minority reduced participation by the Chinese but not by the Caucasians (Li, Karakowsky, & Siegel, 1999). The researchers attributed this difference to the lower social power of Chinese relative to Caucasians in Canada. Similarly, the relative status of men and women and the degree to which a given context is defined as gender appropriate may mediate the effect of group proportions (Tolbert et al., 1999; Yoder, 1994). High-status token women do not seem to have the same problems as low-status token women, and when token women are unwelcome newcomers to all-male groups, the group's reaction to them is different than when they are part of a newly formed group (Eagly & Johnson, 1990; Moreland & Levine, 1995).

Intercultural Approach to Diversity in Groups

In 1996, Milliken and Martins characterized diversity as "a double-edged sword, increasing the opportunity for creativity as well as the likelihood that group members will be dissatisfied and fail to identify with the group" (p. 403). At this point in the chapter, it should be clear to you that diverse groups may perform better, or worse, than homogeneous groups. The group must successfully master the intricacies associated with managing a diverse membership. It often takes extra effort to override the negative effects of diversity so that the positive effects can be realized. As McLeod et al. (1996) note, proper management of diversity, not simply increasing diversity, is the key to maximizing group performance.

You have already learned some strategies for increasing the effectiveness of the heterogeneous group. In this section, you will learn about the **intercultural approach** to managing diversity. This approach emphasizes helping people to understand, accept, and value the cultural differences between groups, with the ultimate goal of reaping the benefits of diversity (Ferdman, 1995). The goal is to both celebrate differences and emphasize the dimensions of commonality or inclusion that supercede these differences (Devine, 1995). On the one hand, emphasizing differences without also finding common ground between diverse members is likely to further separate group members. On the other hand, em-

Intercultural approach
Perspective that emphasizes helping people to understand, accept, and value the cultural differences between groups.

phasizing common ground and ignoring member differences may require that members suppress important identities and deny the group the benefits of varied perspectives.

Subtractive Multiculturalism and Additive Multiculturalism

Acculturation strategies

The variety of ways in which individuals and groups can respond to diversity, ranging from the isolation of minority group members to integration.

Subtractive assimilation (subtractive multiculturalism)

The idea that people should give up their unique cultural attributes to fit with the majority culture.

Additive multiculturalism (integration)

The idea that we should respond to diversity by working to understand and appreciate other groups and integrate diverse perspectives.

Individuals and groups can respond to diversity in a number of different ways. These **acculturation strategies** can range from the isolation of minority group members (separation) to the formation of a new group identity that incorporates the diversity of all members (integration or additive multiculturalism) (Ferdman, 1995; Triandis, 1994). Many people, especially Americans, are attracted to the melting pot idea—the idea that groups that are not in the mainstream should "assimilate" by giving up their unique cultural attributes and becoming just like the majority. This idea is also known as **subtractive assimilation, or subtractive multiculturalism,** because people need to subtract or lose some of their original cultural elements in order to fit in (Triandis, 1994). Although you might be attracted to the idea that we should strive for groups that are blind as to differences between members, the truth is that there are often real differences between group members (Worchel & Austin, 1986). Furthermore, group members may not want to give up their unique identities, as these are often an important part of who they are. For instance, one's cultural heritage may be a source of identity and pride. Remember too that a heterogeneous membership usually has advantages, such as increased creativity. Also, given our natural and unconscious tendencies to process people schematically, it is probably unrealistic to expect that we will always be able to process members individually, and not according to their social categories (Devine, 1995).

Additive multiculturalism, or integration, is the addition of skills and perspectives that allow for increasing understanding and appreciation of other groups (Triandis, 1994). The multicultural approach to managing diversity rejects the melting pot metaphor in favor of a "salad" metaphor, emphasizing a diversity-within-unity theme. Imagine a good salad. It has a number of diverse elements, and even a variety of lettuces. Each element retains its flavor and yet contributes to the salad as a whole. The salad would not be as good if it were all lettuce or if we tried to turn nonlettuce elements into lettuce. Were we to put it into a food processor to blend all the elements and make them the same, the salad would lose both flavor and texture. The multicultural approach goes beyond mere tolerance of differences and aims for a mutual respect and appreciation of differences.

Intercultural Competence

One of the first steps we can take toward additive multiculturalism is to become interculturally competent. **Intercultural competence** is the ability to interact effectively with people from other cultures. It depends on understanding

---

Apply It! ••• **Think About the Difference Between Tolerance and Appreciation**

To experience the difference between tolerance and appreciation, think of a time when you felt tolerated in a group and a time you felt appreciated. How did it feel to be tolerated, and how did it affect your relationship with the tolerant persons? How did it feel to be appreciated, and how did that affect your relationship with those who appreciated you? (adapted from Carr-Ruffino, 1996).

Intercultural competence

The ability to interact effectively with people from other cultures.

the influence of culture on behavior, overriding ethnocentrism, accepting and transcending cultural differences, and understanding other members' behavior in the context of their culture.

Intercultural competence includes an awareness of culture and the influence of culture on behavior. We learn our culture's values, norms, and conventions so well that it often influences us without conscious awareness. Indeed, culture is something that we often think of as something that people from other countries or communities have. It often takes contact with other cultures to sensitize us to the influence of culture on behavior. If you have traveled or moved to another culture or a part of the United States that is culturally very different from the community you came from, you are probably aware of the influence of culture to a greater extent than someone who has not. For instance, I moved from a white suburban middle-class community to an inner-city African American lower-income community when I was 11. Before this time, I was unaware of the ways in which my suburban white culture affected how I related to other people. When I moved from Virginia to California at age 20, I discovered yet again that there are cultural differences in the United States.

Intercultural competence also requires that we acknowledge, and make an effort to override, our **ethnocentrism.** Ethnocentrism is the belief that the customs, norms, and values of our ingroup are universally valid and correct (Triandis, 1994). Understanding and appreciating cultural differences is initially difficult for most people because humans are naturally prone to ethnocentrism. Therefore, it is important to be aware of your tendency to be ethnocentric and to understand how your culture, stereotypes, and attitudes influence your interactions with members of other cultures. The idea is to open your mind enough to recognize that there are other valid ways of doing things and of looking at the world. In short, it means coming to understand that what is "normal" and "correct" often varies by culture and that our way is not necessarily the only right way.

Ethnocentrism

The belief that the customs, norms, and values of our ingroup are universally valid and correct.

Triandis (1994) suggests that when confronted by cultural differences we can do one of four things: (1) ignore the differences; (2) bolster our position by seeking others from our own culture to agree that our way is right; (3) differentiate—deciding it is okay for them to do it their way and us to do it our way; and (4) transcend—agreeing that both are correct under some conditions. Triandis (1994) recommends that we suppress the first two responses and use the last one most frequently. For instance, I once read of a hotel that employed both Ethiopian and American males to park guests' cars. The Ethiopians often greeted one another by kissing each other on the cheek. Initially this cultural difference in greetings caused conflict. Some of the American workers began ridiculing the Ethiopian workers and demanded that management stop the Ethiopian greetings. Fights erupted between the two groups of coworkers. The hotel management called a meeting at which the two groups discussed their differences, voiced their concerns about working with the other, and shared information about their cultures. Both groups agreed that the kissing should not go on in front of hotel guests, but otherwise it was okay. After this, the groups were able to work together without incident. Some of the Americans even began to greet their Ethiopian coworkers in the Ethiopian way, and the Ethiopians learned to greet their American coworkers in the American way.

An important part of additive multiculturalism and intercultural competence is to become familiar with the ways in which cultural differences can affect group members' behavior. Most experts on intercultural training and diversity recommend that we learn about the cultures of other group members so that we can correctly interpret their behavior and avoid behaving in ways that are offensive to them. It is important to be mindful of the fact that people from different cultures, environments, and subgroups may have different values and assumptions, and these can affect the way that people lead, cooperate, compete, communicate, plan, organize, and are motivated (Tung, 1997). **Box 8-2** contains a student story about the influence of culture on group behavior.

Sometimes learning about other cultures is done formally through workshops offering intercultural training. Many international corporations offer such training to employees before sending them to work in other cultures. **Box 8-3** presents an example of an **intercultural sensitizer (ICS).** An ICS is a programmed training exercise that presents individuals with descriptions of various situations and possible responses to them in order to teach that different behaviors have different meanings in different cultures (Bhagat & Prien, 1996). The ICS presents short vignettes (stories) in which individuals from different cultures interact and experience a clash of cultures. The reader is asked to select from a number of alternatives that may explain the problem from the other's point of view (Cushner & Landis, 1996). The point is to encourage individuals to learn about the subjective elements of a culture, such as values, norms, and attitudes.

The influence of culture on various group processes such as conflict is discussed throughout this text. This information can be used to improve your intercultural competence. Most of these discussions refer to dimensions proposed by Hofstede (1980). Hofstede studied approximately 117,000 IBM employees in 40 countries and concluded that four types of culturally relevant value dimensions affect group member and leader behavior: (1) power distance, (2) uncertainty avoidance, (3) individualism/collectivism, and (4) masculinity/femininity.

Intercultural sensitizer (ICS)

A programmed training exercise designed to teach that different behaviors have different meanings in different cultures.

BOX 8-2 / STUDENT STORY

Lori's cultural heritage affects her behavior in groups.

My culture has a big impact on how I work in groups. Both of my parents are of Japanese descent. My grandparents were born in Japan and immigrated to the United States. They taught my parents the values from their collectivist culture. Whereas the American culture is more individualistic, the Japanese culture is more group-oriented. The Japanese hold loyalty and honor as extremely important values. These were instilled in me at a very young age. Both of my parents were very young when they were placed in internment camps during World War II. I always admired my grandparents' and parents' courage not only to survive the harsh conditions but to remain loyal to the United States. I asked my parents why after the camps they did not have negative feelings toward our country and why they put up with the forced internment. They responded by saying, "We did what we had to do for our country, even if it meant restructuring our lives." Whenever I am involved in a group setting, I think about this. People are relying on me to do my best and give my all, and I feel loyal toward them. When I feel something is worth my time, I am dedicated to that something. I will do everything I can to make my group proud and to work toward our success.

BOX 8-3 / THE INTERCULTURAL SENSITIZER (ICS) OR CULTURAL ASSIMILATOR

Below is a much-abbreviated sample of an ICS vignette. Read the story, and choose one of the explanations at the end.

> The Russian employees at the American firm were very serious and looked down and sped up when their American coworkers smiled or waved at them as they passed in the hall. Consequently, the American workers felt that the Russians were strange and did not want to work with them. How would you explain the Russians' behavior to the Americans?

1. The American workers have probably offended them in some way.

2. In Russia, it is considered unprofessional to smile, laugh, or joke at work.

3. The Russians dislike other cultures and distance themselves from others.

The correct answer is 2. Think about how your behavior in the situation would be influenced by this interpretation versus the other interpretations of the Russians' behavior.

Power distance

In a culture, the amount of respect and deference less powerful (subordinate) members generally give to more powerful (superior) members.

These dimensions are described briefly in the following paragraphs. **Box 8-4** gives you a chance to score your own culture on Hofstede's dimensions.

According to Hofstede (1980, 1991), **power distance** is the amount of respect and deference less powerful (subordinate) members give to more powerful (superior) members. In contrast to low power distance cultures, in high power

[handwritten margin note: Amount of respect lower members give to superiors compared to other subordinate]

BOX 8-4 / EVALUATE YOUR CULTURE ON HOFSTEDE'S DIMENSIONS

For each of the pairs below, choose Statement 1 or Statement 2.

Pair One

1. In my culture, most employees are hesitant to express disagreement with managers.
2. In my culture, many people will break rules if they think that it is in the best interest of the company, or if they believe a rule is "stupid."

If you chose 1, then it is likely you are from a high power distance culture; if you chose 2, it is likely you are from a low power distance culture.

Pair Two

1. In my culture, people are comfortable with spontaneity and do not feel the need to do much planning ahead of time.
2. In my culture, there are clear rules governing behavior in most situations and people follow them.

If you chose 1, you are probably from a low uncertainty avoidance culture; if you chose 2, it is likely that you are from a high uncertainty avoidance culture.

Pair Three

1. In my culture, relationships with others are to be preserved despite their costs.
2. In my culture, people are more likely to think of what's best for them and to act on this basis, rather than considering what is best for the group.

If you chose 1, you are probably from a collectivist culture; if you chose 2, yours is probably an individualistic culture.

Pair Four

1. In my culture, people care less about work and more about general quality of life than they do making a lot of money and achieving at work.
2. In my culture, achievement at work is one of the most important things.

If you chose 1, you are probably from a feminine culture; if you chose 2, yours is probably a masculine culture.

distance cultures, there is a greater respect for authority, more comfort with more directive and authoritarian leadership, and greater fear about disagreeing with leaders. Hofstede's research indicates that power distance is higher in Latin American countries (such as Brazil, Mexico, and Panama) and East Asian countries (such as Indonesia, India, and Thailand) than in the United States and non-Latin European countries (such as Denmark, Germany, and Great Britain). The power distance of our culture may affect how we respond to authority and how much we wish to be consulted by leadership. It may also affect our responses to inequities in groups. For instance, we might expect that those from low power distance cultures will be more likely to react and seek redress if they perceive they are getting less than other group members.

Uncertainty avoidance is the degree to which individuals in a society feel uncomfortable with situations that are unstructured, unclear, or unpredictable. High uncertainty avoidance is reflected in an emphasis on ritual behavior and rules; members from such cultures may prefer situations in which the rules and norms are very clear. Unlike those from low uncertainty avoidance cultures, who are more comfortable in situations where the norms are unclear and believe that "bad" rules are meant to be broken, people from high uncertainty cultures take rules very seriously. They also prefer planning versus spontaneity. According to Hofstede's research, high uncertainty avoidance cultures include Japan, Argentina, France, Panama, Spain, and Turkey. Low uncertainty avoidance cultures include Sweden, Denmark, India, Canada, and the United States.

Individualism/collectivism is the extent to which individuals in a society view themselves as individuals or as part of a group. In collectivistic cultures, individuals emphasize the needs of the group over their individual needs, and harmony in relationships is very important. In contrast, individuals from individualistic cultures behave more according to self-interest. They are also more likely than those from collectivist cultures to sever a relationship when the costs exceed the benefits. The United States, Great Britain, and Australia rate especially high on individualism, and Brazil, Panama, and Indonesia are among the more collectivistic cultures.

In groups, this dimension influences behavior in conflict situations, cooperativeness versus competitiveness, "slacking behavior," and the importance to members of receiving personal credit for their contributions. For instance, people from individualistic cultures probably engage in more competitive behavior in groups, slack more in group situations, and desire personal recognition for the group's success more than do those from collectivist cultures. In conflict situations, collectivists are very concerned with maintaining a good relationship and therefore are more likely to use less confrontational styles than those from individualistic cultures. In comparison to individualists, collectivists may also prefer to work in groups rather than alone. This dimension is probably the most widely known and studied of the four dimensions and is the one that will be referred to most frequently in later chapters. Hofstede's (1980) study suggests that the United States, Canada, Great Britain, Australia, and The Netherlands are individualistic cultures, and Panama, Brazil, Indonesia, Thailand, and Japan are collectivist cultures.

Masculinity/femininity refers to the extent to which a society's dominant values emphasize assertiveness and materialism (masculine) versus concern for people and quality of life (feminine). Individuals from masculine cultures are more concerned with achievement, whereas persons from feminine cultures are more

---

Uncertainty avoidance

The degree to which individuals in a society feel uncomfortable with situations that are unstructured, unclear, or unpredictable.

Individualism/collectivism

The extent to which individuals in a society view themselves as individuals or as part of a group.

Masculinity/femininity

Whether a society's dominant values emphasize assertiveness and materialism (masculine) or other-centeredness and quality of life (feminine).

concerned with working in a pleasant, friendly environment. Also, in contrast to those in masculine cultures, feminine cultures prefer shorter hours to high salaries and can be said to "work to live" rather than "live to work." Gender roles are also more defined in masculine cultures. According to Hofstede's research, Japan, Mexico, Indonesia, and the United States are examples of more masculine cultures, and Sweden, Denmark, and The Netherlands are examples of feminine cultures.

Ecological fallacy

The mistaken belief that because two cultures differ, that any two members of those cultures must necessarily differ in that same manner.

Although it is often recommended that we familiarize ourselves with other cultures in order to better understand and respond to fellow group members, it is very important to understand that members carry their own personal experience of their culture. In other words, we should not assume that something that is generally true of a culture is true for every member of that culture. To do so is to commit the **ecological fallacy** (Smith & Bond, 1999)—the mistaken belief that because two cultures differ, any two members of those cultures must necessarily differ in the same manner. In reality, there is considerable diversity within any culture and subtle yet distinct group distinctions among people who initially appear to be from the same culture (Hurtado, Rodriguez, Gurin, & Beals, 1993). We can offend others if they feel "typecast" by our generalizations about who they are because of their culture (Ferdman, 1995). I remember one of my students was adopted in Korea as an infant by Euroamerican parents and reared in Euroamerican culture. Her behavior is consistent with Euroamerican culture (California-style), not Korean culture. She felt offended when some people made assumptions about her because of her Asian features. There are also many biracial and bicultural individuals with complex cultural identifications. The bottom line is that it is important to understand how other individuals construct themselves as cultural beings—that is, what parts of their culture are part of who they are (Ferdman & Brody, 1996). Although our stereotype of another culture may be positive, generally correct, and even useful at times in terms of understanding and responding to others, we should be careful. People are not always members of the cultures that we think they are, and even when they are, they may be imperfect embodiments of it.

Increasing Your Multicultural Group Skills

Your multicultural group skills may be improved by following the recommendations given earlier in the chapter. For instance, it is a good idea to look for commonalties with group members from other cultures. Reminding yourself and others of the rewards of diversity and taking the time to form accurate impressions are also important. Taking actions designed to increase cohesion, such as socializing together and emphasizing superordinate goals, are also useful in the multicultural group. The previous section on multiculturalism suggests a few more strategies as well:

1. Recognize and override your ethnocentrism.
2. Do not demand that others assimilate. Instead, differentiate (decide it is okay for people to be different), transcend (discuss with the other the conditions

under which each is correct), and integrate (create a group identity that includes elements important to all members).

3. To improve communication and to be inclusive, learn about the cultures of other group members.

4. Be aware of your culture's influence on you so that you can share it with other group members, especially when conflicts result from miscommunication or others seem puzzled by your perspectives or behavior.

5. Encourage other members to appreciate diversity by your reactions to member differences.

6. Encourage other members to share their culture. Greater knowledge of other cultures increases positive attitudes and interpersonal effectiveness.

7. Remember that cultural differences may make the "platinum rule" (treating others the way they want to be treated) more effective than the "golden rule" (treating others the way that you want to be treated).

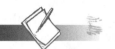

Concept Review

Defining Diversity

- **Diversity** refers to how similar (**member homogeneity**), or different (**member heterogeneity**) group members are from one another. Different types of diversity include **demographic** or **social category diversity, personal diversity, ability and skill diversity,** and **informational diversity.** Two general diversity categories are **surface-level diversity** (demographic and physical characteristics) and **deep-level diversity** (attitudes, values, and beliefs).

Our Discomfort With Diversity

- According to the **similarity attraction paradigm,** we are more comfortable in homogeneous groups because the rewards of interacting with similar others are greater and the costs lower. Similar others provide consensual validation and **reciprocal liking.**

- Similar others are more familiar, and familiarity breeds liking. The more often we are exposed to something, the more we like it (the **mere exposure effect**). We may even experience **intergroup anxiety** when exposed to people who are very different from us—especially when **cultural distance** and **social distance** are great, because these contribute to lack of familiarity.

- The **social categorization approach** suggests that our categorization of people like us as "ingroup" and people unlike us as "outgroup" interferes with unity in the diverse group. The approach emphasizes that stereotypes operate as **schemas** and lead to biased processing of people who are different from us. This schematic processing means that we have difficulty perceiving diverse others fairly and may act toward them in ways that contribute to self-fulfilling prophecies.

Group Process Challenges in Heterogeneous Groups

- Group heterogeneity may reduce member satisfaction and commitment and increase turnover because members may perceive that they lack the shared experiences and identity to fully identify with the group.
- Homogeneous group members may communicate more easily and therefore more frequently. This may lead to exclusionary communications between similar members. Miscommunication may be more likely in the heterogeneous group because of language and communication style differences.
- Conflict may be more likely in the diverse group because of differences in style and perspective, culture clashes, and biased processing of dissimilar others. The development of ingroups and outgroups within the group may also be a source of conflict in the diverse group.

The Value-in-Diversity Hypothesis

- Diversity can enhance group performance by increasing the range of knowledge, skills, and contacts that enhance group problem solving.
- Heterogeneous groups may outperform homogenous groups on tasks requiring creativity and innovation.

Contextual Influences on Diversity and Groups

- The type of task and the type of diversity both affect the influence of diversity on a group.
- Although homogeneous groups may perform better on tasks relying on motor and perceptual skills, for tasks high in difficulty and for nonroutine tasks requiring coordination, heterogeneous groups may be more effective.
- Diverse groups have performance advantages over homogeneous groups on creativity tasks involving different cultures. Diverse groups are better able to develop products, services, and marketing campaigns that appeal to a wider variety of people.
- Some types of diversity may be more relevant in some situations than in others, depending on such factors as job-relatedness, status differences, and cultural stereotypes.
- The relative proportion of members from different subgroups also influences the effects of diversity on a group. Smaller subgroup minorities may experience social isolation and be more likely to experience dissatisfaction and

leave the group. Larger subgroup minorities may be more comfortable because of increased support and more likely to assert themselves regarding perceived inequalities. Larger minorities in the group may also be more threatening to majority subgroups.

Intercultural Approach to Diversity in Groups

- The **intercultural,** or multicultural, **approach** to diversity emphasizes helping people to understand, accept, and value the cultural differences between groups with the goal of reaping the benefits of diversity.
- The idea that groups that are not in the mainstream should give up their culture and become like the majority is called **subtractive multiculturalism** (assimilation). The multicultural approach rejects this idea in favor of **additive multiculturalism,** the addition of skills and perspectives that allow for increased understanding and appreciation of other groups.

melting pot vs salad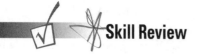

- To become more **interculturally competent,** we need to become aware of the influence of culture on our behavior and recognize that there are other valid ways of doing things and of being in the world. **Ethnocentrism**—the belief that the customs, norms, and values of our culture are universally valid and correct—interferes with intercultural competence.
- **Intercultural competence** requires that we learn about the cultures of other group members so that we can correctly interpret their behavior and avoid offensive behavior.
- Hofstede identified four types of culturally relevant dimensions that are often studied for their effects on group member and leader behavior. These dimensions are **power distance, uncertainty avoidance, individualism/collectivism,** and **masculinity/femininity.**
- It is recommended that we familiarize ourselves with the cultures of others so that we may better understand and respond to group members, but we should avoid the **ecological fallacy**—the mistaken tendency to assume that what is generally true of a culture is true of every member of that culture.

✓ ✱ Skill Review

Increase Similarity and Familiarity

- Work to identify and create similarities with other members.
- Override the tendency to avoid dissimilar others because this just keeps them unfamiliar.
- Do not assume that different others will not like you. Openness and warmth will be reciprocated with openness and warmth.

- If you experience intergroup anxiety, learn more so that differences are no longer anxiety provoking.

Reduce Biased Social Categorization

- Be aware of and question your stereotypes.
- Work to form accurate impressions of individual group members by getting to know them.

Increase Cohesion and Commitment

- Create opportunities for members to have positive experiences together and get to know one another.
- Make an extra effort to solicit the input of new and minority group members.
- Create a superordinate identity through shared goals, a group name, or logo, or a common opponent. Unite the group by creating a shared understanding of the group's issues, concerns, and tasks.

Manage Conflict

- Listen to opposing positions, and work cooperatively to integrate these into a final group position.
- Talk about the group's process and performance and how it can be improved.

Increase Intercultural Competence

- Recognize and override your ethnocentrism.
- Differentiate (decide it is okay for people to be different), transcend (discuss with the other the conditions under which each is correct), and integrate (create a group identity that includes elements important to all members).
- Develop a group culture in which members work to listen and understand others' unique perspectives and experiences.
- Be aware of your culture's influence on your group behavior, especially when conflicts arise from miscommunication or others seem puzzled by your perspectives or behavior.
- Model an appreciation of diversity to other group members.
- Encourage other members to share their culture. Greater knowledge of other cultures increases positive attitudes and increases interpersonal effectiveness.
- Follow the "platinum rule" (treat others the way they want to be treated) rather than the "golden rule" (treating others the way that you want to be treated).

Study Questions

1. What are the different types of diversity studied in group dynamics?
2. How does the similarity attraction paradigm explain our common discomfort with diverse others? How can this information be used to improve group effectiveness?
3. What does the social categorization approach contribute to our understanding of the difficulties facing the group with a diverse membership? What can we do to override our natural tendency to categorize and stereotype group members?
4. Why is member heterogeneity a challenge to member commitment and group cohesion? How can we increase cohesion and commitment in the diverse group?
5. How does member diversity influence conflict? What can be done to reduce conflict in the heterogeneous group?
6. What is the value-in-diversity hypothesis? When is diversity a benefit to the group?
7. What does it mean to say that the influence of diversity on a group depends on the type of task and the type of diversity?
8. How can the proportions of different subgroups in a group affect the group? How are "solos" treated in a group?
9. What is the intercultural approach to diversity? Why have diversity and multicultural theorists rejected subtractive multiculturalism in favor of additive multiculturalism?
10. What are the different ways in which we can respond to diversity? Which ways are the recommended ways according to the intercultural approach?
11. What are the four types of culturally relevant dimensions identified by Hofstede, and how do these affect group behavior? What is the ecological fallacy, and why should it be avoided?
12. What recommendations were given in the chapter for enhancing our intercultural competence?

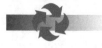

Group Activities

Activity 1: Create Marketing Focus Groups by Considering Diversity and Context

You and your three colleagues have a marketing consulting firm. Companies come to you with their soon-to-be-marketed products, and you conduct focus groups to get feedback to be used in marketing. Your focus groups usually consist of about six people that meet at one time and provide reactions to the new product. With your colleagues, decide the "diversity makeup" (gender, age, ethnicity, skills, and so on) of focus groups for each of the following products: (1) a women's razor, (2) a men's razor, (3) dog food, (4) motor oil, (5) women's cologne, (6) men's cologne, (7) a cruise line, (8) a new cola drink, (9) a fruity snack for lunches, and (10) an action movie. Provide a rationale for your choices.

Activity 2: Discuss Intercultural Experiences

Before meeting in your five- to six-person group for discussion, take twenty minutes to do the following: (1) List those times that you moved from one community to another very different one or traveled to a place culturally different from your home. (2) Choose the one about which you have the most to say, and write down what the experience taught you about the influence of culture on behavior. Did you experience "culture shock"—that is, did the cultural differences create stress or anxiety for you? Did you find that the "new" culture had different ways of thinking and doing things than you were used to? What problems did you encounter as you tried to get your needs met in the new culture? (3) Did you bolster, differentiate, or transcend? (4) Based on your experience, what would you say about the new culture in terms of individualism/collectivism, power distance, uncertainty avoidance, and masculinity/femininity.

Activity 3: Similarity Attraction and Social Categorization in Your Class

In the first part of this activity, you sit in a circle with ten to twelve students. Try to get into a group with people you do not know and who seem somewhat different from you. Have each person make a nameplate for his/her desk by folding a piece of paper into a three-dimensional triangle that will stand up on the desk. Go around the circle and have each member respond *briefly* to the items listed below. Go through the items one at a time; that is, all members first say their ages, then they go around again and all say their majors, and so on.

1. What is your age?
2. What is your major?
3. Do you work for pay? What is your job title?
4. What is your current career goal?
5. Where were you raised?
6. What is your ethnic heritage? Is it an important part of how you define yourself?
7. What skills do you possess?
8. What do you like to do in your spare time?
9. What is your religious background? Is it important to you now?
10. What kind of music do you listen to? Is music important in your life?

When all group members have answered all questions, members individually write down answers to the following questions:

1. Which members do you think you would have the easiest time working with on another group task? Why?
2. Which members do you think you would find more challenging to work with on another group task? Why?
3. The similarity attraction paradigm suggests that your answers to the first two questions would be influenced by your perception of similarity to other group members. Looking back at your answers, does this explain your answers?
4. Which members most surprised you—that is, were not quite what you expected? What lesson can you take from this?
5. Look back at the people you thought might be challenging to work with, and try to think of (a) at least one advantage a group would experience having them as a member and (b) what working with them might be able to teach you.

If your group has the time and the courage, share your answers.

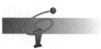

InfoTrac College Edition Search Terms

To do research for your papers and assignments, use InfoTrac that's provided free with new copies of this book. Go to http://infotrac.thomsonlearning.com and enter the following search terms:

- Diversity in Groups
- Similarity-Attraction
- Social Categorization

- Group Composition
- Diversity Training

Chapter 9 Group Productivity

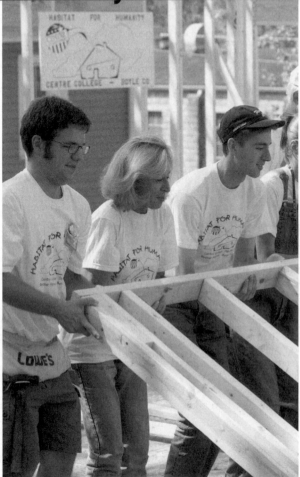

© AFP/CORBIS

Chapter 1 noted that one reason why groups are so common is that groups can accomplish things that individuals cannot. Indeed, it is often the case that a product, service, or goal cannot be created, provided, or reached without the combined efforts of group members. It is likely that your career will require your participation in a workgroup and that your workgroup will receive rewards, financial and otherwise, based on productivity. Group productivity is also important because it assures the future of our economy, the stability of organizations, and a sense of well-being for group members (Pritchard & Watson, 1992). Each chapter of this text discusses topics that have important implications for group productivity. For instance, group members must engage in constructive rather than destructive conflict, lest conflict disrupt their ability to work interdependently and cooperatively. An effective group structure also influences group productivity. Clear group norms and roles promote productivity because members know what is expected of them and whose job it is to do what. Effective leadership and decision making also positively influence group productivity. These two topics are explored in detail in later chapters.

Defining Group Productivity

Efficiency and Effectiveness

Group performance (group productivity)
The quantity or quality of the outcomes produced, or the time required for task completion.

Productivity has been defined in various ways, including the group's output, performance, motivation, efficiency, effectiveness, competitiveness, and work quality. Weldon and Weingart (1993) define **group performance (group productivity)** as the quantity or quality of the outcomes produced, or the time required for task completion. This definition includes both *efficiency* and *effectiveness*, and it makes sense to consider both when speaking of group productivity.

Efficiency
The ratio of inputs to outputs; how much time and resources it takes a group to produce or achieve something.

According to Pritchard and Watson (1992), **efficiency** has to do with the ratio of inputs to outputs—in other words, how much time and resources (including personnel) it takes a group to produce or achieve something. How many meetings does it take a group of students to complete a project? How many practices does a team have to have before it can win a certain number of games? How much money does a group of software engineers have to spend before they perfect a new piece of software? How many nurses are needed to take care of patients when all hospital beds on the unit are full? The fewer the inputs and the greater the outputs, the greater the group's efficiency is.

Effectiveness
The ratio of outputs to goals or expectations; whether the group met or exceeded expectations or goals.

Effectiveness is the ratio of outputs to goals or expectations—in short, whether the group met or exceeded expectations or goals (Pritchard & Watson, 1992). Did the students get the "A" on the project they were striving for? Did the team win the number of games it set out to? Did the software engineers successfully create a software package with few "bugs"? Were the nurses able to take

---

Apply It! ••• Was Your Group Productive?

Think about your most recent job or student project group. Was your workgroup efficient? Did the group accomplish its goals with relative speed and good use of resources? Was your group effective? In general, did the group accomplish its "mission" successfully?

care of all the patients without error and update their medical charts? If the group met or exceeded expectations or goals, the group is effective. Productivity, then, is an index of the output of the group relative to inputs (efficiency), relative to goals (effectiveness), or relative to both.

Group Productivity Is More Than the Sum of Members' Productivity

Workflow interdependence

The extent to which the behavior of one member influences the performance of others and members must cooperate to perform the task.

When you first think of group productivity, you are likely to think of the productivity of individual group members. Indeed, most of the research in psychology on productivity has focused on the productivity of individuals. It is true that the productivity of the group is affected by the productivity of individual members. Also, there are cases in which the group's productivity does not require members to coordinate their efforts and is therefore a simple combination of each member's productivity. However, production of a group product frequently requires that members function *interdependently*, and this requires cooperation and coordination (Pritchard & Watson, 1992). The term **workflow interdependence** refers to the extent to which the behavior of one group member influences the performance of others and the extent to which group members must actually work together to perform the task (Weldon & Weingart, 1993). When workflow interdependence is high and members are unable to coordinate their efforts, productivity will be lowered.

Process loss

Loss of productivity that results from motivational or coordination losses.

Potential Productivity and Actual Productivity

Coordination losses

Process losses that occur when group members do not optimally synchronize their efforts.

Motivational losses

Process losses that occur when members reduce their efforts because they do not value the group or goal or do not think their efforts matter.

Actual productivity

A group's potential productivity minus process losses (*AP = PP − PL*), what they actually accomplish compared to what they could have.

Steiner (1972) suggested that potential productivity is a function of member resources (members' knowledge and skills, availability of tools and other resources) and task demands (such as quantity or quality, simple versus complex). However, according to Steiner, few groups reach their full potential for productivity because of **process loss**. Process loss results from coordination losses and motivation losses. **Coordination losses** occur when group members do not organize their efforts optimally. **Motivational losses** occur when the motivation of individuals is reduced in a group—for instance, because they do not value the group's goal, believe that they are not important to the group, or reduce their efforts because they believe that others are not working hard. Therefore, the **actual productivity** (AP) of a group equals its potential productivity (PP) minus process losses (PL) such as motivational and coordination problems (Steiner, 1972). Steiner summarized this relationship in the following equation:

$$AP = PP - PL$$

Steiner's (1972) elegant formula focused researchers' attention on motivational and coordination problems as well as on the conditions under which groups seem to perform better than individuals. Much of this chapter focuses on increasing group productivity by reducing motivational and coordination losses.

Process gain

When group work increases productivity because it causes members to work harder or more efficiently.

Ideally, we seek a **process gain** from group work as a result of members' mutual encouragement, learning from one another, more efficient workload sharing, and better error capturing because team members are able to cross-check one another's work (Bowers, Pharmer, & Salas, 2000).

Preventing Motivational Losses With Group Goals

People are motivated by goals. In Chapter 1, you learned that one feature of groups is that they have goals that direct the behavior of the group and give the group purpose. Group goals are goals that group members perceive as having been consensually agreed upon or imposed by group members (Cartwright & Zander, 1968). Group goals are especially important to productivity because effectiveness requires that groups set group goals that all members commit themselves to cooperate in achieving. This idea is an old one in the field of group dynamics. Both Lewin (1935) and Festinger (1950) suggested that group locomotion (movement forward of the group) requires that group members agree on where they want to go and how they are going to get there. Looked at in terms of Steiner's definition of actual productivity, it may be said that under the right conditions, group goals reduce motivational losses and therefore increase actual productivity. According to Locke and Latham (1990), goals energize and direct human behavior by focusing our attention on those activities relevant to goal attainment. Group goals improve group performance because group members work faster and longer on the task, focus more attention on it, and are less distracted by irrelevant stimuli (Locke & Latham, 1990).

Many studies have demonstrated that group goals enhance productivity. These studies show that the group goal effect holds across tasks, settings, the method used to set the goal, and goals for quantity, quality, or speed (Weldon & Weingart, 1993). For instance, positive effects of group goal setting have been found in studies on hard rock mining (Buller & Bell, 1986), group papers for class assignments (Klein & Mulvey, 1989), the performance of safe work behaviors (Komaki, Heinzmann, & Lawson, 1980), the quality of restaurant performance (O'Leary et al., 1989), truck loading and unloading (Runnon, Johnson, & McWhorter, 1978), harvesting and hauling lumber (Latham & Locke, 1975), and raising money for the United Way (Zander, Forward, & Albert, 1969). In a qualitative review, Locke and Lathams (1990) found positive effects of group goal setting in 93 percent of the forty-one group goal setting studies available. Using meta-analysis, O'Leary-Kelly, Martocchio, and Frink (1994) statistically combined results of twenty-nine studies and found a strong positive effect of group goal setting (versus no goal setting) on group performance.

Given the importance of goals in directing a group's activity, it is perhaps not surprising that many group productivity problems may be traced to problems with the group's goals. If your group is not making progress, this may signal a problem with its goals. Sometimes groups are unclear as to what their goals are and do not know what they are supposed to accomplish. Ambiguous goals do not provide the group with direction. How can the group perform when members do not clearly understand what their goal is? You may have seen this in student learning groups when professors or teachers provide the group with minimal instruction. Task forces, committees, and project groups may also experience this problem if given only a general mission. New groups may also suffer from a lack of productivity because of confusion about the group's goals. Attendees at a meeting may spend precious meeting time fooling around because they are unclear about the goals of the group or the goals of the meeting. Until the group's goals are specified, the group's meetings are likely to be chaotic and unproductive.

Group productivity problems may also arise when members do not agree about the goals for their group or because members make different assumptions about what the goal of the group is. This could happen if some group members think the goal is quantity, whereas others believe the goal is quality. In a student project group, some might think the goal is to get the project over with, while others think the goal is to get an "A." Too often, groups do not explicitly talk about goals, and this may reduce productivity because the group does not know where to direct its energies, or because members do not agree on the goals of the group.

Commitment to Group Goals

If there is no commitment to goals, then goal setting will not work (Locke, Latham, & Erez, 1988). Commitment to group goals means that group members feel an attachment to the goal, and group members are determined that the group should reach the goal (Weldon & Weingart, 1993). The two major determinants of goal commitment are thought to be *attractiveness of goal attainment* and *belief that goals can be met* (Hollenbeck & Klein, 1987; Locke & Latham, 1990). In other words, reaching the goal has to have some attraction for members, and they have to believe that the group will be successful in reaching its goals if members put forth the effort to do so. Figure 9-1 summarizes the factors influencing commitment to group goals.

 Weldon and Weingart (1993) identify four important factors that influence the attractiveness of goal attainment: (1) satisfaction of individual desires, (2) identification with the group, (3) procedures used to set the goals, and (4) compatibility with personal goals.

Satisfaction of individual desires   Group members will find goal attainment attractive if it validates their sense of self-worth. Being a member of a successful group may boost self-esteem. Achieving the group goal may bring positive regard from members outside of the group. Desirable rewards may be received or punishments avoided only if the group's goal is attained. Imagine the commitment of a basketball player to the goal of winning a game. He or she might think, "I

Figure 9-1

Factors Influencing Commitment to Group Goals

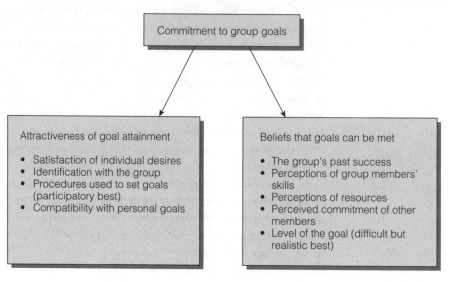

am special, I am a member of a winning team. Others are impressed by the fact that I am a member of a winning team. I want the positive attention that comes with winning, and I want to avoid the coaches' disappointment and the public humiliation that would come with losing."

Identification with the group   Group goals become individual goals when members identify strongly with a group. Recall social identity theory and the notion of collective self-esteem. If being a member of the group is a central part of your identity, then group success is going to be important to you. Members of cohesive groups are more committed to group goal attainment. In such cases, the individual works hard for "us" not just for "me."

Procedures used to set the goals   Attractiveness of the group's goals is greater when the goals are perceived as legitimate. Legitimacy has to do with whether the person who sets the goal is perceived as having the right to do so, whether the goal is believed to be consistent with the group's mission, and whether the goal was determined in an ethical and unbiased way. Imagine, for instance, a district manager delivering to subordinates a set of sales goals for the group in her or his territory. He or she does this without consulting the subordinates and sets sales targets that are unrealistic given that another company has seriously undercut their prices. The group believes that to keep sales numbers steady, they are going to have to work harder than ever. The group members resent the outside imposition of goals by a person they feel is unqualified to set their goals, and thus they do not comply with them.

Take the case of my student Kristin, a video store employee who checked videos in and out for customers. Corporate headquarters assigned Kristin and her fellow employees the task of selling America Online subscriptions to customers renting videos. Management assigned them a goal of selling 5000 new memberships. If they did so, managers would reap a $1000 bonus, and employees like Kristin would receive fifty dollars. The problems with the plan were numerous. For one, had she been consulted, Kristin would have told the higher-ups that this goal was very likely unattainable; customers were generally in a hurry at checkout, making signing up for AOL unlikely. Second, had they consulted Kristin, they would have learned that the goal was unattractive to those required to make it happen; fifty dollars was not enough to motivate the employees to sacrifice their dignity to make a pitch to customers likely to respond with irritation. The project was a disaster, and the store and AOL lost money on it.

In general, research on assigned (by a supervisor or leader) and participative (set after consultation) goal setting has found that both strategies enhance performance, but participative goal setting is somewhat more advantageous. For instance, a review of the group goal literature by O'Leary-Kelly and her colleagues (1994) found that a positive effect was found in 78 percent of the studies using an assigned group goal and 100 percent of the studies that used a goal set with members' participation. A study by Erez, Earley, and Hulin (1985) found that when the goal was perceived as difficult or undesirable, participative goal setting enhanced goal acceptance, and subsequently performance, in contrast to assigned goals. They note that when goals are not especially difficult or undesirable, members may accept them whether they have participated in setting them or not. They concluded that if group members feel that the group's goals were derived through a fair and democratic process, they are more likely to accept the goals, even if they initially rejected them as unreasonable or too difficult. Other studies have also found that self-set goals are more effective than assigned goals when the task is complex and strategies for reaching the goals are developed (Chesney & Locke, 1991; Durham, Knight, & Locke, 1997).

Many researchers and theorists advocate member participation in the setting of group goals. In most cases, it is wise to include members in the determination of goals that affect their work, especially if the goal is difficult or the leader lacks credibility with the group. There are other advantages as well. Lewin (1951a) suggested that **participative decision making** (PDM) increases knowledge and understanding of the task. Similarly, it has been suggested that participation in goal setting clarifies expectations and results in the discovery of information relevant to task performance, thereby enhancing performance (Latham, Winters, & Locke, 1994; Locke & Latham, 1990; Scully, Kirkpatrick, & Locke, 1995). In other words, the discussion of goals provides knowledge of the strategies needed to perform the tasks to attain the goal, without which performance will be low. Some have suggested that participation in goal setting increases individuals' sense of control over the goal,

Participative decision making

The involvement of group members in the setting of goals or making of decisions.

leading to greater acceptance of the goal and, ultimately, greater performance (Erez et al., 1985; Erez & Kanfer, 1983). Others believe that PDM increases commitment to the goal (Lawler & Hackman, 1969) and results in the setting of higher goals (Zander, 1979), although others disagree that PDM has these motivational effects (Latham et al., 1994; Locke & Latham, 1990; Wagner & Gooding, 1987).

Talking about group goals not only ensures that group members are "all on the same page," it also increases commitment to their achievement. Ideally, goals should be talked about until consensus is reached and everyone feels a sense of ownership and a commitment to cooperate. Group discussion and agreement regarding group goals also ensures that goals are communicated as group norms, or expectations regarding appropriate behavior in the group. As you already know, most people are motivated to conform to group norms to avoid social rejection, or because they need information from the group. In addition to clearly identifying goals and obtaining consensus regarding their importance, group discussion also motivates and directs task behavior as the group plans how to achieve the goals. London (1997) recommends that each member's goals and commitment to those goals be measured before group performance to be sure that members agree.

Compatibility with personal goals   Group members are more committed to goals that are compatible with their personal goals. Personal goals are compatible with group goals when working toward one ensures progress toward the other. Conversely, attractiveness to the group goal decreases when meeting the official goal will interfere with personal goal attainment. For instance, an employee's goal of doing as little as possible may be incompatible with the group's goal of increasing productivity.

Weldon and Weingart (1993) suggest that commitment to goals is strongly influenced by members' beliefs that the group can meet the goals. Simply put, members are not going to commit to goals they do not believe they can reach. The group's past success, the skills of group members, other demands on the group's resources, the perceived commitment of other group members, and the level of the goal all influence these expectations regarding the group's potential success. If group members do not believe they have adequate resources or skills to reach a goal, then commitment is reduced. Likewise, members are unlikely to commit to a goal if they believe other members are not committed to it. This is more of a problem in the noncohesive group. In cohesive groups, members are more likely to be committed to the group's goals, and when some members are not committed, they may experience pressure from committed members (Klein & Mulvey, 1995; Weldon & Weingart, 1993).

Specific and Difficult (Yet Realistic) Goals

It is well established that goal setting works best when the goals are specific and difficult, yet realistic (Latham & Locke, 1990; O'Leary-Kelly et al., 1994; Weldon & Weingart, 1993). Individuals and groups work harder when they set specific goals as targets for productivity. "We will do our best" and other general goals do not motivate group performance to the extent that specific goals do. A performance plan outlining a strategy for reaching larger group goals (with target dates for the completion of tasks) is far more effective than simply vowing to work harder or setting a goal without thinking about the specific strategies for reaching it.

Ideally, the goal must be a moderate challenge—hard enough to provide satisfaction when it is achieved, but not so hard that it is never met. Groups that consistently fail to reach their goals may feel shame or lose interest. Also, disharmony may result if group members blame one another for the lack of success. Unfortunately, according to Zander (1982), many groups choose goals more difficult than they have hopes of achieving and, for this reason, fail to reach their goals more often than they succeed. Groups choose difficult goals because they will get more done and feel more pride if they succeed (or come close). Also, group members will not feel embarrassed if their group falls short of a very difficult objective. However, goals that are too difficult will result in the group's failure and lead to discouragement.

Groups are often the best judges of what a realistically challenging goal is for them. However, groups may face external pressures to set unrealistic goals that lead to group failure (Zander, 1982). People or other groups may pressure the group to raise its goals. Customers may demand increased production of a scarce item, and quality may suffer. Comparison with a rival group can lead to higher goals, as when a company compares its sales figures to those of a similar company. Outside commentators may criticize the group or communicate high expectations for the group, pressuring them to set higher goals. Imagine, for instance, a columnist on the business pages of a well-respected newspaper commenting about how long it is taking a company to bring out a new product. Such a public statement would put pressure on the research and design team to push the product's development. Some organizations bring in "efficiency consultants" who evaluate the group's work and sometimes push the group to raise their goals to unrealistic levels. Superiors who are distanced from the day-to-day workings of the group and the constraints they experience may also demand that the group achieve an unrealistic goal.

Feedback Regarding the Group's Progress Toward the Goal

Research indicates that without feedback about the group's progress toward goal attainment, group goals are not very effective in increasing performance. In other words, group members need clear information regarding their progress toward attaining the goal. Zander (1996) recommends that the group's past performance on the task (or ones like it) be reviewed so that clear and challenging yet reasonable goals can be set. The group's goals then need to be stated in measurable terms so that it is possible to monitor progress and provide feedback (Zander,

Feedback cycle

A cycle in which group members set success criteria, perform, compare the performance with criteria, and set new goals or procedures, before beginning again.

1996). Weldon and Weingart (1993) suggest that feedback is important to the success of goal-setting interventions because it allows members to adjust their behavior when monitoring suggests that the goal will not be met. For instance, group members can increase their effort, change their plans, offer additional help to members, divert resources from competing demands, and engage in morale building. Zander (1996) calls this a **feedback cycle.** In a feedback cycle, members set criteria for success of an activity, perform the activity, compare the group's performance with the criteria, decide what to do in light of this evaluation, set new goals or procedures, and move through the cycle again.

Using Group Goals to Enhance Productivity

To summarize, group goals enhance productivity, especially when goals are specific and somewhat difficult, group members are committed to the goals, they receive feedback regarding progress, members believe the group is capable of achieving the goals, and the group understands how the goals can be achieved. Given these guidelines, here are some suggestions for the use of group goals.

1. Obtain accurate measures of the group's past performance, and consider this when setting goals.
2. Set specific rather than ambiguous or general goals; attainment of the goals should be measurable in some way.
3. Set challenging but not unrealistic goals.
4. In most cases, goal setting should involve consultation with group members so they agree with and are committed to the group's goals.
5. Break large projects into subgoals (objectives), and set realistic deadlines for their completion. Make sure that the group has a strategy or performance plan for reaching the goals.
6. Have a method for determining how well a goal is being accomplished, and provide feedback to the group regarding progress toward goals.
7. Make sure members understand the value of a group goal—that is, the pride and approval the group will experience if successful.
8. Encourage outsiders to place realistic demands on the group.
9. Make sure that members are trained in the proper task strategies to reach the goals.
10. Encourage members to recommend changes in equipment or organization that will increase effectiveness.

Apply It! ••• **Improve Productivity With Group Goals**

How could group goal setting be used at your job, in a student project group, or in a membership organization (sorority or fraternity, hobby or sports group, or community activism group) to increase group productivity?

Social Loafing: A Common Motivational Loss

Social loafing

The tendency for individuals to reduce their effort on group tasks, especially common when individual efforts cannot be identified or are not identified.

Group members who do not do their share frustrate us and create resentment. We think it is unfair that such individuals share equally in the group's rewards when they have not made a significant contribution to the group's product. You may call such people "slackers," "leeches," or "freeloaders," but the official term in group dynamics is "social loafers." **Social loafing** is defined as the tendency for individuals to reduce their effort on group tasks. It is most likely on collective tasks where an individual's contributions are pooled with those of other group members and individual efforts cannot be identified, or are not identified.

The study of social loafing is important because so many group tasks are collective tasks that require the pooling of individual efforts to produce a group product (Karau & Williams, 1993). Task forces, committees, sports teams, orchestras, bands, and juries are just a few of the types of groups that fall into this category. Social loafing is one reason why actual group productivity may fall short of potential productivity (George, 1995). In some cases, group productivity is lowered because members who exert maximum effort are unable to fully compensate for loafers' reduced efforts. Group productivity may also suffer if other group members lower their efforts so as not to be "suckers" or feel taken advantage of (Jackson & Harkins, 1985; Kerr, 1983). Understanding social loafing is important so that we can reduce it in everyday groups and organizations.

Social loafing is one of the most studied motivational losses experienced by groups. A French agricultural engineer by the name of Ringelmann conducted the original social loafing studies in the late 1800s and early 1900s. Ringelmann (1913, cited in Kravitz & Martin, 1986) found that individual output declined when people were working in a group on such tasks as rope pulling or cart pushing. In the 1970s, research on social loafing resumed as researchers tried to determine whether individuals exerted less effort when working with others or whether the problem was one of coordinating group members' efforts. Ingham, Levinger, Graves, and Peckham (1974) replicated Ringelmann's work using a rope-pulling machine that determined how hard each member pulled. They blindfolded participants and led half to believe that they were pulling alone and the other half that they were pulling with a group (all participants were actually pulling alone). They then instructed participants to pull as hard as they could. Participants pulled almost 20 percent harder when they thought they were pulling alone, suggesting that the problem was not one of coordination. They termed this behavior "the Ringelmann effect."

It was Latane and his colleagues who coined the term "social loafing." In a classic study, Latane, Williams, and Harkins (1979) found that social loafing occurred in clapping and cheering tasks. College student participants cheered and clapped alone and in groups of two, four, or six persons (each person performed in each condition). They were told to clap or cheer as loudly as possible at specific times, ostensibly so that the researchers could determine how much noise people make in social settings. Although larger groups made more noise, the amount of noise generated by each participant dropped as group size increased. Two-person groups performed at only 71 percent of the sum of their individual capability, four-person groups at 51 percent, and six-person groups at 40 percent. The researchers suggested that members of a group perceive themselves as sharing equal responsibility for the group's task, and when the size of the group increases, each individual's share of the responsibility diminishes proportionately. They concluded that social loafing might be regarded as a kind of "social disease" in that it may have negative consequences for individuals, social institutions, and society.

Since the 1970s, more than eighty social loafing studies have been conducted. Many of these are reviewed in a meta-analysis conducted by Karau and Williams (1993). They conclude that the social loafing effect is reliable and generalizes across tasks and different types of research participants. For instance, social loafing has been found to occur in relay-race swimming (Miles & Greenberg, 1993; Williams, Nida, Baca, & Latane, 1989); evaluation of poems, editorials, or jobs (Petty, Harkins, Williams, & Latane, 1977; Weldon & Gargano, 1988); and generating uses for objects (Harkins & Petty, 1982). Veiga (1991) found social loafing in work teams to be widespread among a sample of 571 managers working for U.S. business organizations.

Explaining Social Loafing

Why would people fail to do their share of a group's work when it is likely that they may be perceived as lazy or uncaring? As you will learn in this section, the causes of social loafing are variable and cannot be reduced to personality alone.

Evaluation potential   One of the most accepted explanations for social loafing is that individuals do not believe that their individual efforts will be evaluated. In short, they think that their individual efforts will go unnoticed or unrewarded and that lack of effort will not be punished (Latane et al., 1979). The idea is that people can "hide in the crowd" and get away with poor performance when their individual outputs are not identifiable and that they are unmotivated if they will not receive credit for their efforts (Williams, Harkins, & Latane, 1981). Indeed, lack of identifiability of individual efforts is an important cause of social loafing. For instance, a study of retail salespeople found that when supervisors recognized employees individually for work effort, social loafing was lower (George, 1995). When individuals think that their efforts will be identifiable to others and may be evaluated, social loafing is less likely (Harkins & Jackson, 1985; Harkins & Szymanski, 1988, 1989).

Dispensability of effort   Social loafing may also occur because individuals do not believe that their contributions will make a difference in the group's performance. If members know that the task will be accomplished without their assistance and that they will enjoy the rewards despite their low participation, they may rationally choose not to waste their energy. For instance, my son's math teacher has the students work in small groups to solve problems. All that is required for success is for one child to come up with the right answer. The children in his group have discovered that my son is usually that person; therefore, they are content to just let my son do it. Kerr and Bruun (1983) found that when participants were led to believe that their efforts were dispensable, they loafed. These effects are often called **free rider effects.** A free rider is one who withholds contributions and benefits from the contributions of others who they believe can and will provide for task success.

Free rider effects

When some members are "free riders" benefiting from others' efforts, usually because they believe that their own efforts are dispensable.

At first glance, the behavior of the free rider appears rational. However, free riders often fail to take into account the possibility that others may elect to be free riders as well, such that the group's task is not accomplished. Free riders may also contribute to the **sucker effect.** A sucker is a group member who provides for task success when other capable members make little or no effort. The sucker effect occurs when "suckers" reduce their efforts because they do not want to "carry" capable free riders any longer (Kerr, 1983; Kerr & Bruun, 1983). Often, they are tired of being taken advantage of and want to teach the free riders a lesson. Kerr (1983) suggests that the sucker effect happens for several reasons. First, it violates a social norm of equity: It is not fair that some do more than others and all receive equal rewards. Second, it violates the reciprocity norm: You are benefiting from my contributions, and I should benefit from yours. Third, it violates the social responsibility norm: It is the responsibility of all members to contribute to the group. Kerr found that in many cases the feelings of exploitation aroused by free riders were so strong that suckers would make the seemingly irrational choice to fail on the task rather than carry a free rider.

Sucker effect

When group members who previously compensated for loafing members reduce their efforts because they are tired of being taken advantage of.

Together, free rider and sucker effects may create social dilemmas. A **social dilemma** occurs when the pursuit of rational self-interest leads to collective disaster (Kerr, 1983). In other words, if able group members loaf and others respond by reducing their contributions so that they are not suckers, then some or all of the group's work may go undone. Kerr gives the example of soldiers in their foxholes who stay in their foxholes (free riders) because they reason that someone else is bound to lead the charge against the enemy (suckers). Now imagine that the suckers decide that they are being taken advantage of and that they are not going to risk their lives for the benefit of the free riders. They too stay in their foxholes, and the battle is lost. Likewise, the battle for a clean house may be lost if some roommates are free riders, others are suckers, and the suckers stop cleaning in an effort to restore equity, the renters lose their security deposit when they leave because of the damage.

Social dilemma

When so many members act selfishly that the group and its members are harmed and productivity is negatively affected.

The Collective Effort Model of Social Loafing

Recently, theorists such as Karau and Williams (1993) and Shepperd and Taylor (1999) have integrated the various explanations for social loafing into a model known as the **collective effort model.** This explanation relies on an extension of

Collective effort model

Suggests that social loafers slack because they do not think their efforts will increase group performance, increase rewards, or lead to valued outcomes, so they slack.

Expectancy

In expectancy-valence theory, a belief that increased effort will lead to increased performance.

Instrumentality

In expectancy-valence theory, a belief that increased performance will be rewarded and recognized.

Valence

In expectancy-valence theory, whether the rewards or outcomes from increased performance are valued.

expectancy-valence theory—a theory of individual motivation. Expectancy-valence theory (Porter & Lawler, 1968) predicts that effort motivation will be high when individuals (1) believe that increased effort will lead to increased performance (**expectancy**), (2) believe that increased performance will be recognized and rewarded (**instrumentality**), and (3) value the rewards or outcomes that increased performance brings (**valence**). According to the theory, if expectancy, instrumentality, or valence is zero, then the individual will not be motivated. To get a sense of the theory, think about your motivation in your classes. You need to believe that trying hard will make a difference in your academic performance (high expectancy). If you try hard and you do not get any closer to mastering the material, you will not be motivated to make the effort (low expectancy). You also need to believe that increased performance will lead to better grades or personal satisfaction (high instrumentality). If you believe that better performance will not result in increased rewards, you will not be motivated (low instrumentality). And last, while you may believe that increased effort will lead to increased performance and that increased performance will lead to increased rewards, you must value the better grades or sense of personal satisfaction (high valence) to be motivated to make the effort to get the rewards.

The collective effort model, summarized in Figure 9-2, applies this thinking to social loafing and the motivation to exert effort on a group task. Karau and Williams (1993) point out that in collective settings, where efforts are pooled, to be motivated to exert effort on a collective task, individuals must believe that their increased efforts will increase the *group's* performance. Otherwise, they will not view their efforts as useful and will not be motivated to work hard on the task. They must also believe that increased group performance will lead to desired outcomes for the group and for them personally. Finally, if they do not value the outcomes, they will not be motivated to work hard, even if their efforts would enhance group performance and lead to increased outcomes. Karau and Williams (1993) note that valued outcomes may be objective outcomes such as pay, or subjective outcomes such as enjoyment, satisfaction, feelings of group spirit and belonging, and feelings of self-worth.

Karau and Williams' (1993) meta-analysis of seventy-eight studies provides support for the model. Another, more recent study also found that people in groups will work hard for a valued outcome if instrumentality is high (Shepperd & Taylor, 1999). Perhaps some comments made by my social loafer students will help to explain why. One group of loafers reports that although they may be perceived as loafers by other students, their lack of effort is actually due to the actions of dominant group members. These dominant members take over the task and discourage the participation of others by shooting down their ideas and announcing what is to be done and how. Not wanting to assert themselves, and believing that the self-designated leaders of the group do not want or value their contributions, these individuals retreat. In other words, the actions of dominant group members suggest to less dominant members that their efforts are unimportant

Figure 9-2

The Collective Effort Model

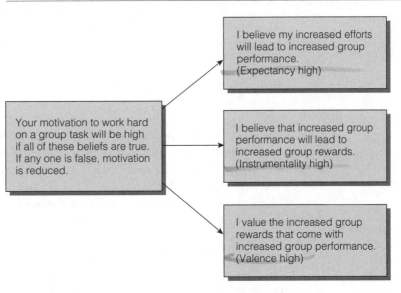

Your motivation to work hard on a group task will be high if all of these beliefs are true. If any one is false, motivation is reduced.

I believe my increased efforts will lead to increased group performance. (Expectancy high)

I believe that increased group performance will lead to increased group rewards. (Instrumentality high)

I value the increased group rewards that come with increased group performance. (Valence high)

to the group's performance, so they have low expectancy. Instrumentality is also low because they are aware that the group receives a grade, and this grade is not connected to their effort.

A second group of loafers does not attribute their loafing to the behavior of dominant group members. They simply believe that their efforts have little to do with the group's performance and the group's grade and, having other assignments to do and feeling little allegiance to this group of relative strangers, choose to loaf. Interestingly, research indicates that group cohesion reduces social loafing (Hardy & Latane, 1988; Williams & Sommer, 1997; Worchel, Hart, & Butemeyer, 1989). A cohesive group is in some ways an extension of the self, and the group's success becomes as important as one's own (Williams & Sommer, 1997). Also, we care more about what fellow group members think when the group is cohesive.

A third group of loafers reports that they will loaf when a grade of "A" is not of high valence to them. In other words, such students may believe that if they put forth more effort the group would perform better, and that increased performance would lead to a better grade for the group, but because they do not value the higher grade, they loaf. For instance, I had a student named Mike who was in a major that required many group projects. He was a student in my group dynamics class during his last term before graduating. He was admittedly a terrible social loafer that quarter, unabashedly saying that he didn't care about his grades as long as he passed and didn't care about his fellow students because he was leaving town.

Apply It! ••• Reflect on Your Loafing

Have you ever been a social loafer who let other group members do the work of the group? Most people can come up with a least one situation in which they have played the loafer. In what situation did you loaf? Was it at work, at home, or at school? Which explanations of social loafing explain your loafing?

Those students who report that they often "end up doing all the work" sometimes acknowledge their own role in making loafers of others. In particular, they admit that they may contribute to the passivity of other group members because they do not trust others to do the job well. They frequently cite previous experiences with loafers. They also report ambivalence about taking over the task. On the one hand, they wish others would participate more to reduce the workload; on the other hand, they dislike the stress of wondering whether the job is going to be done they way they think it ought to be. From an expectancy-valence point of view, these students have high expectancies, high instrumentality, and high valence and low or uncertain expectancies about others.

Gender, Culture, and Social Loafing

Some people do not loaf even when their efforts are unidentifiable or the job will get done without them. Karau and Williams (1993) note that people differ on whether they are more individually competitive, valuing individual over group success, or view collective outcomes as valuable and important. These differences mean that some people are motivated to work hard for a collective outcome even if their individual efforts are not identifiable. Karau and Williams (1993) suggest that gender and culture may influence the degree to which an individual values collective outcomes relative to individual outcomes.

Some theorists suggest that gender roles may affect social loafing. In comparison to males, females are generally socialized to exhibit more communal qualities, such as friendliness, cooperativeness, and a concern for others. In contrast, males are encouraged to develop more agentic qualities, such as competitiveness and assertiveness (Burn, 1996). Karau and Williams (1993) predicted that women would loaf less than men because women place greater value on group harmony, group success, satisfaction of other group members, and other group members' evaluations of one's individual contributions to the group. Consistent with their prediction, they found that social loafing was greatest in studies that used only male subjects. Furthermore, for male groups only, the magnitude of the social loafing was greater as group size increased. The authors suggest that men may pay more attention to the reduced efficacy of their inputs when group size is large, whereas women's efforts are more consistent regardless of group size.

A study of the effects of social ostracism on social loafing also found gender differences (Williams & Sommer, 1997). Social ostracism is the perception of being ignored by others in one's presence. Social rejection evokes strong negative emotions because it violates our need for belonging and our belief that we are good and worthy people. Williams and Sommer (1997) asked participants to generate as many uses as they could for an object, either coactively (working alongside others but producing individual output) or collectively (combining their outputs with the outputs of others to form a single group product). Participants worked with two others who had either ostracized them or included them in an earlier ball-tossing exchange. The researchers found that ostracized females attempted to remedy their sense of exclusion by socially compensating—maximizing their efforts on a group task. In contrast, males who were ostracized were more likely to respond with social loafing, disengaging from a group that appeared to reject them. The researchers offer a gender role interpretation of their findings. Specifically, they suggest that females were more willing to admit that they felt ostracized and to question their desirability as group members. Males, who have been socialized to avoid acknowledging their hurt feelings, reacted by reinterpreting the exclusion as being due to their personal choice and by directing their attention to objects in the environment (tying shoes, looking through a backpack). In addition, the researchers found that the females worked harder in the collective condition than they did in the coactive condition, whereas this made no difference in the effort of the male participants. In the collective condition, females reported feeling significantly more responsible to their groups than did males.

Karau and Williams (1993) also postulated that social loafing would be influenced by culture. In particular, they expected that social loafing would be strongest in studies with research participants from individualistic countries, such as the United States, whose cultures focus on individual achievement and autonomy. Conversely, they expected that participants in studies conducted in collectivistic countries, whose cultures are more group-oriented and place a high value on being a good group member, would loaf less. Their prediction was supported. Research participants in Japan, Taiwan, and China loafed less than did research participants in the United States and Canada.

Although replications of the shouting and clapping social loafing studies in a number of Eastern cultures found some evidence of social loafing, in general, the research indicates that social loafing is less common in collectivistic cultures when more complex tasks are used. Some cross-cultural social loafing studies have even found that participants from Pacific-Asian cultures work harder in groups (Earley, 1989, 1993; Gabrenya, Wang, & Latane, 1985; Matsui, Kakuyama, & Onglatco, 1987). For example, one study conducted by Earley (1989) compared managers from the United States and from China. He found that the American managers worked harder alone than when told they were part of a group of ten, whereas the reverse was true of the Chinese managers. In another study, Earley (1993) found that ratings of actual performance of Chinese and Israeli managers were higher when they believed they were working in a group but lower for American managers in the group condition.

Suggestions for Reducing Social Loafing

Social loafing is potentially costly to group productivity and group harmony, so reducing social loafing is important. The reduction of social loafing may involve confronting loafers and structuring the task in such a way that loafing is less likely. Too often, though, we let loafing go on because it is difficult for us to criticize a group member, and our fear of conflict and others' anger or defensiveness prevents us from doing so constructively. Instead, we are likely to talk behind the loafers' backs, fume in silence, or give them the "cold shoulder." Loafers do not always get these subtle messages, however. In fact, loafers often assume that other group members are comfortable with their low level of participation or "they would say something." Take the case of my student Sasha who, after confronting her roommates about the lack of housework they did, was surprised to hear that they thought she liked doing the housework because she always did it without complaining! Meanwhile, she was so resentful she was thinking about moving out and getting new roommates.

Confronting loafers does not mean launching a personal attack about their laziness or lack of consideration. What it does mean is assuring them that their contributions are important to the group's performance, and that increased group performance will bring greater group and personal outcomes. More specifically, to reduce social loafing, try the following:

1. Persuade members that group performance is dependent on their efforts and their contribution is unique and important (that they are not dispensable).
2. Make sure that group members value the outcomes of increased group performance.
3. Emphasize that valued outcomes are dependent on performance.
4. Build group cohesion so that members value the group and others' impressions of them.
5. Increase the identifiability of individual contributions. For instance, in reports to supervisors, managers, or teachers, describe the division of labor (who did what toward the group's product). If you are the leader, be in touch enough with the group that individuals feel that you will notice their contributions.
6. Constructively confront loafers, explaining that their efforts are important to the group's accomplishing the task, and that their loafing may result in social disapproval from other group members and leaders.
7. If possible, delegate tasks in such a way that members are given tasks that they find personally meaningful and involving.

8. Have individuals work in smaller, as opposed to larger, groups.
9. Provide a standard to which individuals can compare their group's performance.

Improving Group Coordination to Reduce Coordination Loss

Group Coordination

Group coordination
The ways in which group members synchronize their actions in order to successfully complete the group task; who does what, when, where, and how.

The ways in which group members synchronize their actions in order to successfully complete the group task is referred to as **group coordination** (Wittenbaum, Vaughan, & Stasser, 1998). Group coordination includes who does what, when, where, and how. As noted by Steiner (1972), if group efforts are poorly orchestrated, then actual productivity will fall short of potential productivity. In short, coordination losses occur when group members do not optimally coordinate their efforts. The greater the workflow interdependence, the more critical group coordination is to the group's productivity. Think about it this way: If doing your job is dependent on others' doing theirs, then workflow interdependence is high and the coordination of your efforts with the efforts of others is especially important.

Tacit Coordination

Tacit coordination
Occurs when members do not specifically discuss how they are going to accomplish the task and operate according to their assumptions.

Tacit coordination, or implicit coordination, is a frequent cause of process loss. Many groups tacitly coordinate their efforts; that is, they never specifically discuss how they are going to accomplish the task. Instead, members come into the group with expectations regarding the task, other group members, and the work environment and operate according to these (Gersick, 1988). Productivity suffers if members proceed according to differing "mental models" of the group and the task (Rouse, Cannon-Bowers, & Salas, 1992; Wittenbaum et al., 1998). Wittenbaum et al. (1998) identify a number of potential coordination problems that may arise from such incorrect assumptions. For example, members may duplicate one another's work while leaving other tasks undone.

Another problem with tacit coordination is that the group may incorrectly identify the most and least capable members for various tasks on the basis of stereotypes (Wittenbaum et al., 1996, 1998). As discussed in the chapters on status and diversity, people often make mistaken assumptions about other group members based on diffuse status characteristics such as ethnicity, age, and gender. Prejudice can lead to process loss when some group members duplicate the efforts of others because they assume that others are not capable, or when they assign someone less capable to perform a task because their stereotypes prevent them from seeing a qualified member from a stereotyped group as more capable.

Tacit coordination does not always lead to process loss. If unspoken assumptions made by members are congruent (match one another), then coordination should not be a problem. This is more likely in a group that has some history together, for they are better able to assess their own and other members' skills, abilities, and expertise (Moreland, Argote, & Krishman, 1996). For instance, think about a long-standing work team that has successfully completed many similar projects together. These experiences make it likely that members' assumptions about one another and the task are harmonious. Discussions of strategy would be an inefficient use of time that could be better spent on task completion. However, as Wittenbaum et al. (1998) caution, the more tacit the group members' roles, the more difficult it will be to replace members and maintain a functioning group. In groups that operate tacitly, recruitment of new members may be difficult because members may be vague on the role and tasks performed by the departed member.

Another problem with the tacitly coordinated group is that membership change may lead to production losses because new members may not have access to the group's implicit assumptions. The group may not think to articulate and share these assumptions. After all, in their memory, the tasks were always accomplished without explicit coordination. I saw this happen when I was a department chair. Most of our faculty members had worked in the department for more than twenty years and had tacit understandings about how to conduct various committee tasks. However, as "junior" members of the department advanced and were placed on these committees, we had some problems because it was unclear to them how the tasks were to be accomplished. Meanwhile, "senior" members who were used to carrying out these duties almost unconsciously, with little explicit coordination, were puzzled and frustrated when junior members did not carry out a task in the expected way. This experience demonstrates how membership change can render previously effective tacit coordination systems ineffective. It also shows how "unconscious" these systems may be and how important it is to make them conscious when socializing new members into the group.

In summary, the following are situations in which tacit coordination systems are effective and taking the time to explicitly plan or coordinate members' efforts may reduce the group's effectiveness because the time could be better spent on task accomplishment.

1. The group has already established an accurate tacit understanding about how a task is to be accomplished.
2. The group is working on simple tasks that require little coordination.
3. There are effective pre-plans (discussed in the next section).
4. The group has a history of tacit coordination that works.

In the following cases, tacit coordination is risky; explicit coordination planning will probably yield a better group result.

1. Workflow interdependence is high and the group is inexperienced in working together.
2. Workflow interdependence is high and there are no pre-plans to follow.

3. A group is working on a new or uncertain task whose accomplishment requires that members work interdependently.
4. New members have joined the group and are unclear on the tacit coordination understandings among existing group members.
5. Existing tacit coordination systems are not working well because of changes in organizational policy or technology, or because a different configuration would better fit new member skills.

Explicit Coordination

Explicit coordination

Occurs when members discuss how they will coordinate their actions and make conscious their plans for executing tasks.

Performance plans

Specific descriptions of time-and-function-linked series of actions designed to lead to a specific goal or outcome; who will do what, when, where, and how.

Pre-plans

Job descriptions, policies, schedules, and standard operating procedures.

Now that you know when tacit coordination works and when it does not, it is appropriate to think a bit harder about the alternative: explicit coordination. **Explicit coordination** requires that group members discuss how members will coordinate their actions and make conscious their plans for executing tasks. Explicit coordination often involves performance plans or pre-plans. **Performance plans** are descriptions of time-and-function-linked series of actions that, if executed, will lead to a specific goal and outcome (McGrath, 1984). **Pre-plans** include job descriptions, policies, schedules, and standard operating procedures (Wittenbaum et al., 1998). The more complex the task, and the more workflow interdependence, the more important it is for efficiency and effectiveness that the group plan who will do what, when, where, and how (Durham et al., 1997; Weldon & Weingart, 1993). Goals should be set for each task to be performed by the group (Pritchard, Jones, Roth, Struebing, & Ekeberg, 1988).

Pre-plans and performance plans increase the likelihood that members will share similar conceptions of which members should do what and how, and how member efforts relate to one another. Recall that the problem in my department was that these descriptions and standard operating procedures were in the heads of senior group members, who did not clearly describe them to junior members. The solution to the problem in my department was to develop explicit pre-plans for major committee activities. These were essentially recipes for accomplishing the tasks according to university guidelines and department culture. These recipes clearly identified the tasks of the committee chairs and members and how these fit together, and provided approximate deadlines for the completion of subtasks. The idea was to provide the department with an explicit tacit coordination system. With the input of senior department members, draft documents for each major committee assignment were created. Then, the full faculty reviewed, modified, and approved the documents.

In-process planning

Ongoing planning that occurs during the group's work; important when tasks are difficult and variable.

Coordination losses are also prevented by good communication. When tasks are complex and workflow interdependence is high, ongoing communication is necessary to coordinate members' efforts. High task variability and difficulty mean that planning may have to occur on an ongoing basis. Called **in-process planning,** this ongoing communication takes place in both formal and informal meetings

(Wittenbaum et al., 1998). Communication is also important so that plans can be changed as more is learned about what it will take to accomplish group goals and so that members can encourage one another. A good example is a busy hospital emergency room. Pre-plans will be of some use, but the day-to-day variation in the number of patients and their conditions requires ongoing communication and coordination among staff.

Finally, although tacit and explicit coordination are presented separately here, it is important to realize that they are not mutually exclusive. Indeed, many groups have multiple tasks and coordinate tacitly or explicitly depending on the task. Also, many groups fail to find the time to review and change outdated pre-plans and standard operating procedures, and consequently, are not as productive as they could be.

Meetings

Group meetings are intended as vehicles for group members to share information and ideas, plan, coordinate, and make decisions. Meetings in which participants are involved can increase commitment to group goals and provide important information and contacts with other group members. Unfortunately, meetings often fail to live up to their potential as group development and productivity tools. If you are like most people, you have sat through many meetings that you felt were a waste of your time. Indeed, dread is the emotion often experienced by group members prior to a group meeting. Attendance is often low unless members have a large stake in decisions made at the meeting, are required to attend the meeting, or receive some incentive to do so.

Common complaints about meetings are that they are too long and boring, dominated by a few influential people, poorly organized and/or led, called too frequently or not frequently enough, diverted by members with hidden agendas, subverted by members whose behaviors are destructive, and not focused on important issues (Milstein, 1983; Mosvick & Nelson, 1983). These potential pitfalls can be averted through preparation and thoughtful structuring of the meeting situation. With effective meeting norms, clear meeting goals, and good meeting leadership, meetings can be meaningful encounters in which people work hard, produce important outcomes, and leave with positive feelings about the group and its work.

Norms for Meetings

Productive and satisfying meetings depend on the establishment of meeting norms consistent with task accomplishment and positive member relations. Groups need meeting norms that encourage arriving on time to the meeting, beginning the meeting on time, participating appropriately (not too much or too little), handling conflict and disagreement constructively, and using discussion and decision-making methods that prevent domination by a few members and ensure that all pertinent information is heard and processed. Unfortunately, unproductive meeting norms often develop. For instance, once some members come late without consequence, others begin to do so as well. If the group waits for latecomers, the meeting start and ending times tend to become later and later. Groups can also develop negative meeting norms such as going off on tangents and using meeting time for socializing instead of task accomplishment. They may also develop a norm that high-status members say what they think and everyone else just goes along.

For a new group, it is useful to explicitly discuss norms for the group's meetings at the outset. What time will the meetings start and end? What is the group's policy regarding missing meetings or arriving late? How does the group want to handle disagreement? What meeting behaviors are desirable and acceptable? What behaviors are undesirable and unacceptable? How are decisions to be made, by consensus or by majority vote? Does the group want to run the meetings according to standard meeting rules such as Robert's Rules of Order (Robert, 1915/1971)? Who will set the agenda? Who will take meeting minutes or notes so that the group can track its progress and have a record of agreements?

Existing groups may benefit from an analysis of their meeting norms. Otherwise, inertia may lead the group to continue its familiar but dysfunctional meeting patterns. Sometimes a meeting is needed (!) to discuss why the group's meetings are unproductive and what can be done about it. Explicit discussion and analysis of the group's meetings often makes members more conscious of their own meeting behavior and how it fits in with the group's agreed-upon meeting norms. Consequently, members behave better. Observers may be brought in to comment on the group's meetings, or the group may be divided into smaller discussion groups to consider the meeting process (Zander, 1998). Zander also recommends the use of post-meeting reaction questionnaires. These questionnaires are relatively simple surveys in which members rate the meeting on qualities that members have decided are important. The ratings are summarized and reported to the group for discussion. As Zander notes, the numbers themselves are not as important as the group's discussion about why a given quality is rated high or low and what, if anything, should be done about it.

Box 9-1 provides an example of a post-meeting reaction questionnaire that can be used or adapted to improve group meetings. Often, a group will come up with improvement strategies that mirror the suggestions given in the previous paragraphs. Other times, they may come up with creative solutions like the fraternity that chose to increase attendance at their meetings with a meeting raffle. Each attendee contributed one dollar, and at the end of the meeting, a random drawing awarded the money to one attending member.

BOX 9-1 / POST-MEETING REACTION QUESTIONNAIRE

Instructions: Use the scale below to indicate agreement with each of the following statements.

Strongly Agree	Agree	Neutral	Disagree	Strongly Disagree
5	4	3	2	1

1. Our time was well spent.
2. The agenda items were important.
3. A few outspoken people dominated the meeting.
4. The meeting was rushed.
5. The meeting was useful.
6. The meeting began on time.
7. The meeting ended on time.
8. The meeting provided members with important information that could not be effectively conveyed in an email, phone call, or memo.
9. The group stayed on task during the meeting.
10. Group members supported and encouraged the participation of other members.
11. Differences among members were handled respectfully.
12. The meeting contributed to the accomplishment of the group's mission.

Goals for Meetings

Throughout this book, the importance of goals to groups is emphasized. Group meetings are also a case where goals are important for group productivity. Groups that have specific objectives to accomplish in the course of a meeting get more done than groups that have only general goals for the meeting. Specific meeting goals focus the group's work during the meeting, keeping members on track and less distracted. When members are unsure what they should accomplish during meeting time, they tend to do a lot of fooling around because they are not exactly sure what they should be doing. This is why formal or informal group leaders should identify goals *before* the meeting and share them with meeting participants in a written **agenda.**

Agenda
A written list of specific meeting goals and objectives.

The agenda should include the date of the meeting and a list of specific objectives, prioritized by their urgency. It is often a good idea to allocate an approximate amount of meeting time to each agenda item to help keep the group on track. Enough time should be allotted for each agenda item so that alternatives can be carefully considered, most group members can participate, and some decisions can be made or some tasks accomplished. Because meetings take people away from their work and other activities, they find it a waste of time for meetings to be spent reading lists of announcements and prefer that meeting time be used for matters that cannot be taken care of without a meeting. Therefore, agenda items should not include simple informational items. These should be conveyed via memo, electronic mail, or as "announcements" listed at the bottom of the agenda to be read by the participants.

If you are responsible for constructing the agenda, keep in mind that it is often appropriate to consult with group members about meeting objectives—for instance, by sending out the meeting agenda ahead of time for feedback. This also ensures that attendees and leaders are prepared for the meeting. For instance, when I was department chair, I sent out a tentative meeting agenda by electronic mail at least three days before the meeting. I included a few sentences of background information on agenda items so that members could be more prepared for discussion and could alert me to other information that might be needed for the meeting.

Meeting Leadership

Productive meetings are usually led by leaders who serve both task and socioemotional functions. Meeting leaders are task-oriented when they run the meeting efficiently. This means starting and ending on time, preventing the group from getting off topic, and keeping the group focused on meeting goals. Meeting leaders are socioemotionally oriented when they encourage participation, manage conflict and disagreement constructively, and promote positive relationships between meeting attendees.

Meetings that run late cause anger and resentment. People resent having meetings cut into the time they have allocated for other things and often stop paying close attention once the designated ending time has come and gone. A task-oriented meeting leader has a well-organized agenda and conducts the meeting so that the most important business is taken care of within the allotted time. This means that members are not allowed to explore new topics before completing the agenda. Unless it is clear that a new topic is of overriding importance, the leader assertively redirects the discussion back to the agenda. For instance, a meeting leader may interrupt a tangent by saying something like "We're getting off topic, and we only have 30 minutes left to take care of these pressing agenda items. I will make a note of these other issues, and I promise we'll discuss them at a later meeting, or at the end of this meeting if we finish all of today's work with time to spare."

Keeping the meeting on track also means controlling group members who distract the group from its meeting tasks. For instance, some members repeat themselves or go off on long-winded tangents. A task-oriented meeting leader should interrupt these members, saying something like "I think we're clear on your position, but in all fairness, we should hear from others" or "What you have to say is interesting, but it's off topic and we have a lot we still need to accomplish. For the rest of our meeting, we need to limit discussion to things that are directly related to our work today." It is the leader's place to address members who engage in side conversations, often whispered, so that the meeting can continue without distraction. For instance, I turn to the "side talkers" and say "I'm sorry, but I am distracted by your side conversation, and I am having a hard time hearing the larger discussion. I would be grateful if you would finish your conversation later or, if it is related to our topic, that you share with the whole group."

Task-oriented meeting leader behavior is important, but a meeting leader should not be so task-oriented that little space is left for members to share and process opinions and information. In other words, skilled meeting leaders also display socioemotional and relational behaviors. Meeting leaders are socioemotional when they act to make sure that member participation is largely equal and members feel listened to. This means, for example, that meeting leaders must control dominating group members such as the those who constantly interrupt others. The leader can interrupt the interrupter with a statement like "Wait a minute, let's let her finish her thought," or after the interrupter finishes, the leader might say "Suzy, you were in the middle of your thought when James spoke up, but we want to hear what you have to say. Could you finish sharing with the group now?" Ensuring more equal participation also means soliciting input from a variety of members. Sometimes dominating members figure they might as well speak up because no one else is saying anything. Quieter and lower-status members do not speak up because they figure their input is not welcome and they do not want to compete with more verbal members. A skilled meeting leader invites participation from a number of meeting attendees. For instance, a leader can ask those who have not participated to contribute by saying something like "Dion, we haven't heard from you, and I think I can speak for the group when I say that I am interested in what you have to say." Leaders can also structure the meeting to solicit equal participation. For example, when I am leading a meeting, I will sometimes ask each participant to make a one- or two-minute statement about his or her position on the issue, or I'll ask each person to make a list of ideas and then have each member share his or her favorite one with the group. Chapter 11, Group Decision Making, discusses several structured techniques that promote equitable participation.

A good meeting leader also manages conflicts that arise in the meeting, keeping the climate cooperative and preventing differences from becoming destructive conflicts. Applying the information contained in Chapter 7, Understanding and Managing Conflict, a meeting leader may have to emphasize goals the disputants have in common (superordinate goals) and lead them through problem-focused negotiations. What are the major concerns of those who disagree? How can we all work together to create a solution that satisfies all sides' major concerns and needs?

Apply It! ••• Are Your Meetings Productive?

Analyze the meetings at your last job, in a student project group, or in a membership organization (such as a sorority or fraternity, hobby or sports group, or community activism group). Were the meetings productive? Why or why not? What could be done to make them more productive?

The meeting leader may also need to intervene and remind participants to express disagreement respectfully: "Emotions are running high here, and I want to remind everyone to express disagreement without making any personal attacks," or "I want to remind the group that we all need to make an effort to try and understand others' perspectives." The leader may rephrase potentially destructive participant comments before others have a chance to counterattack. For example, "We see you're upset David, but I'm worried the way you put your message is interfering with others' understanding of it. Are you just trying to say that you are concerned that this tight deadline will increase employee injury?"

Groups generally manage to perform adequately despite their inattention to factors that contribute to group productivity. But there is a difference between "okay" group performance and excellent group performance, a difference explained by attention to these factors. With a little effort, actual productivity can closely approximate or even equal potential productivity. The suggestions for improving group meetings are a good example of how much difference a little preparation and attention to group goals and norms can make in promoting group productivity and a positive group experience.

Concept Review

Defining Group Productivity

- **Group performance** is the quantity or quality of the outcomes produced or the time required for task completion. It is a combination of **efficiency** (the ratio of inputs to outputs) and **effectiveness** (whether the group met or exceeded goals).
- **Workflow interdependence** is the extent to which the behavior of one group member influences the performance of others and the extent to which group members must actually work together to perform the task.
- **Potential productivity** is a function of member resources and task demands. **Actual productivity** of a group equals its potential productivity minus process losses such as motivational and coordination problems. Coordination losses occur when group members do not optimally organize their efforts. Motivational losses occur when the motivation of individuals is reduced when they are in a group.

Preventing Motivational Losses With Group Goals

- Group goals are goals that group members perceive as having been consensually agreed upon or imposed by group members. Group goals improve group performance because group members work faster and longer on the task, focus more attention on it, and are less distracted by irrelevant stimuli.
- For goals to work, group members must be committed to them. They must find the goal to be attractive and must believe that the goal is attainable.
- Group members will find goal attainment attractive if it validates their sense of self-worth, if the group is cohesive and valued by them, if they participated in the setting of the goals, and when working toward group goals is compatible with personal goals.
- Members are committed to attainable goals. Expectations regarding the group's potential success are influenced by the group's past success, the skills of the group members, other demands on the group's resources, the perceived commitment of other group members, and the level of the goal.
- Goal setting works best when the goals are specific and difficult, yet realistic.
- Goals should be stated in measurable terms so that it is possible to monitor progress and provide feedback.

Social Loafing: A Common Motivational Loss

- **Social loafing** is the tendency for people to reduce their effort on group tasks. Social loafing may lower group productivity if members who exert maximum effort are unable to compensate for loafers' reduced efforts or if other group members lower their efforts so as not to feel taken advantage of.
- Lack of identifiability of individual efforts is an important cause of social loafing. Social loafing may also occur when individuals feel their efforts are "dispensable," or unimportant to the group's success.
- **Free riders** contribute little and benefit from the work of others (suckers). The **sucker effect** occurs when suckers reduce their efforts because they do not want to "carry" capable free riders. Free rider and sucker effects may create **social dilemmas.**
- The **collective effort model** suggests that to be motivated to exert effort on a collective task, individuals must believe that their increased efforts will increase the group's performance and that increased group performance will lead to desired outcomes for the group and for them personally.
- Gender and culture affect social loafing. Research indicates that women loaf less than men do. This may be because women tend to place greater value on group harmony, group success, satisfaction of other group members, and other group members' evaluations of their individual contributions to the group.
- Social loafing is strongest in studies with research participants from individualistic countries like the United States. Conversely, participants in studies

conducted in collectivistic countries, such as Japan, Taiwan, and China, loaf less. Some cross-cultural social loafing studies have even found that participants from Pacific-Asian cultures work harder in groups.

Improving Group Coordination to Reduce Coordination Loss

- **Group coordination** is the way in which group members synchronize their actions in order to successfully complete the group task. Poor coordination is a source of process loss and reduced productivity.
- **Tacit coordination** is a frequent cause of process loss. Productivity may be reduced when members proceed according to differing "mental models" of the group and the task.
- Tacit coordination does not lead to process loss when unspoken assumptions made by members are accurate and congruent. This is more likely in a group that has some history together. However, the more tacit the group members' roles, the more difficult it will be to replace members and maintain a functioning group.
- **Explicit coordination** requires that group members discuss how members will coordinate their actions. Explicit coordination often involves **performance plans** (descriptions of a time-and-function-linked series of actions) and **pre-plans** (job descriptions, policies, schedules, and standard operating procedures).
- Explicit coordination is needed when workflow interdependence is high and the group is inexperienced in working together, when the group is working on a new task, when there are no pre-plans to follow, or when new members have joined the group and are unclear on the tacit coordination understandings among existing group members. Explicit coordination is also called for when existing tacit coordination systems are not working well because of changes in organizational policy or technology, or because a different configuration would better fit new member skills.
- **In-process planning** is often needed when tasks are highly variable and difficult, necessitating planning on an ongoing basis.

Skill Review

Evaluate and Improve Group Productivity

- To measure and improve productivity, ask: Was the group efficient? Did the group accomplish its goals with relative speed and good use of resources? What changes would increase efficiency? Was the group effective? In general, did the group accomplish its "mission" successfully? What could be done differently in the future to make the group even more effective?

- Identify sources of process loss, such as coordination loss and motivational loss, and act to address them.

Set Specific Group Goals

- Have group members participate in the setting of specific and challenging (yet attainable) goals.
- State the group's goals in measurable terms so that progress can be monitored, provide feedback on progress, and make adjustments in process as needed.

Prevent and Treat Social Loafing

- Show members that their contributions are needed, important, and identifiable.
- Emphasize the valued outcomes that are connected to enhanced performance.
- Build group cohesion, so that members value the group and others' impressions of them.
- Constructively confront loafers.
- Give members tasks that they find personally meaningful.
- Keep group size small.

Reduce Coordination Loss

- Examine the coordination system used by the group. In new groups, or in old groups facing membership, organizational, or technology changes, consider the use of pre-plans and performance plans.
- When tasks are complex and workflow interdependence is high, engage in planning on an ongoing basis.

Increase Meeting Effectiveness

- Develop effective meeting norms, such as beginning and ending the meeting on time, respectful disagreement, and equitable participation.
- In a new group, take the time to create effective meeting norms. In an existing group, evaluate and improve the group's meetings.
- Have specific meeting goals (objectives), prioritized by urgency, that appear on a meeting agenda that is distributed before the meeting.
- When leading a meeting, display task behaviors such as keeping the group focused on the meeting's goals *and* socioemotional behaviors that promote constructive controversy and equitable participation.

Study Questions

1. What are efficiency and effectiveness?
2. Why is actual productivity often lower than potential productivity? What are the sources of process and motivational losses described in the chapter?
3. What is goal setting, and how does it work to reduce motivational losses? What guidelines were given in the chapter regarding the use of goal-setting techniques?
4. What is social loafing? What explanations were provided for it in the chapter? What suggestions were provided for its reduction?
5. How can free rider and sucker effects lead to social dilemmas?
6. What is the relationship between workflow interdependence and the importance of group coordination?
7. What is tacit coordination? When is tacit coordination likely to reduce a group's productivity? What can be done to solve problems created by tacit coordination?
8. What is explicit coordination, and how are performance plans and in-process planning used to accomplish it?
9. What is the role of feedback in increasing group productivity?
10. What guidelines were given in the chapter for increasing meeting effectiveness?

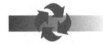

Group Activities

Activity 1: Productivity Consulting Team Activity

You and your four "colleagues" have a business that specializes in team productivity. Your business has been hired by a middle school. The principal has come to your group for advice. She says that her district has ordered her teachers to have students do much of their work in groups. According to the district, children need be prepared to work in groups because this is likely to be their reality as adults. The problem, the teachers say, is that usually one or two children in the group do the work while the others fool around and contribute little. The principal wants you to provide an easy-to-use set of recommendations for the teachers so that students will learn how to be good team members and will actively participate in learning academic content. Before beginning, each member of the "consulting team" should take fifteen minutes to think about how the consulting team can operate efficiently and effectively and prevent motivation and coordination losses (write down your recommendations to share with the group and your instructor). After your group has created the recommendations, evaluate its productivity.

Activity 2: Analyze Productivity Case Studies

With your group, analyze the following case studies. Identify chapter concepts and provide recommendations to improve productivity: What should the group or organization have done to improve productivity? Come up with a title for each case that represents the lesson it teaches.

CASE 1   What I find hardest about being in groups is dealing with different people's expectations of what is to be done. My ideas are almost never the same as everyone else's. Patience helps me get through these times, but sometimes success of the group is just not possible. To be honest, this is why I hate groups in general. Normally I find it easier to just do it myself. This way I don't have to deal with people who don't have the same ideas I do.

This was probably the biggest problem I had when I was in a band. Everyone in my band seemed to have a different idea of what the band was about. Some of the members just liked to jam and hang out, and others, like me, wanted to get a record deal and make a living. It was a constant battle. Another problem was that we never seemed to make much progress. For example, we would say we wanted to play more gigs but assumed that someone else would make it happen; we never really talked about how many gigs or how exactly we were going to get these gigs. Or we would agree we should practice more, but that's as far as it went. We also never really took the time to find a way to schedule our practice sessions around all of our different work schedules. Every time we talked about a practice session, it would take forever to come up with a time.

I should have been able to detect these problems and do something about them, but I guess that is what learning is all about. Unfortunately, I didn't have the tools to make it work, and our band eventually "disbanded."

CASE 2   I used to work at a clothing store. Every day, the team of workers had a sales goal that needed to be met. On the days when I knew that other staff members were irresponsible slackers, I would work extra hard to cover for their lack of effort. I would not be very happy on those days, but I got the job done. I was moody and had to work harder than I was paid for. I also found myself bossing others around and trying to delegate work, although I had no authority to do so. On days when I worked with more dependable staff members, I was less efficient and sometimes downright lazy. I could tell I irritated the other workers on these days, and I have to admit that I felt ashamed and bored.

Most of these work habits stemmed from lack of interest and the unimportance of the job. And although our sales were tracked in the computer, there were no consequences for lack of effort. And even if someone didn't do his or her share of work, there wouldn't be a big difference in overall group performance. I'm glad I don't work there anymore.

Activity 3: The Paper Chain: A Coordination and Goal Activity

Your six-person group will need a stack of paper (from a recycling bin is fine), at least one pair of scissors, and two glue sticks for this activity. Your mission is to construct a paper chain "as long as possible" in thirty minutes. You don't have much time, so get started quickly. Do not read the rest of these instructions until your group has worked together on the task for fifteen minutes, at which time you should stop and follow the instructions in the next paragraph.

Now that your group has worked together for fifteen minutes, take note of your productivity (look around at other groups as well as considering your group's efficiency and effectiveness). Before getting back to work, take five minutes to do two things with your group: (1) Set a specific goal for the next fifteen minutes regarding the length of your chain; for instance, specify how many links you want it to be or the distance you want it to stretch. (2) Discuss with your group whether you are optimally coordinating your efforts and whether you should change your strategy before continuing. In fifteen minutes, when your group is done, follow the instructions in the next paragraph.

Now that your group has completed the task, again evaluate your group's efficiency and effectiveness. Did your group meet its goal? Was the goal specific and challenging but not too difficult? Did setting a goal improve your group's productivity? Why or why not? At the beginning, was the coordination of group members' work tacit or explicit? How was productivity affected by making it explicit?

InfoTrac College Edition Search Terms

To do research for your papers and assignments, use InfoTrac that's provided free with new copies of this book. Go to http://infotrac.thomsonlearning.com and enter the following search terms:

- Group Effectiveness
- Goal Setting
- Social Loafing
- Effective Meetings

Chapter 10 Leadership

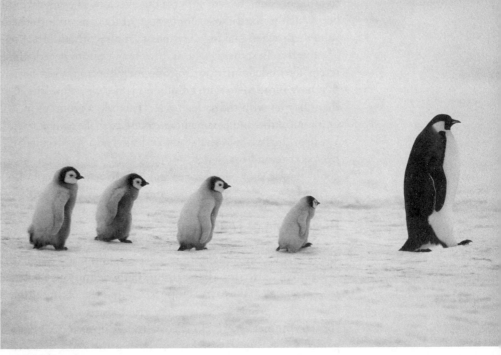

Many people express an interest in becoming better leaders. As one of my students said, "I would like to develop my leadership skills. My major problem right now is that I'm too 'chicken' to initiate a change or ask an uncomfortable question without first having someone else take the lead." Or as another said, "I know I tend to grab the leadership role in the group and can dominate other group members rather than inviting their input. Although I tend to be the leader, I am not so sure that I am a good one."

Leading a group is an important and sometimes challenging job. Leaders are responsible for directing and coordinating the activities of the group, for making sure group goals are achieved, and for addressing members' feelings, attitudes, and satisfaction. Leaders are often relied upon to motivate group members, turn a group into a team, and solve problems and conflicts. Formal leaders (those officially designated by an organization) often have the additional responsibilities of evaluating group members and providing feed-back to them.

Being a group leader is difficult for other reasons as well. Because of their visibility, power, and status, other group members often critically scrutinize the behavior of leaders. Members' perceptions of the leader affect the leader's ability to influence members to support change, as well as member productivity. Members watch to see if the leader treats members fairly and whether the leader consults them when making decisions that affect them or are relevant to their area of expertise. In some situations, they may want to be led, and in others, they will resent the leader's intrusion. Group members may even have reactions to leaders that have more to do with childhood issues with family leaders (such as parents) than they do with the actual leader. Leading a group of individuals with diverse opinions, skills, and personalities can be as challenging as herding a group of cats. Unsurprisingly, then, the study of leadership has resulted in many theoretical perspectives and many definitions of leadership. In this chapter, you will learn about these major perspectives and how to apply them to leadership practice.

Definitions of Leadership

There are dozens of definitions of leadership, each emphasizing a different dimension of leadership (Bass, 1990). Early definitions looked at leadership as the *focus of group processes;* they emphasized that leaders are at the center of the group and serve as primary agents in the group's structure, activities, goals, and atmosphere. Another early focus was on leadership as *personality.* These definitions regarded leadership as a matter of having the right personal traits or qualities. Many definitions emphasize various aspects of influencing others. For example, leadership may be viewed as the *art of inducing compliance* (getting others to do what you want them to do). Similarly, some definitions define leadership in terms of the *exercise of influence* and as an *instrument of goal achievement.* In other words, leadership is about influencing people toward goal setting and goal achievement. Definitions of leadership as a *form of persuasion* also emphasize a leader's ability to influence others but stress that leaders do this with persuasion and inspiration, rather than coercion. Conversely, the *power relations* between leaders and followers has also been the focus of some definitions. Such definitions emphasize the source, amount, and use of power by leaders. Leadership has also been defined as an *act or behavior;* theorists with this approach emphasize what leaders do when they act to direct the group's activities.

These definitional differences reflect great disagreement about the nature of leadership. There is also some controversy regarding the overlap between leadership and management (Yukl & Van Fleet, 1992). For instance, some view managers as those who merely carry out position responsibilities and exercise authority, whereas leaders inspire, shape ideas, and change the way people think about what is possible (Northouse, 1997; Yukl & Van Fleet, 1992). As Kotter (1990) put it, managers provide order and consistency to organizations through planning and budgeting, organizing and staffing, and controlling and problem solving. Leaders produce change and movement through vision building and strategizing, aligning people, communicating, and motivating (Kotter, 1990). In reality, the distinction is not entirely clear-cut; there are times when leaders manage, and managers lead (Yukl, 1989).

Leadership
A process that includes influencing the choice of goals and strategies of a group or organization, influencing people to accomplish goals, and promoting a group identity and commitment.

Yukl and Van Fleet (1992) suggest that it is best to define leadership broadly and to look at the various conceptions of leadership as a source of different perspectives on a complex, multifaceted phenomenon. They define **leadership** as "a process that includes influencing the task objectives and strategies of a group or organization, influencing people in the organization to implement the strategies and achieve the objectives, influencing group maintenance and identification, and influencing the culture of the organization" (p. 148).

Trait Theories of Leadership

Do you have the personality to be a leader? When we look at history and think about great leaders, we are inclined to believe that there was something special and distinctive about them, something that set them apart from their followers. For instance, many people were working for civil rights in the United States in the 1960s, but no one inspired and galvanized the movement like Martin Luther King, Jr. Likewise, many parents who have lost a child to a drunk driver have responded with activism. However, few have been as successful as Candy Lightner, a woman whose daughter was killed by a drunk driver in 1980. She founded Mothers Against Drunk Driving (MADD) and built it into a large national organization that lobbies for stricter penalties for drunk driving.

Trait approach to leadership
A leadership perspective emphasizing the unique characteristics and personality traits possessed by effective leaders.

Leadership research began in the early 1900s, and until World War II it focused on identifying the personality traits associated with leadership (Chemers, 1983). The assumption was that great leaders have in common certain unique characteristics or traits. This view came to be known as the **trait approach to leadership,** although at times you may hear it called the *great man theory of leadership,* or more recently, the *great person theory of leadership.*

Early Research on the Trait Approach

Take a moment to make a list of the personal qualities exhibited by the best leaders you've experienced. What kind of people were they? Researchers spent the first half of the twentieth century trying to relate personal characteristics (traits) to leadership behavior. The general strategy they used was to compare leaders and nonleaders on personality, intelligence, height, and a number of other qualities. Although they found some difference between leaders and nonleaders on a handful of traits, they were unable to determine what type of person is a successful leader. This fact became all the more evident in 1948 when Ralph Stodgill reviewed 124 research studies on individual traits and leadership.

Compare your list to what Stodgill found in 1948. His review concluded that leaders consistently differed from nonleaders on only a few traits. These included intelligence, alertness, insight, responsibility, initiative, persistence, self-confidence, and sociability. A 1974 review by Stodgill of 163 new studies added five more traits: willingness to accept the consequences of decision making, readiness to absorb interpersonal stress, willingness to tolerate frustration and delay, ability to influence others' behavior, and the capacity to structure social interaction systems to the purpose at hand. Stodgill (1948) concluded that having these traits does not guarantee that one will be a leader and that the traits one possesses must be relevant to the leadership situation. He added that the trait approach is likely to be limited because effective leadership in one situation with one group of followers may not be effective with another group of people in another situation. For example, organizations and sports teams sometimes hire a successful leader from elsewhere, only to find that person's leadership success cannot be duplicated in their group. Stodgill's conclusions triggered a new approach to leadership that focused on leadership behaviors and situations, one that will be discussed in this chapter as the situational or contingency approach.

The Resurgence of the Trait Approach

The trait approach to leadership was abandoned for a time by researchers as other approaches gained favor, but in the 1980s and 1990s it came back into vogue. As Kirkpatrick and Locke (1991, p. 59) put it, "Leaders do not have to be great men or women by being intellectual geniuses or omniscient prophets to succeed, but they do need to have the 'right stuff' and this stuff is not equally present in all people." According to Kirkpatrick and Locke, leaders rate higher on *drive,* the desire for achievement coupled with high energy and resolve; *self-confidence,* a belief in themselves; *cognitive ability,* or intelligence; *leadership motivation,* the desire to be in charge and exercise authority over others; *integrity,* the quality of adhering to a strong set of principles, being trustworthy, loyal, and dependable; and *expertise,* specific knowledge of technical issues relevant to task completion. Several studies indicate that a leader's integrity may be the most important factor in members' ratings of leader effectiveness, whereas bosses' ratings of leader effectiveness appear to be guided more by perceptions of technical competence (Hogan, Curphy, & Hogan, 1994).

Flexibility is another important quality. Leaders who possess the ability to "read" the situation and change their leadership behavior to fit the needs and goals of the group members are most effective (Zaccarro, Foti, & Kenny, 1991). Several other traits have also been associated with managerial effectiveness and advancement; these include high energy, stress tolerance, and emotional matu-

Apply It! ••• **Do You Have the Personality for Leadership?**

Do you have the personality traits associated with leadership? Evaluate yourself according to the "big five" personality traits of leaders described previously. Does your evaluation fit with your past leadership behavior? In other words, if you tend to assume a leadership role, do you have the qualities that the research suggests that you would? If you usually do not assume a leadership role, on which of the "big five" are you low? Can you do anything to modify these traits such that you better fit the leader profile?

rity (Yukl & Van Fleet, 1992). Yukl and Van Fleet explain that high energy level and stress tolerance help people cope with the intense pace and demands of most managerial positions as well as the frequent role conflicts and decision pressures. Leaders must be emotionally mature in order to maintain cooperative relations with members, peers, and superiors, because mood swings, impulsiveness, and defensiveness create problems in relationships. If you have ever experienced an emotionally immature leader, you can probably remember thinking that person had no business being in a leadership position.

Many of the leadership traits identified fit into the big-five model of personality structure endorsed by many modern personality theorists (Hogan, 1994, Hogan et al.). Several studies have examined how leaders compare with nonleaders on these personality traits (Barrick & Mount, 1991; Ones, Mount, Barrick, & Hunter, 1994). These studies find that leaders in organizational settings tend to score high on *extraversion* (outgoing and sociable), *friendliness* (warm and likable), *conscientiousness* (dependable), *emotional stability,* and *intelligence* (intellectually able and open-minded).

Transactional and Transformational Leadership

At this point in our discussion of trait theories of leadership, you may feel that something is missing. After all, when we think about what makes a great leader, it is hard not to conclude that great leaders have a "spirit" or "fire" that sets them apart from their followers and lesser leaders. In the latter part of the twentieth century, leadership researchers were thinking the same thing. For example, political scientist James McGregor Burns (1978) wrote about leaders who inspire followers to transcend their own needs in the interests of a common cause (transformational leaders) versus leaders who influence follower behavior by rewarding them for doing what the leader wants (transactional leaders). Around the same time, House (1977) described a charismatic theory of leadership that has become practically synonymous with transformational leadership.

Your average, everyday leader or manager is a transactional leader. Most of the leaders in your experience have probably been transactional leaders.

Transactional leadership

An "ordinary" leadership that is focused on the immediate situation and getting the job done.

Transactional leadership is more focused on the immediate situation and getting the job done. Essentially, transactional leaders develop exchanges with their followers regarding what the followers will receive if they do things right, or wrong (Bass & Avolio, 1994). The dynamics of a quid pro quo ("I'll do something for you if you do something for me") dominate the transactional exchange. The leader's role is to clarify task requirements and rewards for compliance (Hater & Bass, 1988). Transactional leadership theories suggest that the role of leaders is to provide what members need to perform effectively and achieve their goals (House, Woycke, & Fodor, 1991). Transactional leadership is not especially inspirational although it does focus on getting the job done.

According to Bass (1997), a major figure in the study of transactional and transformational leadership, transactional leadership may take four different forms. These are listed below in order of effectiveness.

1. **Contingent Reward.** The leader motivates by setting goals and rewarding goal achievement, rewards effort by providing support and help to members.
2. **Active Management by Exception.** The leader monitors performance and acts when there are mistakes or rule violations; control is maintained largely by enforcing rules.
3. **Passive Management by Exception.** The leader is largely "hands off," intervening only when a problem is brought to his/her attention.
4. **Laissez-faire Leadership.** The leader is uninvolved and largely unavailable and unresponsive to requests for help. This is really the absence of leadership.

Transformational (charismatic) leadership

A charismatic and intellectually stimulating leadership that inspires members to create and achieve new visions.

If transactional leadership is an "ordinary" type of leadership, **transformational (charismatic) leadership** is "extraordinary." Whereas transactional leadership is largely concerned with helping followers reach existing goals and duties, transformational leadership focuses on creating new goals and going beyond the call of duty. Bass and his colleagues (Bass & Avolio, 1990; Hater & Bass, 1988) asked people in a variety of business, military, education, and government settings to describe the most outstanding leaders they knew. The descriptions revealed four essential characteristics, known as the "Four I's," of the transformational leader.

1. **Idealized Influence (Charisma).** The leader has a vision and is respected and trusted by followers who strongly identify with and want to emulate him/her. Followers deeply respect and trust the leader.
2. **Inspiration.** The leader's communications increase optimism and enthusiasm for the tasks. Followers share the leader's vision and confidence that they can do the job.
3. **Intellectual Stimulation.** The leader fosters creativity among followers and stimulates them to look at things in new ways.
4. **Individualized Consideration.** The leader gives personal attention to members, acting as an adviser and coach, giving personal feedback, and stimulating personal development.

Another difference between transactional and transformational leaders has to do with how they interact with the organization. According to Bass and Avolio (1994), transactional leaders work within the organization following existing rules, procedures, and norms. They are often part of a group culture in which everyone has a "price" for his/her motivation to work or cooperate and self-interest dominates. In contrast, transformational leaders change the organizational culture. In a study of ninety leaders, the "transforming" leaders had a clear vision of the future state of their organizations, were social architects for the transformation of their organizations, and built others' trust in their vision and their ability to enact it (Bennis & Nanus, 1985).

Transformational leadership appears to have some significant benefits over transactional leadership. Transformational leadership is positively related to members' perceptions of leader effectiveness, how much effort members are willing to expend for a leader, how satisfied members are with a leader, and how well members are rated by a leader (Hater & Bass, 1988; Howell & Frost, 1989). Also, in one study, those managers identified as top performers were rated higher on transformational leadership than a group of "ordinary" managers (Hater & Bass, 1988). Collectively, findings from more than 100 studies from many settings demonstrate that leaders described as charismatic, transformational, or visionary have positive effects on their organizations and followers (Fiol, Harris, & House, 1999).

Can a leader be effective without being transformational? Bass (1997) concluded that transformational leaders are more effective than transactional leaders but that transformational leaders who use a contingent-reward approach are especially effective. In situations where routine performance is required, the transactional leader may be adequate. However, in situations where extraordinary effort is required, as is the case with social change or organizational or product innovation, a transformational leader is probably needed.

Before we leave the topic of charismatic and transformational leadership, it is important to note that not all charismatic leaders act in the best interests of their followers or the organizations that they are a part of. As Yukl (1998) notes, for every Franklin D. Roosevelt, Mohandas Gandhi, and Martin Luther King, Jr., there is a Charles Manson, David Koresh, or Adolph Hitler. Although charismatic leaders are often hailed as the heroes of management (and, we might add, social change movements), charisma can lead to blind fanaticism in the service of the power-hungry or unethical leader (Howell & Avolio, 1992). Clearly, then, there is a difference between the "ethical charismatic" and "unethical charismatic," sometimes called positive and negative charismatics (Conger, 1989; Howell & Avolio, 1992). **Ethical (positive) charismatics** have moral standards that emphasize the collective interests of the group, organization, or society. Ethical charismatic leaders are interested in contributing to the welfare of their followers, are receptive to feedback from their followers, and stimulate the personal development and leadership skills of others. **Unethical (negative) charismatics**

Ethical (positive) charismatics
Charismatic leaders who use their power to achieve the collective interests of the group, organization, or society.

Unethical (negative) charismatics
Charismatics who manipulate their followers into obedience to promote their own self-interests.

control and manipulate their followers into obedience and subservience, promote what is best for themselves rather than their followers or organizations, and have moral standards that promote their own self-interests.

Improving Leadership Practice With the Trait Model

It is often assumed that transformational leaders are born, not made. However, a study by Howell and Frost (1989) suggests that individuals can be trained to exhibit transformational leadership behavior. Their work suggests the following if you wish to work on this aspect of your leadership behavior:

1. Share with followers an overarching goal—for instance, the importance of the project and followers' contributions, its innovative nature, and its connection to the individual's goals.
2. Communicate high performance expectations and exhibit confidence in followers to meet these expectations, saying for example, "I have every confidence that if you use your creativity and skills you will be successful at this challenging task."
3. Project a powerful, confident, and dynamic presence by maintaining direct eye contact, showing you have energy by pacing slightly, leaning toward followers when you are communicating with them, and having a relaxed posture and animated facial expressions.
4. Work to have a captivating, engaging voice tone.

Additionally, Bass and Avolio (1990) and Yukl (1998) suggest that to become a transformational leader you should:

1. Give pep talks aimed at increasing optimism and enthusiasm and reminding followers of the "vision."
2. Encourage creativity and intelligent problem solving among followers.
3. Give personal attention to all members.
4. Provide feedback in ways that are easy to accept, understand, and use for personal development.
5. Empower people to achieve the vision by asking them to determine the best ways to attain objectives, reducing bureaucratic constraints, and providing adequate resources.

Behavior Theories of Leadership

Behavior theories of leadership

Leadership theories that focus on leader behavior and leadership styles.

If you do not possess the traits associated with leadership and find yourself in a leadership role nonetheless, you will be especially interested in knowing what effective leaders *do*. Leader behavior and leadership styles are the focus of the **behavior theories of leadership.** These theories became popular after World War II and were a primary focus of leadership research through the 1970s.

The Two-Factor Model of Leader Behavior

Two-factor model of leader behavior

A behavior theory of leadership emphasizing two dimensions of leader, task, and socioemotional behaviors.

Task behaviors

Leadership behaviors focused on organizing followers toward task accomplishment; also called *initiating structure* and *production-oriented.*

Socioemotional behaviors

Leadership behaviors focused on reducing tension and enhancing morale; also called *employee-oriented* and *consideration.*

One of most enduring notions of leader behavior is that it falls into one of two primary categories: task or socioemotional. According to this **two-factor model of leader behavior,** some leader behaviors are focused on organizing followers toward task accomplishment (**task behaviors**), whereas other behaviors are focused on reducing tension and enhancing morale (**socioemotional behaviors**). Researchers at Ohio State University (Halpin & Winer, 1957), University of Michigan (Kahn & Katz, 1953), and Harvard University (Bales & Slater, 1955) all pointed to these two sets of leader behaviors although they used different names for them. The Ohio State researchers used a 150-item scale called the Leader Behavior Description Questionnaire (LBDQ) to measure different leader behaviors. Their results indicated that most leader behavior falls into two categories. Behaviors in the *consideration* category focus on concern for group members and encourage two-way communication, mutual trust, and respect. Behaviors that involve the organization and definition of individual and group activities, such as the assignment of tasks and pushing for production, are included in the *initiating structure* category. The University of Michigan researchers termed the dimensions *production-oriented* and *employee-oriented.* The Harvard researchers found that in leaderless college student discussion groups, one person often took on the role of *task specialist* (organizing, summarizing, and directing task behavior) whereas another took on the role of *socioemotional specialist* (acting to reduce tension, raise morale, and encourage participation). In Japan, Misumi (1985; Misumi & Peterson, 1985) developed the *performance-maintenance (PM) theory of leadership* in which performance represented the leader's task behaviors (including group goals and problem-solving tasks) and maintenance represented leader behaviors oriented toward preserving the group.

One version of the two-factor approach that you may be exposed to in organizational settings is the Leadership Grid, formerly known as the Managerial Grid (Blake & McCanse, 1991; Blake & Mouton, 1964, 1985). Many large organizations hire Scientific Methods, an international organization development company, to conduct seminars based on the grid. Employees and managers do self-assessments and participate in small group exercises to learn what effective leadership is and how to manage for optimum results (Northouse, 1997). The Leadership Grid is based on rating individuals from 1 to 9 on their *concern for production* (horizontal axis) and from 1 to 9 on their *concern for people* (vertical axis) and plotting these scores on a grid to determine which of five leadership styles they exhibit (see Figure 10-1). As you can see by looking at the styles, concern for production is very similar to being task-oriented, and concern for people closely resembles a socioemotional orientation. Blake and Mouton (1985) suggest that although a person may exhibit several styles, each person generally has a dominant style. Furthermore, their research indicates that the 9,9 team management style, in which the leader is high on both concern for people and

Figure 10-1

The Leadership Grid

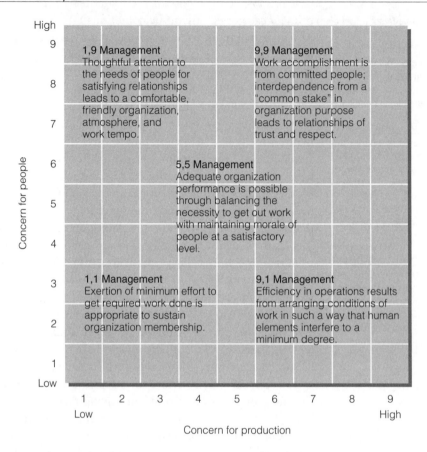

The Leadership Grid is based on rating individuals from 1 to 9 on concern for production *and 1 to 9 on* concern for people *to determine which of five leadership styles they exhibit. The 9,9 style is associated with the greatest managerial success.*

Source: Leadership Dilemmas–Grid Solutions by Robert P. Blake and Anne McCause, p.29, 1991. Gulf Publishing Co.

concern for production, is most likely to lead to increased group performance and to the career advancement of managers (Blake & Mouton, 1964, 1985).

Can you imagine a leader so focused on the socioemotional needs of members that needed task leadership does not occur, respect for the leader is compromised, and performance declines? Can you imagine a leader so focused on the task and its accomplishment that members' personal needs and relationships with the leader suffer and lead to low morale and performance? Indeed, hundreds of studies correlating leader initiating structure and consideration with member

---

Apply It! ••• **Rate a Leader on Task and Socioemotional Behavior**

Choose a leader from your personal experience and rate him or her with the questionnaire in **Box 10-1.** Was the leader more task-oriented or relationship-(socioemotional) oriented? How did this influence the leader's effectiveness in terms of member satisfaction and performance? In what way did the situation (the nature of the task, the skills of the members, and pressures from outside the group) affect the need for task or socioemotional leadership? Can we say that one type of leadership is more effective?

---

satisfaction and performance have yielded inconclusive and contradictory results (Yukl, 1994; Yukl & Van Fleet, 1992). Experimental research in laboratory and field settings finds that increasing relations-oriented leadership usually results in higher member satisfaction and productivity; however, the findings are inconclusive regarding task-oriented leadership (Yukl, 1998). Most leadership researchers now agree that some task-oriented and some people-oriented behavior is necessary for any leader and that the relative importance of these behaviors depends on the situation (Vroom, 1991; Yukl & Van Fleet, 1992).

Specific Leader Behaviors and Effectiveness

In the 1980s, researchers interested in a behavioral approach to leadership turned to the identification of more specific aspects of leader behavior. Yukl (1989) integrated results from that research and came up with fourteen categories of leader behavior (see **Box 10-2**). Leader effectiveness is linked to many of these specific behaviors (Yukl & Van Fleet, 1992). Praise and contingent rewards (rewards based on performance) usually increase member satisfaction and performance (Podsakoff, Todor, Grover, & Huber, 1984). Clarifying, informal and flexible planning, monitoring, and motivating behaviors are also all positively related to managerial effectiveness (Yukl, Wall, & Lepsinger, 1990). Yukl and Van Fleet (1992) point out, however, that in all likelihood these behaviors are complementary and work together to enhance effectiveness. This makes sense when you think about it. For instance, planning and problem solving will not work well unless they are based on good information obtained from monitoring, consulting, and networking. The advantage of identifying the specific behaviors that influence effectiveness is that this information can be used to train managers and leaders, or to develop measures to identify those who are likely to be successful in leadership positions. In fact, formal leadership and managerial training programs are widely used in organizations to increase generic skills and behaviors believed to be relevant to managerial effectiveness and advancement (Yukl, 1998).

BOX 10-1 / LEADERSHIP STYLE QUESTIONNAIRE

Instructions: Read each item carefully and think about how often you (or the person you are evaluating) engage in the described behavior. Indicate your response by circling one of the five numbers to the right of each item.

Never	Seldom	Occasionally	Often	Always
1	2	3	4	5

	Never	Seldom	Occasionally	Often	Always
1. Tells group members what they are supposed to do.	1	2	3	4	5
2. Acts friendly with members of the group.	1	2	3	4	5
3. Sets standards of performance for group members.	1	2	3	4	5
4. Helps others feel comfortable in the group.	1	2	3	4	5
5. Makes suggestions about how to solve problems.	1	2	3	4	5
6. Responds favorably to suggestions made by others.	1	2	3	4	5
7. Makes his/her perspective clear to others.	1	2	3	4	5
8. Treats others fairly.	1	2	3	4	5
9. Develops a plan of action for the group.	1	2	3	4	5
10. Behaves in a predictable manner toward group members.	1	2	3	4	5
11. Defines role responsibilities for each group member.	1	2	3	4	5
12. Communicates actively with group members.	1	2	3	4	5
13. Clarifies his/her own role within the group.	1	2	3	4	5
14. Shows concern for the personal well-being of others.	1	2	3	4	5
15. Provides a plan for how work is to be done.	1	2	3	4	5
16. Shows flexibility in making decisions.	1	2	3	4	5
17. Provides criteria for what is expected of the group.	1	2	3	4	5
18. Discloses thoughts and feelings to group members.	1	2	3	4	5
19. Encourages group members to do quality work.	1	2	3	4	5
20. Helps group members get along.	1	2	3	4	5

Scoring: The style questionnaire is designed to measure two major types of leadership behaviors: task and relationship. Score the questionnaire by doing the following. First, sum the responses on the odd-numbered items. This is the *task score*. Second, sum the responses on the even-numbered items. This is the *relationship score*.

Total Scores: Task _____ Relationship _____

Scoring interpretation

45–50   Very High Range
40–44   High Range
35–39   Moderately High Range
30–34   Moderately Low Range
25–29   Low Range
20–24   Very Low Range

Source: Leadership: Theory and Practice; 2nd ed., Peter G. Northouse, p.49, 2001. Reprinted by permission of Sage Publications, Inc.

BOX 10-2 / YUKL'S (1990) CATEGORIES OF LEADER BEHAVIOR

Planning & Organizing: Determining long-term objectives and strategies, allocating resources (including personnel), and determining how to improve coordination, productivity, and effectiveness.

Problem Solving: Identification and analysis of work-related problems, and action to solve problems and resolve crises.

Clarifying: Assigning work and explaining how to do it, communicating job responsibilities, priorities, deadlines, and performance expectations.

Informing: Disseminating relevant information about decisions, plans, and activities to people who need the information to do their work.

Monitoring: Gathering information about conditions that affect the work, checking on the progress and quality of the work, and evaluating the performance of individuals and the effectiveness of the organizational unit.

Motivating: Using logic or emotion to generate enthusiasm for the work, commitment to task objectives, providing support through the provision of requested resources, information, or assistance.

Consulting: Checking with people before making changes that affect them, encouraging participation in decision making, and allowing others to influence decisions.

Recognizing: Providing praise and recognition for effective performance, special achievements or contributions.

Supporting: Acting friendly and considerate, patient and helpful, showing sympathy and support when someone is upset or anxious.

Managing Conflict & Team Building: Facilitating constructive conflict resolution and encouraging cooperation, teamwork, and identification with the group.

Networking: Socializing informally, developing contacts with others outside of the unit who are a source of information and support.

Delegating: Giving members responsibility and discretion in carrying out work activities.

Developing & Mentoring: Providing coaching and career counseling and doing things to facilitate members' skill acquisition and career advancement.

Rewarding: Providing tangible rewards such as pay increases or promotions for effective performance.

Source: Yukl & Van Fleet, 1992

Another Leadership Style Dichotomy: Autocratic vs. Democratic

Autocratic (authoritarian) leaders

A highly task-oriented, controlling type of leadership in which leaders use their power to coerce others to follow them and allow them little input.

Democratic leader

A consultative, socioemotional type of leadership in which followers are asked for input and leaders attend to followers' personal needs and wants.

The task-socioemotional leadership dichotomy is one of the most enduring in the study of leadership but another important dimension of leadership behavior is the autocratic–democratic dichotomy. **Autocratic** or **authoritarian leaders** use their power to reward or punish others to coerce others to follow them. They are task-oriented and strict and although they closely supervise follower behavior, they are at the same time personally distant and even stern. Members are to do as they are told and are not to ask questions or provide input in decision making. In contrast, the **democratic leader** is likely to consult followers on decisions that affect them. This type of leader is more socioemotionally oriented, attending to followers' personal needs and wants, and there is little interpersonal distance between the leader and followers.

One of the earliest studies on the autocratic–democratic leadership distinction and performance may sound familiar to you if you read the part of Chapter 2 that describes the Lewin, Lippit, and White (1939) study. In that study, the researchers randomly assigned boys in after-school groups to be supervised by an adult that displayed an autocratic, democratic, or laissez-faire leadership style. The democratic style resulted in a high level of productivity that persisted even when the leader was absent. The authoritarian style produced high productivity only in the presence of the leader and seemed to create dependence on the leader and more aggression between group members.

An important component of the democratic style is **participative decision making (PDM).** PDM can vary from no participation (autocratic), to consultation, to joint decision making (power sharing) (Hollander & Offermann, 1990). It may also involve consulting with members individually or making joint decisions with them in a group (Yukl & Van Fleet, 1992). PDM is not to be confused with not providing any leadership at all. Indeed, the leader plays an important role in orchestrating the process by which different views are heard and a decision is made. Peterson (1997) calls this **process directiveness** and found that in a discussion, a leader who insisted that all members be given a chance to participate had a positive effect on the group's decision making and on members' satisfaction with the group and the leader.

Research suggests a modest positive relationship between participation and satisfaction and a small, though significant, positive relationship between participation and performance (Hollander & Offermann, 1990). Meta-analyses suggest that democratic leadership affects satisfaction more for larger groups, and for females more than males (Foels, Driskell, Mullen, & Salas, 2000). Despite the seemingly small impact of PDM on performance, PDM is in most cases a preferable style. One reason is that PDM is related to satisfaction, and satisfaction is linked in many studies to decreased absenteeism and job turnover (people leaving the job or group). Both of these are costly to the group's productivity. For instance, job turnover costs employers millions of dollars a year because job recruitment and job training are expensive in terms of time and money.

PDM is also more humanistic than autocratic leadership. Let's face it, most of us prefer a democratic to an authoritarian leader because democratic leaders lead in a way that is more respectful of us and does not constantly remind us of our lower status. Effective leaders use their power in a subtle, easy fashion that minimizes status differences and avoids threats to the self-esteem of members (Yukl & Van Fleet, 1992). PDM honors followers' knowledge of the work, their skills, the group, and the organization. We are generally the best authorities on our own work and possess substantial knowledge relevant to the task. Therefore, we appreciate having our concerns and input taken into consideration when decisions that affect us are being made. Participation in decision making leads to growth and development of members (Vroom, 1991). It empowers followers, and gives them a sense of ownership for activities and decisions (Yukl & Van Fleet, 1992).

Of course, there are disadvantages to participation. First, participatory decisions are time-consuming (Vroom, 1991). This is a problem in a crisis and may take people from other important work. Second, leaders who use participatory

Participative decision making (PDM)

A leadership continuum reflecting a range of member participation ranging from no participation to joint decision making.

Process directiveness

The way a leader brings out different viewpoints and orchestrates a democratic decision process.

techniques may be perceived as too weak or incapable of making decisions themselves and may lose credibility with followers. Third, sometimes participants lack the skills, knowledge, or intellect to make good decisions. Therefore, it is inappropriate to consult on all matters. Fourth, because participants may disagree, participatory decision making requires a good leader who can manage conflict and keep the group moving toward quick resolution (Crouch & Yetton, 1987). Finally, routine failure to accept follower influence may make followers believe that participation is a sham designed to manipulate them, and this will adversely affect morale and leader–follower relations (Hollander & Offermann, 1990). Participatory decision making is also discussed in Chapter 9, Group Productivity, in the section on goal setting and in Chapter 11, Group Decision-making.

Using the Behavior Model to Improve Leadership Practice

The behavior and style approaches to leadership offer a number of suggestions for improving our leadership behavior.

1. Seek a balance between task and socioemotional leadership. Do not be so focused on the task and its accomplishment that members' personal needs are ignored, leading to lowered morale and performance. Conversely, do not be so focused on personal relationships that you do not provide the structure or direction needed to keep people on task.
2. Use praise and contingent rewards (rewards based on performance) to increase member satisfaction and performance.
3. Honor followers' knowledge of the work, their skills, the group, and the organization by encouraging all members to provide input on important decisions that affect their work.
4. Use power in a subtle, easy fashion that minimizes status differences and avoids threats to the self-esteem of members.
5. Make sure that you make work assignments clear and that followers know how to perform them, understand deadlines, and know performance expectations.
6. Monitor the conditions that affect the work, check on the progress and quality of the work, and evaluate the performance of individuals and the effectiveness of the group.
7. Motivate by using logic or emotion to generate enthusiasm for the work and commitment to task objectives, and by providing support through the provision of requested resources, information, or assistance.

Situational or Contingency Theories of Leadership

By the 1960s, it was apparent that a comprehensive study of leadership would have to consider the conditions under which different types of leadership are effective (Chemers, 1983). This led to the development of leadership theories

**Contingency
(situational) theories
of leadership**

Leadership theories
emphasizing that the
situation determines
whether a given style
of leadership will be
effective.

that would tell us when a given type of leader behavior was likely to be effective. These theories go under the heading of **contingency,** or **situational, theories of leadership.** The point of these theories is that the situation determines which leadership behaviors are most likely to be effective. In other words, in answer to the question "What makes a good leader?" these theories say "It depends on the situation."

Fiedler's Contingency Model

**Fiedler's contingency
model**

A contingency theory
suggesting that the
effectiveness of a
leader's style
depends on leader–
member relations,
task structure, and
position power.

**Least Preferred
Coworker (LPC) Scale**

Instrument used by
Fiedler to classify
leaders as task or
socioemotionally ori-
ented based on their
ratings of a least pre-
ferred coworker.

One of the first contingency theories was Fiedler's (1967) situational theory of leadership. **Fiedler's contingency model** divides leaders into those who are task-oriented and those who are socioemotionally oriented by using an instrument called the **Least Preferred Coworker (LPC) Scale.** When filling out the LPC, you are asked to think of all past and present coworkers and choose the one with whom you had the most difficulty working to get a job done. You then rate this person on sixteen bipolar (opposite) adjectives using an eight-point rating scale. For instance, you would rate the person on "pleasant–unpleasant," "cooperative–uncooperative," and "interesting–boring." Your LPC is the sum of the ratings of the least preferred coworker. The higher your score, the more "relationship oriented" you are in your leadership, meaning that you value good interpersonal relations with members over task success. The lower your score, the more "task-oriented" you are. Task-oriented leaders value the achievement of task objectives over interpersonal relationships.

Fiedler's theory is a contingency theory, meaning that different situations call for different types of leadership. According to the theory, a socioemotional (high-LPC) leader will be more effective in some situations than in others, and likewise for the low-LPC leader. It depends on the leader's *situational control*— the degree to which the leader has influence over the group's behavior. Situational control is determined by three features of the situation: (1) *leader–member relations,* the degree to which members and the leader enjoy a good relationship; (2) *task structure,* the degree to which the task is clear-cut; and (3) *position power,* the leader's power to reward or punish members. A "favorable" situation is characterized by good leader–member relations, high task structure, and strong leader position power. Conversely, a situation is "unfavorable" when leader–member relations are poor, the task is unstructured, and the leader's position power is weak.

Fiedler's theory is complicated, but the bottom line is that Fiedler believes a task-oriented (low-LPC) leader is effective in two situations. First is the situation in which the leader is on good terms with group members, the task is highly structured, and the leader has a position of high authority and power. The reasoning is that when the group is responsive and the task is clear, a firm and directive style works well and a focus on interpersonal relations is unnecessary. The second condition under which the task-oriented leader will be effective is when the leader has poor relations with group members, the task is ambiguous, and the leader has low authority and power. Fiedler (1993) suggests that under such conditions, task leaders focus on task completion and do not waste time worrying about the members' emotional states, thus moving the group forward.

The socioemotional leader is ineffective in situations in which member relations are especially bad because the leader will spend too much time worrying about interpersonal relations that cannot be fixed instead of directing attention to the task (Bons & Fiedler, 1976). Socioemotional leaders are also ineffective when the task is highly ambiguous because they do not provide enough task guidance. The socioemotional leader is effective when leader–member relations are moderately good or moderately bad, when the task is moderately clear, and the leader has moderate authority and power. The idea is that a more considerate, interpersonally sensitive leader results in greater follower involvement and motivation when the task is somewhat unclear or the group somewhat unresponsive (Chemers, 1983).

According to Fiedler, leadership style is hard to change. Therefore, groups should seek a leader whose style matches the leadership situation, or seek to change the situation lest problems arise for the leader and the group (Fiedler & Chemers, 1984). Chemers and his colleagues (Chemers, Hays, Rhodewalt, & Wysocki, 1985) tested this idea in a study of college administrators. They found that mismatches between leader style and situational control were associated with increased job stress, stress-related illness, and absence from work for the administrators.

Fiedler's model has generated a lot of research and critique. In particular, his LPC measure has been criticized as a rather mysterious measure of the leader's orientation that doesn't appear to measure what it's supposed to measure; that is, it lacks what researchers call face validity (Northouse, 1997). At the very least, it is a rather indirect measure, because your score is liable to be greatly influenced by your particular work experiences. For instance, you may have had only minor negative experiences with coworkers and therefore appear more socioemotional than you are. Conversely, you may have worked with the "employee from hell" and therefore look more task-oriented than you are. In either case, your score may not reflect your leadership orientation. More than 150 studies have examined the model, and in general, although laboratory studies provide support, many field studies do not (Peters, Hartke, & Pohlman, 1985).

The theory has also been criticized because it is too complicated for everyday leaders to apply (Northouse, 1997). However, despite the weaknesses of the LPC as a measure and the mixed research support, Fiedler deserves credit for further developing the important idea that different leadership styles may be called for in different situations. Leader–member relations, task structure, and the leader's position power likely influence the effectiveness of task or socioemotional leadership. Our next leadership theory pursues this line of thought.

Path-Goal Theory of Leadership

Path-goal theory of leadership

A contingency theory recommending that leaders vary their style depending on the members and the task, and should clarify how to reach goals.

The **path-goal theory of leadership** is a contingency theory based on the expectancy-valence theory, which you learned about in Chapter 9, Group Productivity. Remember that according to this theory, people are motivated when they believe that increased effort will lead to increased performance and increased performance will lead to increased rewards that are valued by the individual. According to path-goal theorist House (1971, pp. 321–339), "the motivational function of the leader consists of increasing personal payoffs to members for work-goal accomplishment, and making the path to these payoffs easier to travel by clarifying it, reducing roadblocks and pitfalls, and increasing the opportunities for personal satisfaction en route."

Path-goal theorists believe that leaders should adapt their styles to the situation; the impact of leadership is contingent on the characteristics of the task and members. House and Dessler (1974) suggest that interpersonally oriented leader behaviors (called *supportive leadership*) and task-oriented leader behaviors (called *directive leadership*) are helpful depending on the situation. Two important situational variables influence the type of leadership that will be effective: (1) the characteristics of the members, such as skills and personality; and (2) the characteristics of the environment, such as type of task.

For instance, directive leadership such as specifying tasks and goals will be welcomed when members' jobs or roles are unclear, members are inexperienced, and there are few procedures to guide the work. However, it will have negative effects if members already know what the goal is and how to reach it. In such cases, directive leadership may be viewed as unnecessary, disrespectful, and overly controlling. Supportive leadership is important when the task is stressful, unpleasant, or boring. However, if members' tasks are intrinsically satisfying, then a supportive leader has few effects. Individuals high in a need for affiliation also prefer supportive leadership, whereas some employees prefer to be left alone.

A revised version of the theory adds two other leader behaviors (House & Mitchell, 1974). *Participative leadership* involves consulting with members and integrating their opinions and suggestions into decision making. *Achievement-oriented leadership* focuses on setting challenging goals, emphasizing excellence in performance, and showing confidence that members will reach high standards. The conditions under which participative and achievement-oriented leadership are effective are not as well developed or researched as directive and supportive leadership (Yukl, 1998). House and Mitchell (1974) suggest that participative leadership is useful when the task is ambiguous because it helps members learn more about it and how to accomplish it. Participative leadership is also favored by employees with a strong sense of autonomy and a need for control. Achievement-oriented leadership is believed to be most effective in ambiguous situations in which members can benefit from a leader who fosters members' self-confidence about their ability to reach a difficult goal.

Path-goal theory is intuitively appealing. It makes sense that a leader may need to change his or her behavior depending on the task and the members' skills and personalities. Path-goal theory suggests that it is important for leaders to coach, guide, and help members clarify goals and what it will take to achieve them (Northouse, 1997). Despite its appeal, however, research has yielded mixed support for the theory (Podsakoff, MacKenzie, Ahearne, & Bommer, 1995; Wofford & Liska, 1993).

Hershey and Blanchard's Situational Model

Situational theory of leadership

Hershey and Blanchard's contingency theory recommending one of four styles based on the group's level of development.

Contrast a group in which the members are uncommitted or inexperienced with a group whose members are committed, competent, and experienced in working together, and it becomes easier to understand why Hershey and Blanchard (1982, 1988) suggested that the appropriate leadership style depends on the developmental level of the group and its members. Hershey and Blanchard's **situational theory of leadership** is a contingency model frequently used by business for training managers (Blanchard, Zigarmi, & Nelson, 1993; Blanchard, Zigarmi, & Zigarmi, 1985; Northouse, 1997). Like other contingency theories, this one suggests that the style of leadership depends on the situation. In this case, the situational variables of interest are the group's "maturity" (how long group members have worked together) and group members' "readiness" (their ability and willingness to accomplish the tasks).

Hershey and Blanchard (1982, 1988) describe four different leadership styles that are combinations of the now familiar task and socioemotional leadership dimensions. In their system, the *directive (task) dimension* refers to the amount of task-related guidance and direction provided by the leader (what to do, how to do it, and when it should be done). The *supportive (relational) dimension* refers to the amount of social and emotional support the leader provides. Supportive behaviors involve helping subordinates feel good about themselves, their coworkers, the task, and the situation. The four styles are four different combinations of these two dimensions.

The *directing* or *S1 style* (high task, low supportive) is very task focused and somewhat authoritarian. Leaders with a directive style tell members what is to be done and how to do it, and members are supervised closely with relatively little attention to the relational aspects of the group. The *coaching* or *S2 style* (high task, high supportive) is also directive, but more attention is given to the social dimension of the group. The leader is interested in what subordinates are thinking and feeling, explains why things should be done in a particular way, and provides support. The leader with the *supporting* or *S3 style* (low task, high supportive) is strongly participatory, using leadership to direct the group to make its own decisions and focusing on the social dimensions of the group. Last, the leader with the *delegating* or *S4 style* (low task, low supportive) lets the group lead itself, making its own decisions and solving problems without the leader's direction.

As a contingency theory, Hershey and Blanchard's situational theory suggests that leaders should change styles depending on the development level of the group and its members (Blanchard et al., 1993). For instance, a group that is low in maturity because its members have little experience working together, or one that is new to the task, often needs a directive style. However, as the group matures, the leader can gradually ease up on the directiveness, moving from a directive style, to a coaching style, to a supporting style, and then to a delegating style when the group no longer needs the leader to assist with the task or member relations. Similarly, the lower the group is in readiness (competence and commitment), the more appropriate is a directing or coaching style, and the higher the readiness, the more appropriate a supporting or delegating style. For instance, according to the theory, subordinates who are highly motivated but low in confidence are likely to benefit from a supporting style. They need some direction and some social support from their leader. The situational leadership theory calls for even more flexibility than other contingency theories because it suggests that the maturity and readiness of a group frequently change. For instance, a new group may not stay new for long. Even in an established, mature group, the introduction of a new project or task may require a directive style with regard to that task, but a supportive style is appropriate for other group tasks.

As stated earlier, the situational leadership theory is popular in business, most likely because it makes sense to managers. Despite its wide use, however, relatively little research has tested the theory (Northouse, 1997), and available research provides only mixed support. For example, a study of 300 high school teachers and their principals found that the theory's prediction that new members would perform better under directive styles was supported, but it was unclear whether the more experienced teachers benefited more from a coaching, supporting, or delegating style (Vecchio, 1987). Research is also lacking on some of the more questionable aspects of the theory, such as the conceptualization of subordinates' developmental level (Blanchard et al., 1993; Northouse, 1997; Yukl, 1989).

Using the Contingency Models to Improve Leadership Practice

The contingency theories are admittedly complex because they try to specify how leadership should vary based on the situation, and situations are highly variable. However, some basic suggestions for improving leadership behavior can be offered.

1. Use directive (task) behavior when tasks are ambiguous and complex, members are inexperienced, and there are few guidelines to guide the work.
2. Use supportive (socioemotional) behavior when the task is boring, unpleasant, or stressful, and when members appreciate a friendly, group-oriented atmosphere.
3. If members lack confidence about their ability to perform a task, specify the behaviors that will lead to increased performance, and provide any needed instruction on how to perform them.

Apply It! ••• **Evaluate a Leader With the Contingency Approach**

Think about your boss or, if you are not currently employed, a past boss or teacher. Was this person an effective leader in that situation according to the three contingency theories described here? Did this person provide the appropriate level of task and socioemotional leadership, given the subordinates, the task, and the situation?

---

4. Identify and remove obstacles to members' goal achievement. Do what you can to make it easier for their actions to lead to successful performance.
5. Be aware of members' differing personalities and consider "tweaking" your leadership approach accordingly. For instance, members who are highly competent and not very social will resent too much leader intrusion. Other members appreciate leader attention and work harder when they get it.

Leadership, Gender, and Culture

Glass ceiling
Term used to refer to the invisible barriers hindering the promotion of women and members of other groups traditionally underrepresented into high leadership positions.

In the rest of this chapter, you will learn about diversity and leadership and some explanations for the fact that in the United States, women and individuals from nonwhite groups are less likely to be cast in leadership roles. Despite progress, a **glass ceiling**—an invisible barrier to the promotion of women and ethnic minorities—remains in place. A report based on a bipartisan federal panel investigation indicated that although white men make up only 43 percent of the workforce, they hold 95 percent of senior management positions (Federal Glass Ceiling Commission, 1995). Furthermore, of the 3 to 5 percent of women that occupy top management positions, 95 percent are white (U.S. Department of Labor, 1997). The picture is somewhat improved when we include lower and middle management. For instance, in 1996, 15.3 percent of employed white men were in executive, management, and administrative positions, compared with 13.9 percent of white women, 8.3 percent of black men, 9.6 percent of black women, 6.6 percent of Hispanic men, and 8.5 percent of Hispanic women (U.S. Department of Labor, 1997). Powell (1999) suggests that the presence of women in top management positions violates the societal norm of men's higher status and superiority more than does women's presence in lower-status management positions. This may explain why the number of women in top leadership positions remains small despite women's gains in lower and middle management (Powell, 1999).

In this part of the chapter, you will also read about the research on leadership cross-culturally. Most of the research on leadership has been conducted in the United States, Canada, and Western Europe (Yukl, 1998) and there is some question about the generalizability of the research findings to other cultures.

Given the globalization of the world economy and the growth of multinational corporations, leadership researchers have increasingly turned their attention to the study of leadership cross-culturally.

Gender and Ethnic Differences in Leadership Style and Effectiveness

Some people assume that women and others from traditionally underrepresented groups are not found as frequently in leadership roles because they do not lead as well as Euroamerican males. Unfortunately, there are few studies of the leadership performance of racial or ethnic minorities in top management positions, other than detailed biographies of black community and religious leaders such as Martin Luther King, Jr., Frederick Douglass, Malcolm X, and Nelson Mandela (Hooijberg & DiTomaso, 1996). Leadership studies in real-world environments have focused more on leadership in settings dominated by whites, such as large organizations and corporations. Laboratory studies of leadership, conducted primarily with college students, also suffer from the fact that nonwhites are less likely to attend college, or to attend colleges where research is conducted. The truth is that there remains a serious gap in our knowledge of African American, Latin American, and Asian American leadership. In contrast, there is lots of research on gender differences in leadership style and effectiveness, mostly comparing Euroamerican men and women. This may be because in the last 20 years, a large number of Euroamerican women have entered social and organizational psychology and have taken up the study of gender differences.

Available evidence indicates that women are no less effective leaders/managers than men (Eagly & Johnson, 1990; Eagly, Karau, & Makhijani, 1995; Kolb, 1999; Powell, 1990). In fact, female managers often have higher levels of work motivation than male managers (Donnell & Hall, 1980), and female managers are comfortable and capable in a conflict management role (Duane, 1989). A U.S. Department of Labor report on the glass ceiling (1991) cites research finding that a majority of women in both line and staff positions had leader-style management skills and a greater proportion of women in staff positions displayed a leadership orientation than men in line positions. A meta-analysis comparing the leadership styles of men and women found female leaders to be somewhat more likely to use a participative, democratic style and males to use a directive, autocratic style (Eagly & Johnson, 1990). However, both genders were more task-oriented when in a "gender-congruent context." In other words, men were more task-oriented in a masculine context, and women in a feminine context. A meta-analysis by Eagly, Karau, and Makhijani (1995) examined leader effectiveness research and concluded that neither male nor female leaders were more effective. However, they did find that the leaders of each sex were viewed as particularly effective when they were in a leadership role regarded as congruent with their gender. For instance, women were evaluated more favorably when they were in education or social service leadership positions, and in studies of military organizations, men were evaluated more favorably.

The bottom line is that there is no research evidence to suggest that women or others from traditionally underrepresented groups are less suited for top leadership positions (Hooijberg & DiTomaso, 1996), so it is important to explore other explanations for this consistent finding.

Explanations for the Lower Percentage of Female and Nonwhite Leaders

Emergent leadership
The study of who tends to emerge as a leader of a group and how groups choose a leader in an initially leaderless group.

The study of **emergent leadership** focuses on how groups choose leaders. Emergent leadership theory suggests that leadership exists only after other group members acknowledge or accept someone as the leader. In essence, you are not a leader until group members give their consent that they will follow you. Research on leader emergence finds that in mixed-gender groups that do not initially have a leader, white males are more likely than others to emerge as leaders (Eagly & Karau, 1991; Sapp, Harrod, & Zhao, 1996). Carli and Eagly (1999) suggest that men may have a leadership advantage because of their greater tendencies to talk more than women in task-oriented groups, behave in more powerful and authoritative ways, be task-oriented, and show more visual dominance. However, when socioemotional leadership is needed, women's leadership approximates men's (Eagly & Karau, 1991). For example, in a group that needs to negotiate and cooperate to achieve its goals, a woman may be more likely to emerge as a leader. Relatively little research has investigated whether these differences are consistent across cultures and subcultures (Carli & Eagly, 1999). One exception is a study by Filardo (1996) in which mixed-gender groups of African American and Euroamerican adolescents were given a cooperative problem-solving task. Among the Euroamericans, the males emerged as leaders, but this was not true of the African American groups.

Status characteristics theory (discussed at length in Chapter 4, Status and Power Dynamics in Groups) suggests that individuals' diffuse status characteristics—such as gender, age, and ethnicity—affect group members' expectations about different members and that this might explain why Euroamerican males are more frequently chosen as leaders. In regard to leadership, the theory suggests that group members expect and accept that individuals with high diffuse status will behave in a competent, confident manner consistent with leadership, whereas individuals with low diffuse status who behave similarly will be ignored or rejected (Carli & Eagly, 1999). In other words, similar behavior is perceived differently depending on who does it and whether it fits expectations. For instance, Butler and Geis (1990) found that when female leaders offered the same suggestions and arguments as male leaders, the women received more negative responses than men. A number of studies indicate that women must perform better than men to be perceived as equally competent by group members (Biernat & Kobrynowicz, 1997; Foschi, 1992, 1996). Especially for tasks involving analysis and reasoning, group members consider men to be more competent unless presented with clear evidence of female superiority (Carli, 1991). In a study of black MBA graduates from the top five business schools, 85 percent reported that considerations of race had a negative impact on their performance appraisals (Jones, 1986).

Another way to look at it is that whether you are perceived as leadership material depends in part on whether you fit the **leader prototype** common in your culture. **Leadership categorization theory** suggests that matching an observed person against an abstract prototype stored in memory plays an important role in the attributions of leadership (Lord & Maher, 1991). The better the fit between the perceived individual and the leader prototype, the more likely the person will be seen as a leader (Foti & Luch, 1992; Offermann, Kennedy, & Wirtz, 1994). In the United States, if you asked a number of people to imagine a leader, most of them would imagine a (white) man in his 30s to 50s. This prototypical leader image may interfere with the perception of women and non-whites as leadership material. Gender and ethnic stereotypes also affect whether we perceive individuals from various social categories to be suitable candidates for leadership roles. According to several studies, our beliefs that women are inappropriate for leadership positions are so strong that contrary data are often ignored in managerial selection and other managerial decisions affecting women (Freedman & Phillips, 1988; Heilman & Martell, 1986; Ilgen & Youtz, 1986; Morrison & Von Glinow, 1990). Cejka and Eagly (1999) found that gender-stereotypic images of occupations corresponded to sex segregation in employment. Glick (1991) found that jobs are generally seen as "masculine" or "feminine" and that job applicants are seen as more or less suitable for different jobs depending on the applicant's sex.

Although there are no comparable studies with regard to race and ethnicity, we might expect similar findings. For instance, Asian Americans have been very successful in scientific and technical fields and yet are less likely than Euroamericans and African Americans to be found in leadership positions in these fields (Tang, 1997). This could be because common stereotypes of Asian Americans as passive, quiet, reserved, and submissive may interfere with others' perceptions of their appropriateness for leadership positions. Hispanics may be stereotyped as unintelligent, lazy, too emotional, kind, friendly, lively, and passionate (Fernandez, 1991). Some of these characteristics are viewed as detrimental to leadership performance (Landau, 1995). Landau, in a study of a Fortune 500 company, found that being female or black or Asian negatively influenced supervisors' ratings of employees' potential for promotion.

Where do leader prototypes come from? After all, leadership models as well as leadership studies suggest that good leaders are directive and task-oriented (stereotypically male qualities) *and* people oriented and interpersonally skilled (stereotypically female qualities) (Cann & Siegfried, 1990). The stereotype of a masculine leader represents a very narrow view that ignores an important dimension of effective leadership, and yet most people continue to think of leadership as more "male" than "female." The reason may be that our leader prototypes come partly from who we customarily see occupying leadership roles.

Leader prototype
A mental picture of what a model leader should look and be like; the leader archetype.

Leadership categorization theory
A theory suggesting that we compare potential leaders to our leader prototypes and this determines whether we cast them in leader roles.

Apply It! •••	**Compare Ethnic Stereotypes and Leader Prototypes**

Get out a lined piece of paper. Draw a vertical line down the middle and label one column "Female" and one "Male." Down the left-hand margin list the major ethnic groups in your culture, skipping five lines after each one. For instance, Americans might list African Americans, Asian Americans, Latin Americans, Euroamericans. Next, write down common stereotypes of each group, separately for each gender. How well do the stereotypes fit your leadership prototype? Could such stereotypes influence whether individuals from these groups are considered appropriate for leadership positions? Do you think your diffuse status characteristics (age, gender, and ethnicity) influence others' perceptions of your suitability for leadership roles?

In virtually every culture, males of a specific ethnic group occupy the most prominent of society's leadership roles. Individuals from certain groups are seldom seen in prominent leadership positions. For instance, in the United States, Latina, African American, Asian American, and Native American women represent only 4 percent of women in management, leading some to say that such women face not just a "glass ceiling" but a "concrete ceiling" that is virtually impossible to break through (Burn, 2000). This **gender and ethnic job segregation** perpetuates a situation in which certain groups dominate certain roles because people from other groups do not seem right for the job.

Gender and ethnic job segregation

The finding that most jobs are gender typed and that particular ethnic groups are rarely found in some job categories.

Organizational and group practices may also contribute to a situation in which few qualified women or minorities are available for leadership positions. Access to education, training, or experiences that lead to leadership positions is not always offered to those from lower-status groups, such as women and minorities, with the same frequency as it is to Euroamerican males. For instance, it is common to have to work in a particular sequence of jobs to work your way up in the organization—that is, you climb a "job ladder" to the top. Research indicates that women tend to be placed in dead-end jobs, whereas jobs that provide promotion opportunities are designated as male jobs (Baron, Davis-Blake, & Bielby, 1986; Bergmann, 1986; Ragins & Sundstrom, 1989). As noted by the United Nations' International Labour Organization (1998, p. 2), "At lower management levels women are typically placed in non-strategic sections, and in personnel and administrative positions, rather than in the professional and line management jobs leading to the top." Black men and women are channeled into "racialized" jobs—for instance, into liaison jobs linking the company to the black community or into running affirmative action programs—while the more visible and revenue-producing jobs are reserved for whites (Collins, 1993; Jones, 1986).

In addition, women and nonwhites may be less likely to receive mentoring from individuals with advanced experience and knowledge (Ragins, 1999; Thomas, 1990; Thomas & Higgins, 1996). Mentoring is important because protégés receive more promotions, better compensation, and greater career mobility (Ragins, 1999). For instance, women are less likely than men to receive personal support, job-related information, and career developmental support from their supervisors (Cianni & Romberger, 1995; Ohlott, Ruderman, & McCauley, 1994). One study found that 91 percent of female executives surveyed reported having a mentor, and the majority identified mentoring as a key strategy for breaking through the glass ceiling (Ragins, Townsend, & Mattis, 1998).

Leadership Cross-Culturally

There is some controversy around the question of whether the essence of leadership is the same around the world. Some argue that leadership is the same in that it is always about motivating people and aligning them with the organization's mission (see Fulkerson & Schuler, 1992). Others, such as Hofstede (1991, p. 66), argue that "management techniques and training packages have been developed in individualist countries, and they are based on cultural assumptions that may not hold in collectivist cultures." Research studies on a variety of leadership-related topics have been conducted in non-Western countries, but not enough of them to reach definitive conclusions. The truth regarding culture and leadership is understandably complex. This is mirrored in the typical finding of both cross-cultural similarities (cultural universals) and differences (cultural specifics) in cross-cultural leadership studies.

Several studies have examined whether groups in other countries tend to develop separate task and socioemotional leaders, as Bales demonstrated in 1950. Krichevskii (1983), in a study of sports teams and student groups in the Soviet Union, found that they did. Studies of British students and managers (Smith, 1963) and Dutch students (Koomen, 1988) also replicated Bales' findings. No empirical studies are available from more collectivist cultures, although it is widely reported that members of work teams in Japanese organizations are flexible in occupying these roles (Smith & Bond, 1999).

The findings regarding the effectiveness of task and relationship leadership behaviors do show significant cross-cultural variation. You may recall that in the United States, contingency theories of leadership were developed because it appeared that the type of leader behavior that was effective depended on the situation. Studies conducted in Western Europe yielded similar results (Smith & Tayeb, 1988), as did a study conducted in the former Soviet Union (Zhurvalev & Shorokhova, 1984). However, studies in Taiwan (Bond & Hwang, 1986), India (Sinha, 1995), Japan (Misumi, 1985), and Iran (Ayman & Chemers, 1983) showed that leaders simultaneously high on both task and socioemotional dimensions were most effective.

Studies on transformational and transactional leadership find more consistent cross-cultural similarities. Bass and Avolio (1993) found that in the United States, Japan, Singapore, Italy, Canada, Spain, New Zealand, Germany, and India, leaders perceived as transformational were more highly evaluated by their subordinates. Similarly, a study of 62 cultures found that attributes associated with transformational leadership were universally endorsed as contributing to outstanding leadership (Den Hartog, House, Hanges, Ruiz-Quintanilla, & Dorfman, 1999). Contributing to outstanding leadership in all cultures were attributes reflecting *integrity* (trustworthy, just, honest), *charismatic leadership* (encouraging, positive, motivational, confidence builder, dynamic), and a *team orientation* (team builder, communicative, coordinator). Attributes seen universally as barriers to effective leadership included being a loner and being noncooperative, ruthless, nonexplicit, irritable, and dictatorial.

Despite the apparent cross-cultural similarities in their study, Den Hartog et al. (1999) note that how these qualities are enacted may depend on culture. For instance, what constitutes a "good communicator" and how "vision" is expressed are likely to vary greatly across cultures. In China, vision is normally expressed in a nonaggressive manner, whereas in India, bold, assertive styles are preferred to quiet, nurturing styles (Den Hartog et al., 1999). In countries that emphasize egalitarianism, such as The Netherlands and Australia, leaders are expected to inspire high levels of performance but must avoid the appearance of being "above" others (Den Hartog et al., 1999). In Indonesia, transformational leaders boast about their own competence to create pride and respect, but this is unacceptable for transformational leaders in Japan (Bass, 1997). In short, even charisma must be defined within a cultural context.

Recall that in addition to the basic task and socioemotional leadership distinction, four specific leadership styles have also been studied. In general, cross-cultural studies have found some uniformity in the relative effectiveness of the styles. For example, a study of leaders in the United States, Mexico, Taiwan, Korea, and Japan found that supportive leaders who made rewards contingent on performance were rated most positively (Howell, Dorfman, Hibino, Lee, & Tate, 1997). The finding that transformational leaders are more effective than those practicing contingent reward, that contingent reward is more effective than active management by exception, and that active management by exception is more effective than laissez-faire leadership has also been replicated in Austria, Belgium, China, Germany, India, Japan, New Zealand, Spain, Singapore, Sweden, and New Zealand (Bass, 1997). Bass cautions, however, that there were country-based differences in the magnitude of the differences between the leadership styles. Dorfman and his associates (1997) also found cultural universality for supportive, contingent reward, and charismatic leader behaviors. However, they found cultural differences (cultural specificity) for directive, participative, and contingent punishment leader behaviors. Howell et al. (1997) reported similar findings. Directive leadership had more positive effects in Mexico, Korea, and Taiwan than it did in the United States or Japan, and participative leadership had positive effects only in the United States.

Using Diversity Research to Improve Leadership Practice

Although the findings on diversity and leadership are complex and incomplete, it is safe to make the following recommendations to improve leadership practice.

1. Be aware of your leader prototype and the tendency to overlook women and minorities as possible candidates for leadership positions.
2. If you are in a top leadership role, do what you can to make sure women and minorities receive the same training, mentoring, and job experiences to prepare them for leadership positions as Euroamerican males receive.
3. If you are a woman or minority group member, be aware that you may have to perform better in order to be perceived as equally competent, you may have to request assignments to gain leadership experience, and you may have to remind upper management of your qualifications for promotion.
4. When working as a leader in a cross-cultural context, familiarize yourself with the culture's leader prototype and communication norms, and adjust your behavior accordingly. For instance, in some cultures, directive leadership is appreciated; in others, consultative or participative leadership is more effective. In some cultures, leaders are expected to be bold and assertive; in others, a more subtle communication style is expected.
5. Remember that leaders are viewed positively when they exhibit integrity, charismatic leadership, and a team orientation. However, the leadership behaviors that reflect these qualities vary by culture. Therefore, for effective leadership in other cultural contexts, you should pay attention to how the particular culture enacts these qualities.

Concept Review

Definitions of Leadership

- **Leadership** is a process that includes influencing the task objectives and strategies of a group or organization, influencing people in the organization to implement the strategies and achieve the objectives, influencing group maintenance and identification, and influencing the culture of the organization.

Trait Theories of Leadership

- Leadership research began in the early 1900s and until World War II focused on identifying the personality traits associated with leadership. This is known as the **trait approach to leadership** or the *great person theory of leadership.*
- In research reviews, Stodgill (1948, 1974) found only a few traits correlated with leadership effectiveness. The approach was largely abandoned until the 1980s, when leaders were found to rate higher than most people

on drive, self-confidence, cognitive ability, creativity, leadership motivation, expertise, flexibility, energy level, stress tolerance, and emotional maturity. In terms of the "big five" dimensions of personality, leaders tend to score high on extraversion, agreeableness, conscientiousness, emotional stability, and intelligence.

- **Transactional leadership** (ordinary leadership) is focused on the immediate situation and getting the job done. The leader's role is to clarify task demands and rewards for compliance. Four different forms of transactional leadership, in order of effectiveness, are contingent reward, active management by exception, passive management by exception, and laissez-faire leadership.

- **Transformational leadership,** also called **charismatic leadership,** has four characteristics: idealized influence, inspiration, intellectual stimulation, and individualized consideration. Transformational leadership is positively related to perceptions of leader effectiveness, the effort members are willing to expend, and member satisfaction. Unethical charismatics control and manipulate followers and are self-serving rather than leading on the behalf of group members or the organization.

- Where routine performance is required, the transactional leader may be adequate, but where extraordinary effort is required, as is the case with social change or organizational or product innovation, a transformational leader is probably needed.

Behavior Theories of Leadership

- **Behavior theories of leadership** became popular after World War II and were the primary focus of leadership research through the 1960s.

- Research programs at several universities all pointed to two reliable sets of leader behaviors: **task behaviors** and **socioemotional behaviors,** also called *initiating structure* and *consideration.* The two-factor model was important in that it identified two broad classes of leader behavior but limited because it was not clear when each was effective.

- Later, researchers worked to identify specific leader behaviors that are related to effectiveness. Leader effectiveness is linked to praise and contingent rewards, clarifying, and informal and flexible planning.

- Autocratic and democratic leadership styles have also been studied. **Autocratic leaders** use their power to coerce others to follow them. **Democratic leaders** are more consultative and socioemotional. **Participative decision making (PDM)** is an important component of the democratic style. It may involve consulting with members individually or making joint decisions with them in a group. Research suggests a modest positive relationship between participation and satisfaction and a small but significant relationship between participation and performance.

Situational or Contingency Theories of Leadership

- Popular for the past thirty years, **contingency theories** posit that the situation determines which leadership behaviors are most likely to be effective.
- **Fiedler's contingency model** was one of the first contingency theories. Fiedler's **Least Preferred Coworker (LPC) Scale** is used to divide people into socioemotional or task leaders. The task-oriented (low-LPC) leader is effective when the leader is on good terms with group members, the task is highly structured, and the leader has a position of high authority and power, or when the leader has poor relations with group members, the task is ambiguous, and the leader has low authority and power. The socioemotional leader is effective when leader–member relations are moderately good or moderately bad, the task is moderately clear, and the leader has moderate authority and power.
- The **path-goal theory of leadership** suggests that leaders clarify paths to work goals and reduce obstacles. Situational variables, such as member characteristics and the task, influence effective leadership style. Directive leadership is appropriate when members lack the experience or training to perform a task. Supportive leadership is important when the task is aversive or boring. Participative leadership is useful when the task is ambiguous and when members have a strong need for autonomy and control. Achievement-oriented leadership is useful when members need self-confidence about their ability to succeed.
- Hershey and Blanchard's **situational theory of leadership** recommends that leaders provide varying combinations of task and socioemotional leadership depending on the development of the group (its maturity and the commitment and competence of its members). Directing and coaching styles are appropriate when the group's development is low, and supporting and delegating styles are appropriate when its development is high.

Leadership, Gender, and Culture

- There is no research evidence to suggest that women or others from traditionally underrepresented groups are less suited for top leadership positions, yet a **glass ceiling**—an invisible barrier to the promotion of women and ethnic minorities—remains in place.
- For the most part, there are few differences in the way men and women lead. Female leaders appear to be somewhat more likely to use a participative, democratic style and males to use a directive, autocratic style, but both genders are more task-oriented when in a "gender-congruent context."
- In mixed-gender groups that do not initially have a leader, Euroamerican males usually emerge as leaders. Men may have a leadership advantage because of their tendencies to talk more than women in task-oriented groups,

to be more task oriented, to behave in more powerful and authoritative ways, and to show more visual dominance. Men's tendency toward emergent leadership decreases when tasks require relatively complex social interaction.

- **Leadership categorization theory** suggests the better the fit between the perceived individual and the **leader prototype**, the more likely the person will be seen as a leader. In the United States, the prototypical leader is a Euroamerican male, and this may interfere with the perception of women and nonwhites as leadership material.
- Organizational practices may also contribute to the glass ceiling. Access to education, training, or experiences that lead to leadership positions is frequently not offered to those from lower-status groups. Women and minorities are less likely to receive jobs and assignments that lead up the organizational ladder and are less likely to receive mentoring.
- In studies of leadership cross-culturally, it is typical to find both cross-cultural similarities (cultural universals) and differences (cultural specifics).
- So far, research indicates that groups in other countries also tend to develop separate task and socioemotional leaders, as Bales demonstrated in 1950. The findings regarding the effectiveness of task and relationship leadership behaviors, however, show significant cross-cultural variation.
- Studies on transformational and transactional leadership find that attributes associated with transformational leadership are universally endorsed as contributing to outstanding leadership but that charisma must be defined within a cultural context. Cross-culturally, transformational leaders are more effective than those practicing contingent reward, contingent reward is more effective than active management by exception, and laissez-faire leadership is the least effective. Studies have found cultural universality for supportive, contingent reward, and charismatic leader behaviors, but cultural differences (cultural specificity) for directive, participative, and contingent punishment leader behaviors.

Skill Review

Improving Leadership Practice With the Trait Model

- Share with followers an overarching goal.
- Communicate high performance expectations, and exhibit confidence in followers to meet these expectations.
- Project a powerful, confident, and dynamic presence.
- Give pep talks aimed at increasing optimism and enthusiasm and that remind followers of the vision.
- Encourage creativity and intelligent problem solving among followers.

- Give personal attention to all members.
- Provide feedback in ways that are easy to accept, understand, and use for personal development.
- Empower people to achieve the vision by asking them to determine the best ways to attain objectives, reducing bureaucratic constraints, and providing adequate resources.

Improving Leadership Practice With the Behavior Model

- Seek a balance between task and socioemotional leadership.
- Use praise and contingent rewards (rewards based on performance) to increase member satisfaction and performance.
- Honor followers' knowledge of the work, their skills, the group, and the organization by encouraging all members to provide input on important decisions that affect their work.
- Use power in a subtle, easy fashion that minimizes status differences.
- Monitor the conditions that affect the work, and the progress and quality of the work.

Improving Leadership Practice With the Contingency Models

- Use directive (task) behavior when tasks are ambiguous and complex, members are inexperienced, and there are few guidelines to guide the work.
- Use supportive (socioemotional) behavior when the task is boring, unpleasant, or stressful, and when members appreciate a friendly, group-oriented atmosphere.
- If members lack confidence about their ability to perform a task, specify the behaviors that will lead to increased performance and provide any needed instruction on how to perform them.
- Be aware of members' differing personalities, and consider adjusting your leadership approach accordingly.

Improving Leadership Practice With Diversity Research

- Be aware of your leader prototype and the tendency to overlook women and minorities as possible candidates for leadership positions.
- If you are in a top leadership role, do what you can to make sure women and minorities receive the same training, mentoring, and job experiences to prepare them for leadership positions as Euroamerican males receive.
- If you are a woman or minority, be aware that you may have to perform better in order to be perceived as equally competent, you may have to request assignments to gain leadership experience, and you may have to remind upper management of your qualifications for promotion.

- When working as a leader in a cross-cultural context, familiarize yourself with the culture's leader prototype and communication norms, and adjust your behavior accordingly.
- Remember that cross-culturally, leaders are viewed positively when they exhibit integrity, charismatic leadership, and a team orientation. However, the leadership behaviors that reflect these qualities vary by culture.

Study Questions

1. How is leadership defined? What is the difference between leadership and management?
2. What is the trait approach to leadership? On what traits do leaders differ from nonleaders?
3. What four forms may transactional leadership take, and what is their relative effectiveness?
4. What are the "four I's" that characterize transformational leadership? What are the benefits of transformational leadership? What is the "dark side" of transformational leadership?
5. What are the behavior theories of leadership?
6. What is the two-factor model of leader behavior? Which is more effective, task or socioemotional leadership?
7. What specific leader behaviors have been linked to leader effectiveness?
8. What is autocratic leader behavior, and what is democratic leader behavior? What is PDM, and what are its benefits?
9. What are situational or contingency theories of leadership?
10. What are the main features of Fiedler's contingency theory? What does Fiedler say about improving leadership effectiveness?
11. What is the path-goal theory of leadership, and what are its implications for leadership practice?
12. According to Hershey and Blanchard's situational theory of leadership, what are the four leadership styles, and how do you determine what leadership style to use?
13. What does the research tell us about gender differences in leadership style and effectiveness? Why do men often emerge as leaders in mixed-gender groups? According to leader categorization theory, how do leader prototypes affect who becomes a leader? How does gender and ethnic job segregation affect our leader prototypes?
14. How do common organizational and group practices contribute to the situation in which women and minorities are less likely to be promoted into leadership positions?
15. What do we know about leadership cross-culturally?

Group Activities

Activity 1: Collect Data to Evaluate Transformational Leadership

Divide your six-person group into pairs. Each pair is to go out with a tape recorder and ask five people to "describe the most outstanding leaders you have ever known" (30 minutes). When the group meets back, analyze the responses according to the four I's of transformational leadership (that is, write down what each person said that falls into each of the four categories). What did people say that did not fit into Bass' categories? Do those responses fit with other leadership perspectives discussed in the chapter? If time permits, create a set of recommendations for leaders based on the responses. (You can also have each person in the class write a few paragraphs describing the outstanding leaders and then give each group an equal number of responses to analyze.)

Activity 2: Explore Contingency Theories and Leadership Preferences

Contingency theories of leadership suggest that your leadership style should be based in part on the characteristics of the people you are leading and characteristics of the situation, including the task. Put yourself in the situations described below and decide what kind of leader you would prefer: (A) highly directive, low socioemotional; (B) highly directive, highly socioemotional; (C) low directive, highly socioemotional; or (D) low directive, low socioemotional. After you have done this, share your answers with your group. Which contingency theory best explains your answer for each scenario? If time remains, discuss your personal preferences for leadership style. Are there certain styles to which you respond well or poorly, based on your personality or values? Are there certain styles you would have an easier time or a harder time displaying as a leader, based on your personality or values?

SCENARIO 1   You are one of five new interns at a prestigious organization, and you are all are a bit intimidated by the expertise and achievements of the employees there. You are not really sure what you can contribute to this impressive organization, and you are really looking forward to the training you will receive.

SCENARIO 2   You have a master's degree from the same program that your boss does. Although he graduated a year before you did, you had experience in the field prior to entering the program, whereas he did not. You have been on the job for eighteen months now and are comfortable with your job duties and are confident in your ability to perform at a high level on new tasks.

Activity 3: Learn About Coaching as Leadership: A Leadership Fishbowl

From your class, choose a group of six current or former athletes and have them sit in a circle in the middle of the classroom. This group (the "fishbowl group") will discuss their "best and worst coaches" and "what makes a good coach." The rest of the class forms a larger circle around the six-person group so that they can observe and take notes on the conversation. The observers should be on the lookout for things that the fishbowl participants say that are related to (1) the personal qualities and traits possessed by good coaches (Did they exhibit the four I's of transformational leadership? Were they flexible, mature, confident, extroverted, warm, and intelligent?); and (2) the behaviors displayed by good coaches (How autocratic are they? How democratic? How task-oriented? How socioemotional?). The class then forms new six-person groups in which they share their observations and create a definition of a good coach based on the day's discussions. Does your definition apply to some sports more than others? Does it apply to nonsports leaders? Explain.

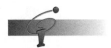

InfoTrac College Edition Search Terms

To do research for your papers and assignments, use InfoTrac that's provided free with new copies of this book. Go to http://infotrac.thomsonlearning.com and enter the following search terms:

- Transformational Leadership
- Leadership Research
- Gender and Leadership
- African American Leadership
- Hispanic American Leadership

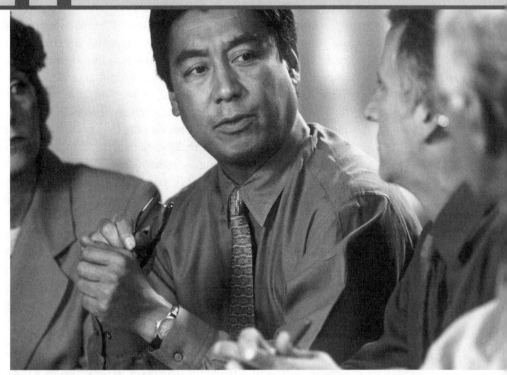

© Jon Feingersh/CORBIS

Acommittee is a cul-de-sac down which promising young ideas are lured and then quietly strangled. A camel is a horse designed by a committee. A committee is a group that keeps minutes and wastes hours. Sayings such as these reflect people's skepticism about the ability of groups to make quality decisions. Are "two heads better than one," as one American saying suggests? Or is another American aphorism, that "too many cooks spoil the broth" more accurate? As with many questions in group dynamics, the answer is "it depends." As Poole and Hirokawa (1996, p. 3) put it, "The unique chemistry of social interaction can distill the best each member has to offer, creating a resonance of ideas and a synthesis of viewpoints. A different chemistry can stop the reaction and contaminate the product." In this chapter, you will learn about the situations that lead groups to make poor decisions and the conditions under which group decisions are superior to decisions made individually. You will read about some common group decision-making errors, models, and strategies, and how you can enhance group decision making. The goal is to understand how groups can make quality decisions efficiently and, during the decision-making process, build the group rather than dividing it.

Many decisions are group decisions. Groups must often decide what they are going to do and how they are going to do it. Through group discussion, group members share and process information to arrive at a decision. A friendship group decides what they are going to do that weekend. A family group plans a wedding, anniversary celebration, or reunion. In the workplace, it is common for a workgroup to decide policies, strategies, and responses to problems facing the group. Peterson (1997) notes that the lone politician, executive, or administrator with the authority to make unilateral decisions is increasingly rare. This is because there is a growing awareness that groups bring more intellectual resources to bear on a problem (presumably leading to a better-quality decision) and, in many cases, decision acceptance is greater when decisions are made more democratically.

We need a better understanding of how group processes affect group decision making because it is challenging for groups to make decisions efficiently and effectively. Groups sometimes make decisions hurriedly and ineffectively because it takes time to share relevant information and perspectives and because conflict is common in decision making. For instance, group members may go along with the recommendations of a dominant group member or leader just to get things over with. Of course, a long process does not guarantee a quality decision. Many groups spend excessive time going off on tangents—sharing information or discussing matters that are largely irrelevant to the decision, or sharing the same information over and over again. This means that groups may not consider all applicable information and members may get bored and frustrated by the repetition. Likewise, many groups do not manage group conflict or dominating members well, and so take longer to resolve differences and reach consensus than is necessary. Another common difficulty is that groups do not have procedures in place to ensure that a few members do not dominate the decision-making process. Members who have been left out may then be less committed to the decision and to the group.

Group Decision Basics

A good way to begin thinking about group decision making is to think about the general group decision process. What is the *ideal* process for a good decision outcome? What types of group process problems and constraints interfere with quality group decision making? Many group dynamics scholars have thought about these questions.

A General Group Decision Process Model

Listed below are the six steps commonly identified as important to the group decision process (see, for example, Hackman, 1990; Hirokawa, 1985; Peterson, 1997), along with the potential process challenges that await the group at each step. These are important because, as you will see when you read the chapter, virtually all work on group decision making refers in some way to one of these steps or one of these challenges.

1. **Define the problem.** Specifically define decision-making objectives. What does the group want to accomplish? Do all members understand the nature of the problem or the decision(s) to be made? Before members can participate in identifying options and generating alternatives, they need to frame the problem clearly. The better informed members are about the problem they are to solve, the better able they are to make a quality decision (Hirokawa, Erbert, & Hurst, 1996).

2. **Identify options.** Carefully review and formulate decision alternatives. What is the range of relevant and realistic options available to the group? How can these be identified? How can the group make sure that dominant members do not restrict the range of options considered? Groups can quickly focus on a narrow range of options and assume those are the only options available to them.

3. **Gather information.** Search for information about the potential consequences of each option. What needs to be known about each alternative in order to make a clear decision? How can all members, not just high-status or dominant members, be encouraged to share what they know about the alternatives? Groups often do not take the time to gather all relevant information and do not have a process that ensures that all members share the unique information they possess.

4. **Evaluate options.** Objectively analyze the information about the different options and their consequences. What are the costs and benefits of each alternative? What process will be used to ensure that the information gathered is fully reviewed? How are the personal biases toward options that personally benefit members to be overridden? How will the group deal with dominant or high-status members who focus the group's attention on the benefits of options they favor and dismiss other options? Bad decisions and serious consequences can result from decisions made without full and objective evaluation of the alternatives.

5. **Make a decision.** Choose an alternative. What is the method for deciding between the options? Does the group vote, does it discuss until there is unanimous agreement (consensus), or do powerful group members decide? The method matters because it affects the decision that is made. For instance, some methods lead lower-status members to vote with higher-status members

even when they disagree. Method also affects members' satisfaction with and commitment to the decision.

6. **Implement the decision.** What is required to implement the decision? Which members will be responsible for the tasks and subtasks required for implementation? The work of the decision group is not really done until the decision is implemented.

Cognitive, Affiliative, and Egocentric Decision-Making Constraints

Decision-making constraints

Factors that inhibit effective group decision making, including cognitive, affiliative, and egocentric constraints.

In theory, a group of people working together, capitalizing on one another's diverse knowledge and perspectives, should produce effective solutions for difficult problems, but this ideal is often unachieved (Rogelberg, Barnes-Farrell, & Lowe, 1992). Indeed, according to research on group decision making and performance, groups perform better than their average individual member but worse than their best individual member (Bottger & Yetton, 1987; Libby, Trotman, & Zimmer, 1987; Yetton & Bottger, 1982). Why is it that groups often fail to capitalize on their potential to make better decisions than individuals? Most of the reasons fall into one of the three categories of **decision-making constraints** identified by Irving Janis (1989). These decision-making constraints are barriers to effective group decision making.

Irving Janis is an important figure in the study of group decision making, and you will see his name a number of times in the chapter. In 1989, after years of studying real-world decision-making groups, Janis categorized the factors that inhibit quality decision making into three types of constraints: (1) cognitive constraints, (2) affiliative constraints, and (3) egocentric constraints.

Cognitive constraints

When a group does not consider all relevant information when making a decision, most commonly because of limited time.

"We don't have time for a lot of discussion; we have to make a decision and make it quickly." "How are we expected to decide this in two weeks?" "In the past, we cut staff positions, and that worked fine. Let's just do that again." Comments like these suggest that a group is operating under **cognitive constraints.** These are an issue for the group when members are unable to consider all relevant information because they do not have access to it, do not have the time to get it and consider it, or are unaccustomed to the level of complexity of the problem and are unable to process it fully. Cognitive constraints can interfere with the group's accurate framing of the problem as well as the generation and evaluation of alternatives. Groups facing cognitive constraints often take decision-making shortcuts, such as following standard operating procedures even though they are inadequate to deal with a new or changed situation. For instance, the group just does what it did in the past in seemingly similar situations. The group may also quickly adopt the first halfway decent solution proposed, a strategy called **satisficing** (Janis, 1989). When satisficing, the group seizes upon the first alternative that meets minimal requirements and then engages in **bolstering**—convincing themselves it is the way to go by emphasizing its advantages and overlooking disadvantages and alternatives.

Satisficing

When a group seizes upon one of the first decision alternatives that meets minimal requirements.

Bolstering

When group members convince themselves that their quick decision is a good one by emphasizing its advantages and overlooking disadvantages and alternatives.

Ideally, group decision making draws on the combined expertise of the group's members. Unfortunately, members sometimes deprive the group of their input because of concerns about impairing relationships with other group members. This may interfere with the generation, evaluation, and selection of alternatives. "Everyone else seems to be in agreement, so why should I rock the boat by putting in my two cents worth?" "I'd better keep my mouth shut and go along with the boss so I can stay on his good side." "Jerome feels awfully strongly about this, and I don't want to fight about it, so I'll just go along with what he wants." In these cases, members withhold their ideas from the group because of concerns about impairing relationships in the group. Such comments signal the presence of **affiliative constraints.**

Affiliative constraints

When a desire to maintain positive relationships between group members or a reluctance to question powerful members causes members to hold back in decision discussions.

Affiliative constraints arise out of a desire to maintain positive relationships between group members and one's place in the group. For instance, some members may not speak up because they do not want to be the one to introduce conflict into a seemingly harmonious group. This is especially a problem in cohesive groups. Members do not want to ruin a good thing by introducing conflict and are more concerned with agreement than with evaluating alternatives (Janis, 1982). Later in the chapter you will read about groupthink, a decision-making error that occurs in cohesive groups with a strong interest in maintaining harmony. Sometimes group members are so interested in minimizing conflict and keeping the peace that to calm an agitated or insistent member, they adopt or adapt the member's erroneous or narrow thinking and back off from their own correct thinking. Conformity pressures may also operate as affiliative constraints. Remember that groups are notorious for exerting pressure on members to conform to the majority opinion and that individuals are notorious for conforming to this pressure because they want to belong.

CYA rule

("cover-your-ass rule") When members withhold information or opinions that contradict group leaders to avoid retribution and gain leader approval.

Members are also sensitive to status differences in the group and show a reluctance to say things at odds with the positions of powerful group members. This is another affiliative constraint on good decision making because it prevents honest discussion and evaluation of alternatives and is due to a desire to maintain good relations with other members, namely the leaders of the group. Janis (1989) talks about the **CYA rule** ("cover-your-ass rule"). Group members who want to climb the status ladder often rely on this common affiliative rule. Telling the leaders what they want to hear and not being the bearer of information or opinions that contradict them protects you from retribution and makes them like you. Janis (1989, pp. 46–47) gives this synopsis of what dozens of governmental officials in policy-planning roles told him about the CYA rule:

> The first thing you do before you open your mouth is to find out
> what your bosses think should be done. . . . You had better do
> enough detective work to find out what it is they really want so that
> you can keep your ass covered by adopting their position. Arguing
> for anything else could antagonize them so much that your ass will

be carved. If you are quite sure that they have no definite preference and really want more innovative proposals, it's OK to try to earn brownie points by suggesting a new policy that you think will be successful, but be careful to do it in a way that does not expose your behind for a whacking later on. Avoid going all-out in advocating any new policy because if it fails, you will be the fall guy; it will be your ass that will be in a sling.

Janis (1989) reminds leaders that the CYA rule means that they may have to do their own homework because subordinates may be reluctant to report unpleasant facts and may withhold or distort information in order to protect themselves. To encourage information and idea sharing, leaders must be careful not to "shoot the messengers" of ideas that challenge or contradict their own thinking.

Egocentric constraints

When members withhold information or opinions because controlling or self-interested members control the discussion.

Egocentric constraints are apparent when some group members are so desperate to control the group's decision that they belittle the ideas offered by others and present themselves as the experts on the situation at hand. They bolster their own ideas by emphasizing supportive evidence and criticize competing ideas. In these ways, they shut down discussion and participation and contribute to a defensive communication climate (see Chapter 5, Communication in Groups). Sometimes such individuals have a personal interest in the groups, making a particular decision because they will benefit personally from one avenue as opposed to another, but other times they simply have a need to be in control and to be right. Often these people come from an extremely competitive orientation and view the group decision as a battle to be won. Whatever the motivation, the effect is to bully the group into considering only a narrow range of alternatives, bias the evaluation of alternatives, and pressure the group to make a choice that might not otherwise have been made.

Reducing the Impact of Cognitive, Affiliative, and Egocentric Constraints

Gouran and Hirokawa (1996) suggest that, being human, we can hardly expect to eliminate these constraints. The best we can do is to manage them so that they do not prevent groups from making informed decisions. Here are their suggestions for doing this.

Suggestions for Reducing Cognitive Constraints

1. Look for differences between what appear to be similar situations to avoid the trap of applying an old solution that might not work in a new situation.
2. Identify deficiencies in information, and come up with realistic possibilities to overcome them. Ask, "What do we know?" "What do we need to know?" and, "How are we going to find out?"
3. Motivate the search for information by reminding the group of the consequences of a poor decision.

| *Apply It!* ••• | **Analyze Decision Constraints** |

Describe a time when you were part of a decision-making group that made a poor decision because of cognitive, affiliative, or egocentric constraints. What were the consequences? How could the group's decision making be improved?

Suggestions for Reducing Affiliative Constraints

1. Remind the group of the importance of the decision and obtain a commitment to making the best possible choice, even if this requires some disagreement along the way.
2. Make it clear that the goal is to evaluate ideas and that this requires separating issues from personalities. In other words, we should refrain from personal attacks and should not take others' criticisms of our ideas as personal attacks.
3. Sincerely encourage members to question what the group is considering; remind them that holding back could lead the group astray.

Suggestions for Reducing Egocentric Constraints

1. Remind the group that it is a group decision and that everyone's opinion and information is needed. This serves to remind controlling individuals that others will use their rights as group members, so they had better let others have their say.
2. Gently question controlling members to highlight deficiencies in their position and to reduce their insistence that it is the only viable position. For instance, say, "Could you share more of your thinking?" "Do you have any reservations about the idea?" "Before we go down that path, don't you think we should examine our other options?"

Groups as Collective Information Processors

Our general model of the group decision process points to the importance of groups as processors of information. Information is what makes us aware of a problem, and defines the boundaries and urgency of that problem (Propp, 1997). Identifying and sharing relevant information are central to the identification of options and the evaluation of those options. The establishment of an information base affects all phases of the group decision process (Hirokawa & Scheerhorn, 1986). Janis and Mann (1977) suggest that group members be "vigilant" in processing information in order to avoid faulty decisions.

Collective Information-Processing Model

I sometimes enter a group decision-making situation reluctantly, thinking that it is clear what the group should decide and feeling irritated that we must spend time talking about it. What typically happens, though, is that I quickly realize that others in the group have information or experience that I did not have when drawing my conclusions. Once others share, I arrive at a better solution than I came to on my own. I leave the situation grateful that the decision was made in a group after all.

Collective information-processing model

A model emphasizing that individual members possess unique information relevant to the group decision.

My experience is consistent with the **collective information-processing model** of group decision making. This model emphasizes that each group member is an informational resource to the group and how group members use discussion to retrieve these resources (Hinsz, Tindale, & Volrath, 1997). The **collective memory** of a group, or the combined memory of the group's members, is often superior to the memory of an individual member (Clark, Stephenson, & Kniveton, 1990). The diverse store of information that group members hold is one of the group's richest resources. Think about it. Because of your experiences, training, and role in the group or organization, you possess information other members do not have (called *unshared* or *unique information*). By pooling the decision-relevant information uniquely possessed by each member, the group has the potential to make a better decision (Winquist & Larson, 1998).

Collective memory

The combined memory of the group's members, usually superior to the memory of an individual because members remember different things.

Transactive memory system

The way groups rely on individual members to be the group's memory in regard to particular subject areas.

Over time, it is common for groups to rely on individual members to be the group's memory in regard to particular subject areas. This is known as a **transactive memory system.** For example, as a former department chair, my group looks to me for information regarding policy decisions made during my tenure. Another member, who is active in university government, is the group's memory for policies that come out of this organizational unit. Couples usually have transactional memories also. Watch how when telling a story, one partner looks to the other partner to fill in the pieces s/he cannot remember.

Deficiencies in Information Pooling

The more unshared information that groups share or "pool," the better their decision making. Conversely, poor decisions may result when unique information is not considered (Gigone & Hastie, 1993; Stasser & Stewart, 1992; Winquist & Larson, 1998). Unfortunately, research indicates that many groups do not have procedures to ensure that the unique information held by members is shared with the group. Instead of being an occasion for members to share information that only they possess, group discussion is more likely to be spent sharing information that everyone already knows. This happens partly because the fact that more people know it increases the likelihood of its being shared (Winquist & Larson, 1998).

Affiliative constraints also reduce member sharing of unique information or opinions. Once there appears to be a majority position, people tend to share and discuss information supportive of it, possibly for fear of rejection (Dennis, 1996; Propp, 1997). This is especially true of less assertive and unconfident members. They are disinclined to share their unique information and this really hurts the group when they possess important information, or expertise (Zalesny, 1990). Indeed, some research suggests that a group's decision-making performance depends largely on whether more competent group members (those with the best skills, experience, or analytical abilities) are able to influence the group process (Bottger & Yetton, 1987). Unfortunately, group discussions are frequently a series of two-person conversations between the leader of the discussion and a few very vocal participants (Zander, 1982). As Zander notes, this dampens the interest of others and causes them to withdraw. The group is thus deprived of decision-relevant information and perspectives.

Cognitive constraints also inhibit information sharing in decision-making groups. Humans are limited in their information-processing abilities and have difficulty remembering and focusing on several ideas at a time. They get distracted by the discussion and start viewing the problem through the lenses of other group members. Members with unique information may forget or suppress it because it seems less relevant given the focus of the discussion (Dennis, 1996).

Deficiencies in Processing Available Information

Not only are groups not generally very good at getting members to share their unique information, but even when they do groups may not consider this information equally. In other words, simply increasing the amount of information is not enough to improve a group's performance because how the group processes that information depends on attitudes toward the information and its source (Shaw & Penrod, 1962).

As suggested in earlier chapters, information from high-status members may be given more attention. Also, group members will rely on others to help them determine whether a given piece of information is important or useful (you might recognize this as informational pressure). We listen more to members we like, members we respect, and members who have power over us (an affiliative constraint). Cognitive constraints are also an issue. In this case, we listen more to members who confirm what we already believe because information consistent with our prediscussion preferences (how we were leaning before the group's discussion) is more easily processed and therefore more memorable and influential (Dennis, 1996; Propp, 1997).

Egocentric constraints also affect the evaluation of information because members may interpret information in ways that support the decision outcome they want. A now famous example was NASA's decision in 1986 to launch the shuttle *Challenger* despite information from the engineers that an

---

Apply It! ••• **Evaluate Your Groups Collective Information Processing**

Think of a group you were a member of that had a transactive memory system. Which members were responsible for which parts of the group's memory? Have you been a member of a group that failed to pool all available information because of a cognitive, affiliative, or egocentric constraint?

---

engine component failed in tests when the temperature dropped below 52 degrees Fahrenheit (the temperature at launch time was expected to be 32 degrees). You might predict that this information would lead to a decision to postpone the flight. However, NASA officials, who were heavily invested in the launch, concluded that because the malfunction had not resulted in any serious problems in previous shuttle flights, it would be unlikely to do so in this case (Hirokawa et al., 1996). This decision resulted in the death of seven crewmembers when seventy-three seconds after liftoff, the *Challenger* exploded.

Enhancing Collective Information Processing

How do we enhance the collective information processing of a group? Zander (1982) reminds us to be aware of the informational resources of the group and to take time to gather information from members. This is especially important when a group is relatively new because transactive memory systems take time to develop and the group may be unaware of the informational resources of its members (Littlepage, Robison, & Reddington, 1997). Several other techniques focus on structuring the group experience such that all group members are required to contribute. These techniques include brainstorming, the nominal group technique, and the Delphi technique. The idea is that these techniques are needed because untrained groups do not have the norms or resources to promote equitable participation and positive interaction (Kramer & Kuo, 1997).

Brainstorming

Brainstorming
A technique where group members first offer as many ideas as possible without discussion or evaluation, and then discuss the merits of the ideas.

Research tells us that the more ideas a group generates, the greater the probability that quality ideas will be offered (Diehl & Strobe, 1989). Ask the average person how a group might generate lots of ideas, and you will likely hear the answer "brainstorming." Originated by Osborn in 1957, **brainstorming** requires that group members take five to seven minutes to offer as many ideas as possible without discussion or consideration of their practicality. Members are instructed to defer judgment until everyone has contributed, to say whatever comes to mind, and to build on and combine the ideas of others.

> ## Apply It! ••• Compare Your Experience With Research on Brainstorming
>
> Think about your experience in brainstorming groups. Did you really feel free enough to offer any idea that came into your mind, or were you inhibited by one of the factors described below?

Osborn (1957, 1963) thought that members' tendencies to immediately evaluate and criticize others' ideas stifled creativity and the number of ideas generated. He reasoned that with brainstorming, members would inspire one another to think of things they otherwise might not and would be motivated to outdo one another by offering more and more ideas. Surprisingly, though, laboratory research does not find that brainstorming groups produce more ideas or better-quality ideas than individuals brainstorming alone (see, for instance, a meta-analysis by Mullen, Johnson, & Salas, 1991).

A number of factors that may reduce the performance of brainstorming groups have been identified. These include social loafing (some members leave it up to others to come up with the ideas), evaluation apprehension (some members hold back for fear of looking silly or stupid), production blocking (too many people trying to speak at once causes some members to pull back or distracts them from their own ideas), and social comparison (some members are hesitant to offer ideas that diverge too far from the ideas of others) (Brown, Tumeo, Larey, & Paulus, 1998).

Group Support Systems (Electronic Brainstorming)

Group support systems (GSS)

A technique in which group members use computers to interact, often anonymously; intended to increase the number of ideas and reduce normative pressures and groupthink.

Remember that one of the reasons offered for the ineffectiveness of brainstorming is production blocking—that is, we have a hard time paying attention to what others are saying and generating ideas at the same time. Another reason offered is that fear of judgment and conformity pressures create affiliative constraints. Computer-based brainstorming, in which group members exchange information by typing on their computers, is thought to get around these cognitive and affiliative constraints. Electronic brainstorming is conducted with **group support systems (GSS).** GSS group members interact from their computer workstations by typing ideas that are immediately shared with other members. Dennis (1996) summarizes the potential advantages of GSS. First, because they can all type at the same time, members are less likely to forget ideas they come up with while others are sharing. A second advantage is that the written record of all contributions can be referred to at any point in the discussion. Members can easily pause to process information and do not have to miss anything because they can always read the record. Last, in most cases, group members make contributions anonymously. This should reduce the influence of member status on the evaluation of information and alternatives, and lower-status members and those with minority viewpoints may feel safer participating.

Research on GSS has yielded mixed results but supports the idea that GSS increases a group's use of factual information and reduces the use of information based on normative influence (Huang, Raman, & Wei, 1993). Some studies find that GSS increases the number of ideas generated (Jessup & Valacich, 1993), but other studies do not (Dennis, 1996). Dennis concluded that for GSS to work well, members must be given time to review and consider the information before making a decision. Otherwise, they are likely to fall prey to their limited information-processing abilities in the same way those in face-to-face discussion groups are. Groups using GSS may also need leadership to ensure that all members share unique information. Otherwise, as in non-GSS groups, they tend to share ideas consistent with their prediscussion preferences.

Nominal Group Technique

Nominal group technique (NGT)

A technique where group members first brainstorm individually, and are then polled to ensure all ideas are shared.

The **nominal group technique (NGT)** is another derivation of brainstorming (Delbecq, Van de Ven, & Gustafson, 1975). The main difference between NGT and traditional brainstorming is that NGT group members brainstorm individually, without interaction. NGT also uses a polling technique to ensure that all ideas are shared afterwards. These differences help to eliminate production blocking and the tendency for verbally dominant members to cause less dominant members to retreat. Because the technique requires that all members participate and ideas are voted on privately, inequality in participation due to status differences is also reduced. Because each individual works alone and yet is ultimately accountable to the group, social loafing is lessened.

NGT has four basic steps:

1. **Silent generation of ideas.** Working silently and independently, participants write down their responses to a stimulus question. This question should be simple and specific and, if possible, pilot tested to make sure participants understand what is being asked.
2. **Round-robin recording of ideas.** The leader calls on each member to share one idea at a time and writes these where everyone can see them. Discussion of ideas is not permitted at this time. The leader continues to call on the participants until all ideas have been recorded or until the group determines that they have a sufficient number of ideas.
3. **Serial discussion of the list of ideas.** The participants discuss each idea on the list. Ideas are clarified and evaluated.
4. **Voting.** The participants identify what each of them believes are the most important ideas, they privately rank-order their preferences, the votes are recorded, and the voting pattern is discussed. The highest-ranked idea is chosen.

NGT has been used extensively in business and government, and some research suggests that it is superior to simple brainstorming when it comes to the generation of quality ideas (Diehl & Stroebe, 1989; Roth, 1994; Van de Ven &

Delbecq, 1974). But other research does not. Kramer and Kuo (1997) did not find differences between NGT and brainstorming in the number of ideas generated, and according to their study, neither resulted in a greater number of quality ideas than untrained groups. However, the methods still offered an important communication and teamwork advantage in that they reduced domination by a few members and led to more equitable participation. The methods also led to greater satisfaction with the group process. Interestingly, participants in the Kramer and Kuo (1997) study had different reactions to brainstorming versus NGT. Brainstorming led to more positive and negative reactions from group members than did NGT. This is most likely because NGT is structured in such a way that there is very little room for non-task-related communication, thus controlling emotional responses and interaction in the group. The less structured nature of traditional brainstorming leads to more excitement as ideas are spontaneously thrown out but also leads to more spontaneous responses, both positive and negative, to those ideas.

The Delphi Technique

Delphi technique
A way to collect and synthesize the opinions of a group of experts into a decision using a series of written communications.

Remember that one cognitive constraint for decision-making groups is that they may lack the expertise to understand the information they have and to generate and evaluate alternatives. The **Delphi technique** is intended to help by providing a way to collect and synthesize the opinions of a group of experts into a decision (Dalkey, 1969). Because it can be difficult to assemble experts for a face-to-face meeting, and to avoid the social dynamics that can complicate the evaluation of a problem, the technique relies on written communications. A carefully written letter is sent to each expert, outlining the problem and asking what the expert proposes as a solution. The leader then copies and collates these responses, sends them to the experts, and asks them to comment and propose additional solutions. The leader examines the second set of responses, looking for consensus among the experts. If there is clear consensus, a decision can be made. If not, the process is repeated until consensus is apparent. The conventional Delphi technique takes a lot of time and is not appropriate in cases where a quick decision is needed. A variation, called "real-time" Delphi, uses the same process during the course of a meeting or conference (Clayton, 1997). Very little research on the technique has occurred since the 1970s. At that time, some researchers found that the technique increased group productivity, while others did not (Parks & Sanna, 1999). Despite the lack of research support, the technique is regularly used by educational and health-care organizations. See **Box 11-1** for an example.

Additional Suggestions for Improving Collective Information Processing

You do not have to use these formal techniques to increase the effectiveness of your decision-making group. You may feel that these techniques are unwieldy or would not quite work for your group. However, you can create your

---

BOX 11-1 / USE OF THE DELPHI TECHNIQUE TO IDENTIFY COMPONENTS FOR
ADOLESCENT AIDS PREVENTION PROGRAMS

Adolescents are at risk for contracting HIV through sexual intercourse and/or drug abuse because they often lack knowledge, see themselves as invulnerable, and do not practice safe sex. Most adolescent prevention programs emphasize abstinence and information about how HIV is contracted but do not provide skills training that would help adolescents resist high-risk behavior. Adams, Piercy, Jurich, and Lewis (2001) used the Delphi technique to identify components of a model adolescent AIDS/drug abuse prevention program. The researchers invited fifty-five experts on adolescent substance abuse and AIDS to respond to eight open-ended questions such as "What do you believe to be the most important information to include in a model adolescent AIDS prevention program?" They then took the responses and created 295 statements, each of which represented a possible program component. Next, the experts were asked to use a seven-point scale to indicate how important they believed each item was to a model program. Items receiving strong endorsement, such as skill training in decision making and methods for resisting peer pressure, were summarized and recommended for use in AIDS/drug abuse prevention programs for adolescents.

---

own structure for improving group decision making by keeping the following points in mind:

1. Create a discussion structure that ensures equal participation by group members. This can prevent domination by aggressive or high-status members and reduce social loafing. For instance, use a round-robin approach in which you go quickly around in a circle and everyone offers a two-sentence summary of his or her ideas.

2. Use techniques that prevent the group from rehashing the same ideas over and over again. Some form of individual brainstorming and systematic sharing of brainstormed ideas may increase the likelihood that unique ideas and expertise will be shared.

3. Remember that some disagreement may lead to better decisions but fear of conflict may prevent useful disagreement. Therefore, put in place ways to manage conflict and controversy so that avoidance of discord doesn't stifle participation or evaluation of ideas. For instance, before discussing a potentially contentious topic, introduce the group to the norms of constructive controversy discussed in the chapter on conflict. These can serve as "ground rules" for discussion.

4. Consider ways to discourage conformity pressures from reducing decision-making effectiveness. Put into place ways to assure lower-status members that they can participate without fear of retribution from higher-status members. Encourage the expression of minority viewpoints.

Apply It! ••• Improve Your Group's Collective Information Processing

Choose a group you are a member of that regularly makes decisions. Which of the suggestions given here could be used to enhance your group's collective information processing?

---

5. Avoid satisficing (the quick adoption of the first seemingly viable solution). Structure the discussion in such a way that alternatives must be seriously considered and the relative merits and costs of alternatives are explored.

Groupthink

History abounds with examples of poor decisions made by cohesive groups under stressful conditions. How could the military advisers to President Franklin D. Roosevelt downplay the evidence that Japanese warships were moving toward Hawaii to attack Pearl Harbor? Why didn't President John F. Kennedy and his advisers consult experts on Cuba before launching the ill-fated Bay of Pigs invasion? Why did President Lyndon B. Johnson and his Cabinet choose to escalate a war in Vietnam that the United States had virtually no chance of winning? What were President Richard M. Nixon and his advisers thinking when they authorized the burglary of the Democratic Party's headquarters at the Watergate complex and then tried to cover it up even when it was evident they were caught red-handed? What made President Ronald Reagan and his advisers decide to secretly and illegally sell weapons to Iran and use the profits to fund a group (the Contras) attempting to overthrow the democratically elected government of Nicaragua? Why did Ford build the Edsel car despite evidence it would be a failure? Why did the leadership of the energy corporation Enron make the decision to perpetuate a fraud on their stockholders, and what made them believe that they wouldn't be caught? Each of these decisions was a group decision, issued after a series of meetings of a cohesive group of government officials or business leaders and their advisers. In each case, the group made gross miscalculations about the practical and moral consequences of their decisions. Most likely, they are also examples of a phenomenon called **groupthink.**

Groupthink

The defective decision making that arises in a cohesive group when members seek consensus before fully evaluating alternatives.

Groupthink refers to the defective decision making that arises in a cohesive group when members seek consensus before they have fully reviewed alternative courses of action. This premature consensus-seeking may lead the group to quickly seize upon a proposed solution, at which point members convince one another that the group and its premature decision are right (bolstering). The failures that result may be so disastrous that they qualify as "fiascoes" (Janis, 1982).

Antecedents of Groupthink

According to Janis (1982), cohesiveness is one of the primary features of groups that exhibit groupthink because it leads to premature consensus seeking. Group members want to agree with one another. Cohesiveness may create an affiliative constraint on group decision making when members are so interested in maintaining camaraderie that they fail to share doubts or critique ideas.

Although cohesiveness appears to be a primary factor in the development of groupthink, it alone does not produce groupthink. Indeed, research indicates that not every cohesive group suffers from groupthink (Mullen, Anthony, Salas, & Driskell, 1994; Tetlock, Peterson, McGuire, Chang, & Feld, 1992), and some studies find little research support for the view that cohesiveness plays an important role in groupthink (Aldag & Fuller, 1993; Whyte, 1998). Meta-analyses suggest that cohesiveness does increase the likelihood of groupthink when additional antecedent conditions are present (Mullen et al., 1994). Janis (1982, 1989) has identified four other conditions (antecedents) necessary for groupthink to occur: high stress (serious threats), limited search and appraisal of information, directive leadership, and insulation from outside experts. These are described in more detail below.

Janis (1982, 1989) suggests that a *provocative situational context* is the primary antecedent determining whether cohesion will lead to groupthink. A provocative situational context is one in which the group experiences high stress from an external threat, members believe they stand to lose no matter what they choose, and they have little hope that a better solution will be found. This stress leads to a cognitive constraint because it prevents the group from fully evaluating a range of alternatives. The group feels pressure to make a drastic decision quickly, and the stress makes members more conforming as they turn to each other for social support. Turner and her colleagues (Turner, Pratkanis, Probasco, & Leve, 1992) found that in comparison to cohesive groups not experiencing external threats, cohesive groups facing external threats were much more likely to make poor decisions. For instance, in all the examples at the beginning of this section, the groups felt that they, or what they stood for, were under attack.

Secondary determinants of groupthink fall under the heading of *structural faults of the group,* and contrary to Janis's original thinking, these appear to be more important than a provocative situational context in predicting groupthink (see Schafer & Crichlow, 1996; Tetlock et al., 1992). These antecedents focus on how the way things are done in the group reduces information sharing and inhibits the generation and evaluation of alternatives. For instance, one of these structural faults is *lack of impartial leadership.* When a leader is very directive, has great power over group members, states his or her preferences, and does not encourage an unbiased examination of alternatives, then members are likely to accept this position even if they have doubts. Another structural antecedent, *lack of methodological norms for decision making,* is present when a group does not have norms requiring a systematic approach to the generation and evaluation of alternatives. In such cases, norms favoring agreement among members lead the group to adopt a particular course of action without fairly evaluating it or alternatives. Last, if the group is structured such that it operates in isolation and does not consult experts outside of the group, then information relevant to the evaluation of decision alternatives will not enter into the group's thinking (this structural antecedent is called *insulation from outside experts*). Research suggests that insulation does increase the likelihood of groupthink (McCauley, 1989).

Meta-analysis indicates that in addition to cohesiveness, the most important structural antecedents are directive leadership and the lack of methodological procedures for evaluating decision options (Mullen et al., 1994). Some research also suggests that the more attractive and powerful the leader, the more quickly members will agree with him or her without considering other options (Aldag & Fuller, 1993). The stage of group development may also make a difference in whether cohesion leads to groupthink. Several researchers argue that groupthink may be more likely in a group's earlier stages, when members are insecure about challenging others (Street, 1997).

Symptoms and Consequences of Groupthink

According to the theory, these antecedent conditions give rise to three types of groupthink symptoms (Janis, 1982), although research does not find that all conditions must be present before these symptoms will occur (Turner & Pratkanis, 1998).

The first category of groupthink symptoms includes an overestimation of the power and morality of the group. The group feels invulnerable, which leads to excessive risk taking. The unquestioned belief in the morality of the group causes members to overlook the moral and ethical consequences of their choice.

A second category represents how the group exhibits signs of closed-mindedness. Members rationalize (bolster) the choice, downplaying its negatives and focusing on positives, and avoiding people and information that might make them question it. They may also underestimate their competitors or enemies. They stereotype outgroup members as too weak or stupid to prevent the success of their plan.

The third type of groupthink symptoms reflects the operation of conformity pressures in the group. Members engage is self-censorship, keeping doubts to themselves. There is the illusion of unanimity, and members assume that there is consensus because they assume silence indicates agreement and few members express dissenting views. When members do express dissenting views, they quickly receive the message from other members or the leader that to dissent is to be disloyal to the group (some dissenters may even be booted from the group). Last, there may be self-appointed **mindguards**—members who protect the group from receiving information that might shake confidence in their decision.

Mindguards
Members who protect the group from receiving information that might shake confidence in their decision; a symptom of groupthink.

Figure 11-1
The Groupthink Model

Antecedents

- Cohesiveness
- Provocative situational context
- Structural faults of the group

Symptoms

- Overestimation of the power and morality of the group
- Closed-mindedness
- Underestimation of competitors or enemies
- Censorship of dissenting views
- Self-appointed mindguards

Consequences

- Poor information search
- Biased processing of available information
- Incomplete survey of alternatives
- Failure to critically examine preferred choice
- No back-up plan

Such symptoms of groupthink usually herald the arrival of defective decision making in the form of a poor information search, biased processing of available information, an incomplete survey of alternatives, failure to critically examine the preferred choice, and failure to have a back up plan (Janis, 1982). These are the consequences of groupthink. The groupthink model—antecedents, symptoms, and consequences—is summarized in Figure 11-1.

Reducing Groupthink

Vigilant decision making

Decision strategies intended to reduce groupthink, including a thorough information search and evaluation of alternatives, and impartial leadership.

If groupthink arises from poor search procedures, directive leadership, and the absence of procedures to ensure that alternatives are accurately appraised, then the cure is better search procedures, impartial leadership that encourages the airing of doubts and objections in the group and encourages search for information and evaluation from sources outside the group, and procedural norms supporting systematic consideration of alternatives (Janis, 1982, 1989; McCauley, 1998). This is what Janis (1982) called **vigilant decision making.** Research supports the notion that vigilant decision making is linked to group decision making success (Herek, Janis, & Huth, 1987; Peterson, Owens, Tetlock, Fan, & Martorana, 1998). To make decisions "vigilantly":

1. Leaders must not push their own views. Instead, they should use their influence to encourage genuine debate. All members should be encouraged to take the role of "critical evaluator." To convince members that it is indeed safe to share doubts and objections, leaders have to demonstrate that they can be influenced by others' concerns and avoid verbal and nonverbal communication that punishes those who voice objections.

2. The leader can appoint a "devil's advocate" whose job it is to ask questions like "Haven't we overlooked. . . ?" and "Shouldn't we think about. . . ?" Ideally, this role should be rotated among group members. Care should be taken to seriously consider the devil's advocates' points.

3. Insulation can be avoided by having one or more outside experts or qualified colleagues come to meetings, share their opinions, and critique the group's thinking. This should occur before consensus is reached. Having multiple groups (or subgroups of a larger group) work on the same problem is another safeguard.

4. The group should use a method that requires considering the costs and benefits of proposed alternatives. For instance, the group should generate best-case and worst-case scenarios for each solution so that the positive and negative consequences of the leading alternatives can be foreseen.

5. After reaching preliminary consensus but before a final decision is made, the group should have a *second-chance meeting* at which members rethink the decision one last time. Each member should come to the meeting prepared to talk about the risks associated with the proposed policy. Members should openly discuss any residual doubts or lingering objections.

Some researchers recommend the use of group support systems (GSS) to prevent groupthink (Miranda, 1994). The idea is that GSS technology permits an anonymous exchange of ideas that should prevent self-censorship and the tendency for members to go along with higher-status members. Directive leadership is prevented by the anonymous nature of GSS, and the method promotes the generation and evaluation of numerous alternatives.

Vigilant decision making is not without its critics. The extensive search for information and discussion of alternatives is time-consuming and sometimes time-wasting, and in some cases a quick decision is equally effective (Suedfeld & Tetlock, 1992). Other critics argue that vigilant decision making may not enhance decision making because a group cannot foresee and control all the

---

Apply It! ••• Is Your Group at Risk for Groupthink?

Evaluate your group using the questionnaire in **Box 11-2.** Is your group at risk for groupthink? Has your group made poor decisions as a result of groupthink? What changes does your group need to make to prevent groupthink?

BOX 11-2 / IS YOUR GROUP SUSCEPTIBLE TO GROUPTHINK?

Check all that apply to your group. The more you check, the more susceptible to group-think your group is.

_____ 1. The leader of the group makes his or her views clearly known before the group has a chance to deliberate.

_____ 2. The group quickly seizes on an option offered by a high-status member and does not consider other alternatives.

_____ 3. Members are highly motivated to agree with one another in order to maintain good relationships with one another.

_____ 4. The group is relatively new, and members are uncomfortable challenging other members.

_____ 5. The group is not in the habit of consulting knowledgeable people outside of the group.

_____ 6. Decisions are made without listing the pros and cons of the different alternatives and what would happen were each to be chosen.

_____ 7. The leader is powerful, and members do not wish to disagree with him or her.

_____ 8. The group avoids information that might lead them to question their chosen route.

_____ 9. The group feels as though they are under attack and must make a decision quickly.

_____ 10. The group believes in its moral or intellectual superiority and minimizes its opponents or challenges.

---

possible events that may affect the success of a decision (Peterson et al., 1998). Unanticipated "stuff" happens; what seemed like a good decision given the information available at the time may turn out to be a bad one after all.

Group Polarization

Imagine yourself in the following scenarios. You really enjoyed a new comedy but find yourself thinking that it was even funnier once you talk about it with like-minded friends. You are really aggravated by something another group did to your group and find yourself even angrier once you have a discussion with group members who feel the same way. You are on a jury. It's a murder case in which a woman drowned her five young children. She has pleaded not guilty by reason of insanity. You are leaning toward a guilty conviction because she seemed to know right from wrong at the time of the crime, but there's a bit of doubt in your mind because she was psychotic. However, after you discuss it with other jurors, you are convinced a guilty verdict is the right thing.

Group members often enter into the group discussion situation with some initial thoughts and opinions about the topic. Often, others in the group have similar feelings and ideas about the topic so that there is a general group senti-

Group polarization

The tendency for group discussion to amplify members' initial inclinations so that the average inclination of group members is strengthened.

ment about the issue. Dozens of studies suggest that group discussion reinforces these shared beliefs so that members are even more convinced that this is the way to go. The formal name for this phenomenon is **group polarization.** Officially, group polarization is the tendency for group discussion to amplify members' initial inclinations so that the average inclination of group members is strengthened (Moscovici & Zavalloni, 1969). This means that groups often make riskier or more cautious decisions than individual members would make alone.

Explanations for Group Polarization

Persuasive arguments explanation for group polarization

Suggests that group polarization occurs as members hear additional arguments favoring their prediscussion preferences.

Social comparison explanation for group polarization

Suggests that group polarization occurs when members strengthen their prediscussion preferences because they want to be liked and accepted.

Why is it that following group discussion, members' attitudes and opinions shift in the direction already favored by the group, leading the group to agree on a position that is more extreme than the average opinion of its members? Is it simply a matter of members' being even more persuaded once they hear additional arguments in favor of their prediscussion preference? This is what the **persuasive arguments explanation for group polarization** suggests. Or is it that we want to be liked and accepted in the group, so we adjust our position to fit the group sentiment and take our position a step further so that we can be better than average? The **social comparison explanation for group polarization** suggests this is the case.

The persuasive arguments explanation is based on the assumption that we are persuaded when the arguments in favor of one position outweigh the arguments in favor of another position. When there is a prevailing opinion trend in the group, the group is more likely to hear a number of arguments in favor of that trend. In other words, because a number of members are thinking along the same lines, the average perspective is likely to be expressed by someone. Once the trend is apparent, members tend to share information that is consistent with it. The average perspective is then strengthened as members share additional arguments in favor of it. As members build on the idea, they rehearse and validate it, and publicly speak in favor of it, increasing their commitment to it (Brauer, Judd, & Gliner, 1995).

The social comparison explanation for group polarization emphasizes that in the course of group discussion, members compare their positions with the positions of others and are motivated to modify their positions in the direction of the dominant tendency. Allegedly, they do this because they want to project a favorable image to other members (Lamm, 1988), and because hearing that others think similarly gives them reassurance that they are correct and the confidence to go even further (Williams & Taormina, 1993). Initially, group members are tentative in their attitudes but once they see that others agree with them, they seek to look even better to the group by going even further in the direction of the predominant group attitude (Brauer et al., 1995). If enough members do this, the group ends up taking a more extreme position.

Group discussion provides additional information about the issue at hand, as well as information about the expectations of other group members. Together, these things result in group polarization as members have more arguments and more social support in favor of their initial inclinations. Studies by social identity theorists suggest that this is even more likely when identification with the group is strong. In such cases, other group members are more likely to be seen as valid sources of information, and members are more likely to move in the direction of what appears to be a shared group norm (Abrams, Wetherell, Cochrane, Hogg, & Turner, 1990; McGarty, Turner, Hogg, David, & Wetherell, 1992; Spears, Lea, & Lee, 1990). Think about it like this: The group's discussion promotes the perception of ingroup membership because members feel greater identification with the group as members share similar attitudes. All that sharing may also lead members to perceive the group's norm as more extreme than it is. This leads to attitude polarization as members conform to the more extreme group norm (Mackie, 1986).

Group Polarization and Group Effectiveness

Group polarization isn't necessarily bad. After all, it is often good for a group to reach consensus, and just because the group's decision is more extreme, that does not necessarily mean it is a bad decision. But like the dynamics that lead to groupthink, the dynamics that lead to group polarization can interfere with good group decision making. Alternatives may not be considered because everyone seems to agree. The negatives of the group's inclination may not be explored as everyone seeks to support the group opinion by offering additional arguments in favor of it. Members may share only information they have in common rather than unique information relevant to the decision that only they possess. Many of the suggestions for enhancing group decision making given earlier in the chapter are helpful in preventing these potential pitfalls. For instance, appointing a devil's advocate, encouraging the expression and exploration of minority views, and using a systematic approach that requires careful consideration of the pros and cons of decision options are all useful in avoiding a bad decision made as a result of group polarization.

Decision Styles and Group Decisions

Making a quality decision is an important goal of group decision making, but it is not the only one. As noted in Chapters 9 and 10, when people are involved in making decisions that affect them, they are more satisfied and committed to the decision and to the group. But group decisions take time and are not always necessary. In this section, you will learn when it makes sense to make a decision on your own and when it makes sense to involve the group.

You will also read about members' decision styles and how these affect the group.

Leader Decision Styles (Vroom-Yetton Normative Decision Model)

Decision making is an important leadership behavior, and leaders must often decide whether to make decisions alone or in a group. Imagine what would happen if you decided unilaterally where your family (or group of friends) was going on vacation. It is unlikely that your decision would be accepted, and group members would probably be angry with you for not consulting them. Next, consider employees' likelihood of adopting new and inconvenient safety procedures on which they had not been consulted—not very likely. Of course, consultation is not always necessary. Does a manager really need to consult the group before switching to a new, yet comparable, brand of paper at a lower price? As these examples illustrate, the situation may influence the effectiveness of group decision making. Sometimes there is a big payoff for including the group in decision making, and sometimes it does not make a difference.

Normative decision model

Proposes that how much leaders should consult the group when making a decision depends on decision quality, decision acceptance, and time.

According to Vroom and Yetton's (1973) **normative decision model,** three situational factors need to be considered when deciding how much to include members in decision making. The model is summarized in Figure 11-2. The first factor, *decision quality*, refers to how important the decision is to the functioning of the group. To decide this, leaders need to ask themselves three questions: (1) How significant is this decision? In general, if it is a trivial decision, then it is probably okay for the leader to make it without consultation. (2) Do I have enough information to make this decision? If not, consultation is needed. (3) Is the problem well structured? That is, is it clear what the options are and what information is needed to make the decision? If not, then the ambiguity of the problem requires that the leader interact with members to clarify the problem and how to solve it.

A second factor to consider when deciding how much to consult others before making a decision is *decision acceptance*. How important is it for group members to accept the decision in order for it to be successfully implemented? In general, if employee acceptance is important, then employees should probably be consulted. The third factor to consider is *time*. Consulting others takes time, so in general, if a quick decision is needed, it may be best to make it with no or only minimal consultation.

According to Vroom and Yetton (1973), five types of decision styles represent a continuum ranging from no participation by members to maximum member participation. The three situational factors just discussed determine which is likely to be effective.

1. **AI (autocratic).** Manager makes decision alone, using available information.
2. **AII (autocratic).** Manager asks for information from members but makes the decision alone.

Figure 11-2
Vroom-Yetton Normative Decision Model

Key questions to be asked/answered
about situation or problem

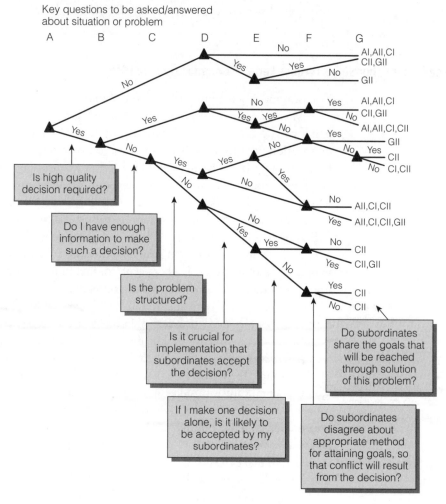

A   B   C   D   E   F   G

Is high quality decision required?

Do I have enough information to make such a decision?

Is the problem structured?

Is it crucial for implementation that subordinates accept the decision?

If I make one decision alone, is it likely to be accepted by my subordinates?

Do subordinates share the goals that will be reached through solution of this problem?

Do subordinates disagree about appropriate method for attaining goals, so that conflict will result from the decision?

Potential Strategies for Making Decisions

According to Vroom and Yetton, leaders often adopt one of the five strategies shown here in making decisions.

Decision strategy	Description
AI (Autocratic)	Leader solves problem or makes decision unilaterally, using available information
AII (Autocratic)	Leader obtains necessary information from subordinates but then makes decision unilaterally
CI (Consultative)	Leader shares the problem with subordinates individually, but then makes decision unilaterally
CII (Consultative)	Leader shares problem with subordinates in group meeting but then makes decision unilaterally
GII (Group Decision)	Leader shares problem with subordinates in a group meeting; decision is reached through discussion to consensus

The normative decision model suggests five different strategies for making a decision, each varying in terms of how much to involve the group. The decision tree guides the leader to the different strategies appropriate for the situation.

Apply It! ••• **Consider Your Leadership Decision Style**

Think about the last time you served in a leadership capacity (if you haven't been in an official leadership position, you may have acted as a leader in a class project group, friendship group, family, or workgroup). How autocratic or participative were you in your dealings with others? What decision procedures did you use more or less frequently? How close did your behavior come to that of the model? What model "rules" did you violate most consistently, and what were the consequences?

3. **CI (consultative).** Manager shares the problem with selected members individually, getting their ideas and suggestions without bringing them together as a group.
4. **CII (consultative).** Manager and members meet as a group, and manager obtains their suggestions. Manager then makes the decision, which may or may not reflect their influence.
5. **GII (group).** Manager and members meet as a group and generate and evaluate solutions. Manager accepts the group's decision.

Vroom and Jago (1988) have since revised the model to take into account the relative priority of the different criteria and to include some additional situational factors, such as amount of member information and the geographic dispersion of members. The revised version is more complete, but also so complex that a computer software program is recommended to make use of it (Yukl, 1998). Research generally supports the model (Field & Andrews, 1998; Vroom & Jago, 1988, 1995; Yukl, 1998).

Although the model can be unwieldy, practically speaking, autocratic decisions (AI, AII) are not appropriate when the decision is important and members possess relevant information. Autocratic decisions should also be avoided when decision acceptance is important and members are unlikely to accept an autocratic decision. In such cases, it is advisable that the decision be made after consultation with the group (CII, GII). This is also true when decision acceptance is important and when members may disagree among themselves, because consultation with the group provides the opportunity to resolve differences through discussion and negotiation. When several different decision procedures are possible, consider other aspects of the situation such as time pressure and leader skill in choosing which style to adopt. For instance, Crouch and Yetton (1987) found that in situations where members disagreed and the leader had good conflict management skills, group procedures were effective. Conversely, for leaders without these skills, consulting members individually was more effective.

Member Decision Styles

Decision styles
Group member differences in approaches to group decision making.

According to some researchers, individual group members may have different **decision styles** (Morrison, Kelly, Moore, & Hutchins, 1998). The decision-style model described by Rowe, Boulgaides, and McGrath (1984) identifies four different styles: directive, analytical, conceptual, and behavioral. Those with a *directive style* like to keep it simple and make decisions quickly without considering many alternatives. They rely on their intuition, the available facts, and what has worked in the past. In contrast, individuals with an *analytical style* like a complex problem and carefully consider a range of alternatives after collecting detailed data. The *conceptual style* describes those that prefer to look at problems creatively. They like to consider new and unusual ideas and focus on the "big picture." Individuals with a *behavioral style* are open to the suggestions of others and like to make decisions in a group. They are concerned with how their fellow group members feel and what is good for the organization.

These styles are interesting to think of in terms of what happens when members of a decision-making group have different styles. You can imagine how members with a directive style might clash with members who have an analytical style because the directive person decides quickly and the analytical person wants to collect information and review it carefully before making a decision. You can imagine how the person with a conceptual style might irritate more directive and analytical members by emphasizing the future and wanting to entertain nontraditional ideas.

It is important to keep in mind that no one style is best and that there are advantages to having decision-style diversity in your group. Sometimes it is fine to make a quick decision without taking the time to generate and evaluate alternatives, but other times it is best to carefully analyze alternatives. Sometimes a creative approach focused on the future is called for, but other times the group has neither time nor enough information to seriously consider unusual ideas. Ideally, people with different styles provide balance to one another. If different decision styles create problems in your group, you may find it useful to talk about your different styles and when each one can best serve the group. Having a better understanding of others' styles can go a long way toward reducing irritations.

Culture, Gender, and Group Decision Making

Decision style diversity is not the only type of diversity that affects group decision making. In this section, you will learn how culture and gender affect group decision making.

Culture and Group Decision Making

Although relatively little research has been done on culture and decision making, Hofstede (1980) found that people in cultures high on "masculinity" favored individual over group decision making. These cultures, such as Austria,

Venezuela, Italy, and Switzerland, value assertiveness, money, and things rather than nurturance and people. Likewise, a seven-nation study found that culture affects how much a leader consults with subordinates in decision making (Reber, Jago, & Bohnisch, 1993, reported in Vroom & Jago, 1995). Managers in Germany, Austria, and Switzerland were the most participative, followed by the United States and France. Managers in Poland and Czechoslovakia were the most autocratic, tending to make decisions on their own, without consulting the group.

We can also consider the relationship between culture and group decision making by asking whether some types of cultures might be more prone to certain types of group decision-making errors. For instance, groups in collectivist cultures that favor more directive leadership and emphasize conformity may be more susceptible to groupthink and group polarization. Groups in individualistic cultures may be more prone to egocentric constraints on decision making because members may be more likely to use the group for personal gain. Groups in collectivistic cultures may be more prone to affiliative constraints because of their greater concern for group harmony. Groups from cultures that are high in power distance (where status differences are large and respected) may be more prone to limited information pooling because lower-status members may be less likely to offer their ideas and information. Keep in mind, though, that these are untested hypotheses. Hopefully, future research will tell us more about the relationship between culture and common group decision-making errors.

One non-Western decision-making technique has received particular attention. In the 1980s, when Japan's economy was strong, organizational psychologists began studying the nature of Japanese organizations. One of these psychologists, William G. Ouchi (1981), described most Japanese organizations as "hierarchical clans" comprised of culturally homogeneous, cohesive workgroups linked together. Decisions are often made using the **Ringi** system, a technique that involves everyone in the organization that the decision affects. In one form of Ringi, a written document is sent from member to member and edited by each person without any person-to-person interaction. This process continues until all members are satisfied (Zander, 1982). In some cases, Ringi involves a small team that talks personally to all of those involved. Each time a significant modification is suggested, all members are contacted again. This process continues until consensus is reached. The advantage of Ringi is that once a decision is reached, everyone is likely to support it (Ouchi, 1981). The disadvantage of the Ringi system is that it takes a long time (Ouchi, 1981). Also, according to Janis (1989), because the method is used in organizations that are culturally homogeneous and emphasize conformity, deviant views may be repressed, and groupthink may be more likely.

Ringi
Japanese group decision-making techniques that involve everyone in the organization that the decision affects.

Gender and Group Decision Making

Most studies on gender and group decisions compare the decision making of all-female groups with that of all-male groups and examine the effects of gender in mixed-gender decision-making groups. For instance, meta-analytic research suggests that female groups are better at incorporating the views of all members into the final decision, presumably because they are more relational and more democratic (Wood, 1987). All-female groups may also be more likely to consider a variety of information when making a decision. In one study of same-sex groups, female groups accepted significantly more information into their final information bases than did male groups (Propp, 1997). Although several European researchers have hypothesized that, because of their greater concern for group harmony, female groups would be more susceptible to groupthink, research has not confirmed this hypothesis (Kroon, van Kreveld, & Rabbie, 1992).

In mixed-gender groups, who would you expect to be more likely to initiate group decision making, a female leader or a male leader? Research to date suggests that female leaders are more likely to adopt a democratic, participatory style and male leaders are more likely to be autocratic (Eagly & Johnson, 1990). This may be because females are socialized to be more communal and other-centered, but it may also be because subordinates do not respond well to autocratic female leaders. According to some research, autocratic behavior on the part of male leaders is viewed as decisiveness, but the same behavior on the part of women is perceived as inappropriate (Vroom & Jago, 1995).

Earlier in the chapter, you learned that groups often make more or less use of information depending on the status of the group member offering it. This is a problem for group decision making because the group may ignore important ideas, information, or suggestions from lower-status group members, and consequently may make an inferior decision. Expectation states theory and status characteristics theory (see Chapter 4, Status and Power Dynamics in Groups) suggest that members make assumptions about what group members have to contribute to the group and how valuable these contributions will be. These performance expectations are often based on diffuse-status characteristics such as gender, age, and ethnicity. Based on past research suggesting that males tend to be accorded higher status in mixed-gender groups, Propp (1995) reasoned that males would be seen as more credible sources of information. Therefore, not only would they be given more opportunities to share information, but the information they shared would be seen as more valuable than that contributed by females.

Propp (1995) tested these hypotheses in a study in which groups had to decide a child custody case and members were given different pieces of information about the case. On the positive side, she found that women contributed as much information to the group discussion as men; their participation was not discouraged by the group. On the negative side, the information that was shared by male members was more likely to be accepted than that introduced by female

Apply It! ••• **Compare Your Experience With Research Findings**

What do you think of Propp's research findings? Is your experience in mixed-gender groups consistent with what she found?

members (Propp, 1995). This was especially true when the female group member was offering information that was not possessed by other group members. In other words, if a male member was the only source of the information, it was more likely to be accepted by the group than if a female member was the only source of the information.

Propp (1995) cautions that groups should be careful to make judgments regarding the credibility of information based on individuals' knowledge and expertise. Assigning credibility on the basis of diffuse-status characteristics such as gender can bias the pool of information the group uses in making a decision. She adds that female group members must demonstrate their competence early in the life of the group so as to increase their credibility. Propp also suggests that computer-mediated group decision making, in which members are unaware of which member is contributing what piece of information, may reduce the impact of diffuse-status characteristics.

Concept Review

Group Decision Basics

- The six common steps important to the group decision-making process are defining the problem, identifying options, gathering information, evaluating options, and making and implementing the decision.
- Because of **decision-making constraints,** groups often perform better than their average member but worse than their best member.
- **Cognitive constraints** occur when group members fail to consider all relevant information because they don't have access to it, don't have the ability to understand it, or don't have time to consider it.
- **Affiliative constraints** happen when members do not share information or concerns because of worries about impairing relationships with other group members.
- **Egocentric constraints** are evident when some group members suppress the input of others and push their own agendas.

Groups as Collective Information Processors

- According to the **collective information-processing model,** each member is an informational resource to the group and it is through discussion that these resources are shared. The more unshared information that groups pool, the better their decision making will be. Decision quality is frequently reduced because groups spend their time sharing information everyone has in common and because they pay more attention to information that comes from higher-status group members.
- **Brainstorming** is intended to increase the number of ideas a group generates. Members throw out as many ideas as they can before evaluating them. Research does not support the idea that brainstorming results in higher-quality ideas. Social loafing, evaluation apprehension, and production blocking may explain this. **Group support systems (GSS),** or electronic brainstorming, is intended to overcome these problems, but research support is mixed.
- With the **nominal group technique (NGT),** group members first brainstorm individually, and then a polling technique is used so that all ideas are shared. Some studies support the effectiveness of NGT, but others do not.
- When group members are not knowledgeable enough to make a good decision, they may use the **Delphi technique** to collect and synthesize information and opinions in written form from a group of experts. Although little research has been conducted on effectiveness, this technique is frequently used in education and health care.

Groupthink

- **Groupthink** describes the defective decision making that arises in a cohesive group when premature consensus seeking leads members to quickly seize upon a proposed solution before they have fully reviewed alternative courses of action.
- Antecedents of groupthink include cohesiveness, a provocative situational context, and structural faults of the group. Research emphasizes the importance of structural faults, such as lack of impartial leadership, lack of methodological norms for decision making, and insulation from outside experts, in increasing the likelihood of groupthink.
- Symptoms of groupthink include an overestimation of the power and morality of the group, closed-mindedness, underestimation of competitors or enemies, censorship of dissenting views, and self-appointed mindguards.
- The consequences of groupthink are a poor information search, biased processing of available information, an incomplete survey of alternatives, failure to critically examine the preferred choice, and failure to have a backup plan.

Group Polarization

- Following group discussion, members' attitudes and opinions tend to shift in the direction already favored by the group, leading the group to agree on a position that is more extreme than the average opinion of its members. This is called **group polarization.**
- The **persuasive arguments explanation** suggests that in the course of discussion, our preexisting opinions are strengthened as we hear additional arguments offered by others.
- The **social comparison explanation** suggests that we want to be liked and accepted in the group, so we adjust our position to fit the group sentiment and take our position a step further so that we can be better than average.
- Social identity theorists add that when identification with the group is strong, other group members are seen as valid sources of information, and members are more likely to move in the direction of what appears to be a shared group norm.

Decision Styles and Group Decisions

- According to the **normative decision model,** leaders should use one of five decision styles, depending on three situational factors: decision quality, decision acceptance, and time. The styles vary in how much they include subordinates in decision making, ranging from no involvement at all to letting them make the final decision.
- Group members may have different **decision styles.** The decision-style model identifies four different styles: directive, analytical, conceptual, and behavioral. Those with a *directive style* like to make decisions quickly without considering many alternatives. Individuals with an *analytical style* carefully consider a range of alternatives after collecting detailed data. People with a *conceptual style* like to consider new and unusual ideas and focus on the "big picture." Individuals with a *behavioral style* like to make decisions in a group and are concerned with how their fellow group members feel and what is good for the organization.
- No one style is best because decision situations vary. There are advantages to having decision-style diversity in your group because people with different styles provide balance to one another.

Culture, Gender, and Group Decision Making

- Culture may affect whether individual or group decision making is preferred.
- Some group decision-making constraints and errors may be more common in some cultures than in others. For instance, groups in collectivist cultures that favor more directive leadership and emphasize conformity may be more

susceptible to groupthink and group polarization. Groups in individualistic cultures may be more prone to egocentric constraints on decision making.

- Meta-analyses indicate that female groups are better than male groups at incorporating the views of all members into the final decision. All-female groups may also be more likely to consider a variety of information when making a decision.
- In mixed-gender groups, female leaders are more likely to adopt a democratic participatory style, and male leaders are more likely to be autocratic.
- In one study, information that was shared by male members was more likely to be accepted than that introduced by female members.

Skill Review

Reduce Decision-Making Constraints

- Have members first brainstorm alone and then use a round-robin approach for sharing ideas.
- Avoid satisficing. Structure the process so that alternatives are fully explored.
- Remind the group that members may disagree but that it is still important to share all ideas if the group is to make a good decision. Have ground rules for discussion that ensure disagreement will be useful.
- Make it clear to lower-status members and members with dissenting views that their input is important and welcome.
- Make judgments regarding the credibility of information based on individuals' knowledge and expertise, not on diffuse-status characteristics such as gender.
- Control dominating members by reminding the group that everyone's input is needed and valued.

Use Vigilant Decision Making to Avoid Groupthink and Group Polarization

- Encourage genuine debate, and encourage all members to take the role of "critical evaluator."
- Appoint a "devil's advocate" whose job it is to question the group.
- Avoid insulation by having outside experts or qualified colleagues critique the group's thinking before consensus is reached. Have multiple groups (or subgroups of a larger group) work on the same problem.
- Use a method that requires the group to consider the costs and benefits of proposed alternatives.
- After reaching preliminary consensus but before a final decision is made, have a second-chance meeting at which members rethink the decision one last time.

Use the Situation to Determine When to Make a Group Decision

- Do not make a decision without consulting group members if the decision is important and members possess relevant information, or when decision acceptance is important and members are unlikely to accept an autocratic decision. It is okay to make the decision autocratically if it is trivial, or if you possess enough information and group members will be willing to accept and implement it even if you make it alone.

Consider Decision Styles, Culture, and Gender

- If problems result from different decision styles within your group, talk about your different styles and when each one can best serve the group.
- If your group leader is from a different culture than you are, understand that s/he may be more or less likely than you to consult the group when making a decision.
- Avoid making assumptions about the value of information based on the gender, ethnicity, or culture of the group member offering it.

Study Questions

1. What six steps are commonly identified as important to the group decision process, and what process challenges do groups often face at each step?
2. What three decision-making constraints are identified in the chapter? What are the symptoms of each?
3. According to the collective information-processing model of group decision making, what is a group's richest resource? How do groups often fail to fully tap this resource, and how does that affect decision quality?
4. How is brainstorming intended to enhance collective information processing? Does it work? Why or why not? Why do some consider electronic brainstorming to be an improvement over traditional brainstorming?
5. What is the advantage of the nominal group technique over traditional brainstorming? What are the four basic steps to NGT?
6. What is the Delphi technique? What decision-making constraint is it intended to reduce?
7. What suggestions were given in the chapter for reducing decision-making constraints?
8. What is groupthink? What are its symptoms and consequences? What antecedents give rise to groupthink? According to research, which ones are especially important? What should a group do to make decisions "vigilantly"?
9. What is group polarization? What explanations are provided for it in the text? How does it impact group effectiveness?

10. According to the normative decision model, how does a leader decide how much to involve subordinates in decision making? What are the five types of decision styles, and when is each one recommended?
11. What is said in the chapter about the influence of culture on group decision making?
12. What do we know about gender and group decision making?
13. What four decision styles are described by the decision-style model? What are their implications for a group?

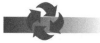

Group Activities

Activity 1: Give and Receive Feedback on Decision Styles

Your small group (four to six members) has 30 minutes to decide whether your school should have a policy about student-faculty dating. When your time is up, review the different decision styles described in the chapter under "Member Decision Styles." Next, using members' behavior during this activity and other activities in which you have observed them, write down which decision style seems to fit each person, and also identify which style you think fits you (15 minutes). Then, all group members share their observations in turn with the group (45 minutes).

Activity 2: Try the Delphi Technique

Pretend that your class group has really come to like one another (hopefully not much pretending is needed), but that this has led to a number of side conversations during large-group activities. Your class leader (your teacher) is also having a difficult time getting the group's attention to begin class and reconvene after break. His/her signal that it's time (switching the lights on and off) is being ignored. In your small group, use the Delphi technique to develop a policy for dealing with students who engage in side conversations and do not stop talking when the leader flips the light switch on and off.

Activity 3: Use a Decision Fishbowl

A group of seven is formed in the middle of the room (the fishbowl group), and others place their chairs in a larger circle around them (the observer group). The fishbowl group has 45 minutes to decide the fate of Davey, a 15-year-old boy. They are to make a recommendation to the judge deciding Davey's case. Here is Davey's case file compiled by a social worker:

Davey is the youngest of three children of parents who divorced when he was 1. His mother remarried a very nice man when Davey was 3. Davey's step-father treated the children as his own and provided well for them. Davey always had lots of toys, nice clothes, and expensive family vacations. He saw his birth father every other weekend, and his father called several times a week.

Unfortunately, the relationship between his mother and birth father remained difficult, and they had frequent loud fights when his father came to pick the kids up. Davey's mother hated Davey's father and constantly tried to turn the children against him. When she was angry at Davey, which was often, she would say he was just like his father. She also drank heavily and told the children it was their fault for "ruining her life." Many times she locked herself in the bathroom, crying hysterically, and told them that she was going to kill herself because they didn't love her enough.

When Davey was 11, he began smoking cigarettes and marijuana, and by 12, he was doing poorly in school and declining to participate in family activities. This resulted in many fights between Davey and his mother, some physical. When he was 13, she threw him out, and made a suicide attempt the next day, saying that Davey had "abandoned her" and "broken her heart."

Davey went to live with his father, who did not provide much supervision; Davey felt neglected and like a burden. He barely passed seventh and eighth grades and wore clothing that made him look like a gang member. In ninth grade, Davey was expelled for selling drugs at school, received probation, and was sent to continuation school. After six months he managed to get readmitted to the regular high school, but within a few months he was expelled permanently for coming to school under the influence of drugs. He went back to continuation school. By this time, he was 15 and was addicted to cocaine. He was arrested for possession of drugs (a pound of marijuana, several hits of acid, and several grams of cocaine). While awaiting his court date, he went to drug rehab, where his counselors were impressed with his commitment to achieving sobriety. He is seeing a therapist weekly, who reports that Davey is working hard to understand his past and "turn over a new leaf." He has been out of rehab for six weeks, and all his drug tests have been clean.

Members of the observer group are to silently observe the fishbowl group while taking notes to answer the following questions. Afterwards, they share their observations with the entire group.

1. Were cognitive constraints operating? (Did the group have enough information, experience, or time?)
2. Were affiliative constraints operating? (Did conformity pressures and status differences influence the process?)
3. Were egocentric constraints operating? (Were there members who dominated the process and seemed intent on getting their way?)
4. Did the group use any techniques, such as brainstorming or nominal group techniques, to ensure equal participation and information sharing?
5. Was there any evidence that the group engaged in premature decision making—that is, that they quickly seized upon a solution and then engaged in bolstering?

6. Were different decision styles evident—that is, differences in how members thought the group should go about making the decision?

InfoTrac College Edition Search Terms

To do research for your papers and assignments, use InfoTrac that's provided free with new copies of this book. Go to http://infotrac.thomsonlearning.com and enter the following search terms:

- Decision-making, Group
- Nominal Group Technique
- Groupthink
- Group Polarization
- Decision Styles

Chapter 12 Teams

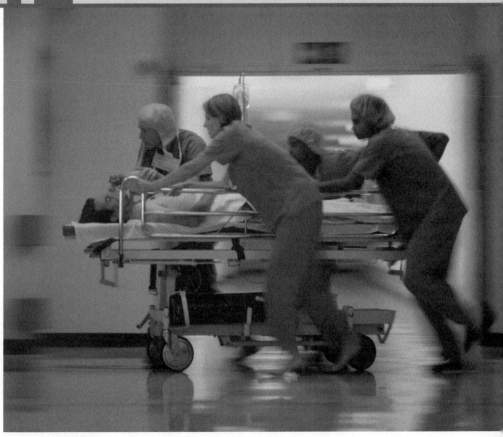

Teams are an important topic as organizations continue to rely on them to improve quality, productivity, customer service, and the work experience (Guzzo, 1995). Teams are the primary unit of performance for increasing numbers of organizations because the kinds of customer service, technological change, competitive threats, and environmental constraints that face today's organizations are beyond the grasp of individual performance (Katzenbach & Smith, 1993). Consider the variety of these teams:

- A hospital is in deep trouble and has lost its accreditation. An interim top management team is appointed to restructure the entire hospital program and select a permanent management team within nine months.

- A community environmental organization creates a yearlong task force to identify county environmental health issues and solutions, especially those associated with the use of agricultural chemicals. The group has members from the county health department, the local farmer's bureau, the farmworkers' union, and a grassroots citizen organization that seeks rights for the chemically sensitive.
- An insurance company seeks to computerize all of its records and hires a team to create and maintain the computer systems it needs. This group will serve as a permanent professional technical support team.
- A performing team, a theater troupe, is comprised of ten regular cast members, has put on at least three performances a year for the past nine years.
- The staff at the group home where children wait for foster home placements is a human service team. They do intake and discharge interviews and work to see that the children are served healthy meals, get enough sleep, receive their medications, and follow the house rules. Meanwhile, a team of caseworkers at the city's social services department works to find placements for the children, and to monitor their progress once they are placed.
- An educational team comprised of a reading specialist, a school counselor, a parent, and a child's teacher meets three times to come up with a plan to help a child adapt to a learning disability.
- At a company that manufactures computer parts, a production team is responsible for making electronic chips.

Teams are used in medical, educational, business, entertainment, military, government, community, social service, and sports organizations. They vary in the tasks they accomplish and range on a continuum from temporary to permanent. The odds are good that you have already spent considerable time on student project teams and that you will spend considerably more time on teams in the course of your work life.

Most of us yearn for that stellar group experience in which the group functions like a well-oiled team machine. The group knows what its work is; the environment and leadership are supportive of the group's work; the group has adequate resources to do its work; the group's members possess the relevant skills needed to get the job done; and members communicate well and cooperate to get it done. Even better, the group experience is a socially positive one in which members feel affirmed, member relations are friendly, and all members care about the group, other members, and the task. What turns a group into a team? How do we foster teamwork? How can team training be used to increase team effectiveness? How do we deal with common team problems? These are some of the questions answered in this chapter.

Teams

Workgroups composed of people with the right balance of skills who cooperate to do a job within a larger organization.

Teams vs. Groups

All teams are groups, but not all groups are teams (Hare, 1992). In group dynamics, **teams** refer to workgroups made up of individuals who see themselves and are seen by others as a social entity, are interdependent because of the tasks

BOX 12-1 / FEATURES OF TEAMS

- Teams are bounded.
- Teams consist of a relatively small number of people.
- Team members have complementary skills.
- Team members are interdependent.
- Team members share a common goal and approach for which they hold themselves mutually accountable.

they perform as group members, are embedded in one or more larger social organizations, who perform tasks that affect others (Guzzo & Dickson, 1996). These features of teams are summarized in **Box 12-1** and described in the following paragraph.

Teams Are Well-Balanced, Cooperative Units

Teams are composed of people with the right balance of skills. They are groups that operate according to norms of cooperation, not competition. Katzenbach and Smith (1993, p. 45) say that "a team is a small number of people with complementary skills who are committed to a common purpose, performance goals, and approach for which they hold themselves mutually accountable." They suggest that this definition summarizes the ingredients for a successful team.

Teams Are Bounded Social Units

Some team researchers emphasize that teams are "bounded social units" doing a job within a larger organization (Guzzo, 1995). Most large organizations are separated into smaller, specialized units that accomplish different jobs fundamental to the organization's mission. "Bounded" means that the membership of the team, along with its tasks, is identifiable. It is known who the members are and whether the job of the group is to monitor something, produce something, provide a service, solve a problem, win a game, or create something new.

Teams Are Small

Teams generally have between two and twenty-five members, though most successful teams have fewer than ten members (Hackman, 1987; Katzenbach & Smith, 1993; Thompson, 2000). Once a team becomes larger than ten members, interaction and consensus become more difficult, participation declines, and more negative group behaviors such as social loafing arise. Although leaders often overstaff teams to avoid excluding anyone and because they assume

---

Apply It! ••• **Was Your Last Project Group a Team?**

Think about a recent group project at school or at work. Evaluate your group according the features of teams described above. Was your project group a team? Why or why not?

---

that bigger teams are better, smaller—even understaffed—teams work harder and are more involved (Thompson, 2000). What is the optimal size for a team? It depends on the task (Klimoski & Jones, 1995). Too few people may have a hard time accomplishing the task and be overstressed. Too many is a waste of resources. Again, bigger is not necessarily better because coordination becomes more difficult as team size increases (Sundstrom, de Meuse, & Futrell, 1990). Teams should generally be staffed to the smallest number that can do the work (Paris, Salas, & Cannon-Bowers, 2000).

Teams Imply Joint Action

To be a team, a group has to have a high degree of task interdependence among group members, who must share information and resources and coordinate their activities to get the job done (Guzzo, 1995). Interdependence means that if one member does not do his or her job, the work of the team is affected. Teams imply joint action (Hare, 1992). Some tasks are not suited for teamwork because they are best accomplished by individuals. Hackman (1998) suggests that tasks such as writing reports, novels, and musical scores are best done by individuals. Teams are great, but they are not always appropriate for the task.

Ways to Classify Teams

Teams vary enormously based on task, their mission, and the organization within which they are embedded. For this reason, theorists have come up with a number of different ways to classify teams.

Classification by Task

Hare (1992) suggests that teams can be classified into four basic types, based on tasks: (1) the *New Discovery Driven Team,* such as the scientific research and development team; (2) the *Rule Driven Team,* which includes sports teams; (3) the *Product Driven Team,* whose purpose is to deliver a product or service; and (4) the *Equipment or Technology Driven Team* that manages a technology, which includes the crews of boats, planes, and spaceships and groups that manage information technologies. These functional specialties are important because they greatly affect the work of the group. For instance, the activities of the airline crew are strongly determined by the demands of the technology, and the activities of the sports team are directed by the rules of the game. Likewise, teams in business, manufacturing, health, and education are tied to a product, an object, or the care or education of people. If the nature of the product or service is changed, the team must be reorganized (Hare, 1992). When thinking about teams, it is instructive to think about the group's task, how it influences the structure of the team, and what will be important for the team's success.

Larson and LaFasto (1989) classify teams into three main categories based on the type of task. *Tactical teams* are tightly organized and execute well-defined plans to carry out focused tasks with clear operational standards. Surgical teams, military teams, and sports teams are examples. *Problem-solving teams* conduct investigations and collect information to resolve problems. For example, crime squads attempting to solve difficult cases and teams of epidemiologists trying to find out what has made people sick are problem-solving teams. The job of *creative teams* is to come up with new ideas, products, or services. Research and development teams fall into this category.

Devine and his colleagues (Devine, Clayton, Philips, Dunford, & Melner, 1999) suggest that while classifying teams according to the type of product they produce is useful, considering temporal duration (whether the team is short-term or long-term) is also important. For instance, they point out that member satisfaction and commitment are more important for long-term than short-term teams. Therefore, they propose four types of teams: (1) the *ad hoc project team* that exists for a finite period of time to solve problems; (2) the *ongoing project team* with a relatively stable membership that solves problems, deals with clients, and makes plans; (3) *ad hoc production teams*—temporary, case-by-case teams that build, assemble, or create products or performances; and (4) *ongoing production teams,* which perform the same tasks as ad hoc production teams but on an ongoing basis.

Classification by Amount of Team Control

Teams vary in how much power and control they have over their work. They vary in how they are led, and in who determines what the goal is and how it will be accomplished. Hackman (1987) has suggested four different team designations based on who determines the group's objectives and how these are accomplished, and who monitors the group's performance (see Figure 12-1). These designations are the manager-led team, the self-managing team, the self-directed team, and the self-governing team.

The traditional team is the *manager-led team,* in which a manager designated by the organization leads the team. This manager is responsible for the group's functioning and for determining its goals and methods. The manager

Figure 12-1

Types of Teams in Organizations

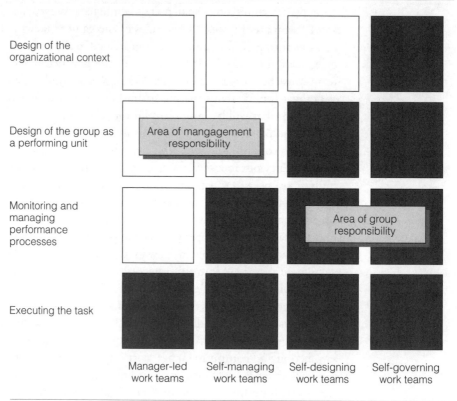

Design of the
organizational context

Design of the group as
a performing unit

Monitoring and
managing
performance
processes

Executing the task

Manager-led · Self-managing · Self-designing · Self-governing
work teams   work teams   work teams   work teams

Source: "The Design of Work Teams" by J. R. Hackman in *Handbook of Organizational Behavior*, edited by J. W. Lorsck, 1987. Prentice-Hall, Inc.

also monitors the team for progress toward team goals and has the power to reward and punish team members. For instance, putting on a theatrical production usually involves a team responsible for sets, lighting, costumes, and staging. A stage manager runs this team, saying what needs to be done, how it should be done, and whether it is done satisfactorily. An airline flight crew is a manager-led team because the airline captain directs the crewmembers. A sports team with a coach who controls the offense and defense is also a manager-led team.

Imagine a team consisting of a social worker, a psychologist, a psychiatrist, a nurse, and a psychiatric technician. This group has been charged with the mental health care of a group of twenty-two institutionalized adults. They are told that they must complete certain assessments and case notes by a certain time every month and that they must meet to do treatment planning for each patient and follow state and national guidelines. However, it is left up to them to decide

Choose a group you are a member of that fits the definition of "team." How would you classify it using the categories described in this section?

how to accomplish these tasks. The hospital has a number of such teams, and each team organizes its work differently. This is an example of the *self-managing* or *self-regulating team.* Although a manager or leader still tells the group what its goal is, the team has the freedom to decide how to accomplish it.

Self-directing or *self-designing teams* are teams that decide what their objectives are and how they are going to achieve them. However, although what they do and how they do it is largely up to them, they still operate within an organizational context that influences their work. For instance, a metals company may have a research and development team that comes up with ideas for new products, and designs and tests them. The group is largely left alone to go about its business as it defines it, but it has little influence over the rest of the organization. The team may design itself, but it does not design the organizational context. In contrast, the *self-governing team* has the power to design the organizational context as well as itself. This type of team is often a top management team or board of directors.

It is not possible to say which of these team types is best because each has its advantages and disadvantages (Thompson, 2000). The manager-led team is often efficient because the group does not have to spend time deciding what to do and how to do it. This type of team seems to do just fine when the goal of the group is clear and the task well defined. However, the lack of autonomy provided by the manager-led team can interfere with commitment to the group and can lower morale. It also does not allow much room for new ideas. If this is a problem, then a self-managing team or a self-directing team may be more effective. However, the more autonomy a team has, generally the more time it consumes and the more conflict there is.

Teams and the Organizational Context

Earlier you read that teams are "bounded social units" that operate within larger organizational units. This is important because it means that teams do not operate in isolation and are affected by the "organizational context." The organizational context determines the team's resources, how much freedom the team is given, how the team will be rewarded, how it obtains information, and how it monitors its work. Teams need a supportive organizational context if they are to be successful.

Figure 12-2

Four Key Supports of the Team Organizational Context

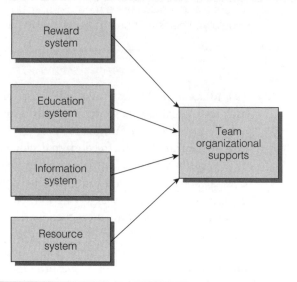

Source: Derived from Hackman, 1998.

Organizational Supports for Teams

Organizational supports

Systems and resources that organizations and leaders provide to support teamwork.

Many organizations designate members to form a team but fail to provide the team with the support it needs to function as one. According to Hackman (1998), key **organizational supports** include (1) a reward system that recognizes and reinforces excellent team performance; (2) an educational system that provides any training or technical consultations that are needed; (3) an information system that helps the team manage its work; and (4) a resource system that supplies the material resources that the work requires, such as equipment, tools, money, or staff. These organization supports are summarized in Figure 12-2.

Hackman (1990) laments that organizations are tuned to support the work of individuals, not teams. Training tends to be provided for individual skill development, not team skill development. Information and control systems provide senior managers with feedback on performance, but teams may not receive the information they need to know how they are doing. Sometimes upper management or administrators claim that they want a workgroup to function as a team, yet they use a reward system that does not promote teamwork. Most organizations have performance appraisal systems that are geared to assessing and rewarding work by individuals, not teams (Hackman, 1998). Unfortunately, comparing and rewarding individuals on the team may result in their competing with one another (Lawler, 1992). In a large study of teams in the United States, only one-third reported that they formally appraised team performance, and even fewer provided material incentives for achieving team goals (Devine et al., 1999).

Team Incentives and Team Recognition

Team incentives

Monetary or material rewards offered to motivate the team to meet production targets.

Team recognition

One-time awards given for good team performance, such as cash bonuses, thank-you notes, time off, and expense-paid trips.

In general, teamwork is stimulated when rewards are given to the whole team rather than to individual members, and when those rewards are contingent on the group's performance. The two most common practices for rewarding and motivating team performance are **team incentives** and **team recognition** (Thompson, 2000). Team incentives typically involve monetary rewards given to the team if it meets a production target. Team recognition is often provided in the form of "spot awards"—one-time awards given for good team performance. One-time cash bonuses, thank-you notes, time off, and expense-paid trips are all types of recognition awards.

Rewarding only team success can create social loafing and free rider effects (DeMatteo, Eby, & Sundstrom, 1998). As discussed in Chapter 9, Group Productivity, some people will slack when they believe that they will share in the group's rewards no matter what they do. For this reason, some experts suggest that two systems be used—one that rewards the team's performance, and another that rewards team members based on their individual performance, expertise, or seniority (Gross, 1995). For instance, Thompson (2000) points out that members vary in skill level and some members contribute more to the group's success than others. Such members may feel it unfair that less qualified or less productive members receive the same compensation, especially if under the old system they would be getting paid more than they are under the new one.

Designing and implementing team-based reward systems is tricky. For more detailed information on this topic, see Gross (1995). Some of the "guiding principles" for team-based pay structures from that text can be found in **Box 12-2.**

BOX 12-2 / SOME GUIDING PRINCIPLES FOR TEAM-BASED PAY STRUCTURES

1. Goals should cover areas that team members can influence. In an effective program, rewards are tied to the team's performance.

2. Balance the mix of individual and team-based pay according to the relative amounts of individual and team-based work members are supposed to do.

3. Consult with team members when designing and implementing the reward program.

4. Avoid "organizational myopia" by considering how the compensation plan will affect relations with other groups and teams in the organization. You do not want to create conflict between organizational units. This could happen if units are in competition for team rewards or feel they are not being treated fairly.

5. Determine the timing of team reports and payments. Keep in mind that members are more motivated by shorter measurement periods and faster payouts.

Source: Gross, 1995

Group Composition

Group composition
The types of people that comprise the team—their knowledge, skills, abilities, and other traits.

Group composition refers to the types of individuals that comprise the team. Team members can vary in knowledge, abilities, skills, experience, personality, and attitude, as well as demographically (such as age or ethnicity). Teams can also be comprised of members from different organizational units. One benefit of a team, as opposed to individuals working alone, is that teams can bring more intellectual and skill resources to bear on a task. The team's membership should be sufficiently diverse (heterogeneous) to enhance team effectiveness (and create a process gain), but not so diverse that members are unable to communicate, coordinate, and agree on the team's mission (a process loss). Meta-analytic research indicates that in general, heterogeneity is a plus for teams working on complex tasks, but homogeneous teams perform better on low-difficulty tasks (Bowers, Pharmer, & Salas, 2000). Chapter 8, Member and Diversity and Group Dynamics, explores this topic in depth and includes a discussion of how to increase commitment and cohesion and reduce conflict in the diverse group.

Regardless of the type of team, care should be taken when choosing the team's members so that the team has the right mix of skills (technical, problem-solving, and interpersonal) to accomplish the task (Katzenbach & Smith, 1993). Members' interpersonal compatibility (compatibility of personalities, styles, and values) is important, but it is only one of the factors that should be considered when putting together a team (Katzenbach & Smith, 1993; Klimoski & Jones, 1995). Indeed, the transformation of a group of individuals into an effective team requires **team competencies**—the knowledge, skills, and attitudes (KSAs) necessary for the performance of the group's tasks (Goldstein & Ford, 2002). These KSAs include the task-specific talents and skills of individual members, the interpersonal and group skills that make coordinated work possible, and a clear understanding of the group's tasks and how group members' work fits together (Cannon-Bowers, Tannenbaum, Salas, & Volpe, 1995). Effective teams have highly skilled members that know how to work together.

Team competencies
The knowledge, skills, and attitudes (KSAs) necessary for team performance.

Taskwork Skills

Taskwork skills
The technical competencies of team members.

When composing a team, it makes sense to consider task-relevant skills and experience. **Taskwork skills** are the technical competencies of team members (Goldstein & Ford, 2002). Members must be competent in their roles if the team is to be effective. Ideally, members have complementary taskwork skills, each bringing to the team unique skills and expertise relevant to the various tasks the group must perform. I thought of this as I recently watched a show on the Discovery Channel called *Monster Garage,* in which the challenge is for a team to convert an ordinary vehicle into a work vehicle and then demonstrate its success with a head-to-head competition against the real thing. In one episode, the team was given a week and a $3000 budget to convert a stretch limousine into a fire engine, capable of running a fire hose that could shoot water 150 feet. In another episode, a different team converted a Ford Explorer into an automated garbage truck. The teams succeed in their missions partly because of the care that is taken in choosing the members. For instance, the limo conversion team included an expert welder, a master machinist, a limo builder, and an engineer who specialized in fire truck design. Each member brought important skills and expertise to the team.

Teamwork Skills

Teamwork skills

Skills related to being able to work as part of a team.

A team may be comprised of talented and competent people and still not be successful if its members do not know how to work as part of a team, or don't want to. **Teamwork skills**—the ability to work together as a team—are as important as technical skills and task-specific knowledge. When a team first comes together, it has to decide what jobs there are to do and which members will do them, and establish norms about how members will work together. As the team proceeds, it is likely that they will have to solve problems, make decisions, resolve conflicts, and coordinate their efforts. Teamwork is difficult if members are not skilled and experienced in interpersonal and group skills such as communication, mutual goal setting, and conflict resolution. These skills promote the group processes necessary for teamwork.

Team mental model

A shared understanding of the team and its work; the team's transactive memory system.

In addition to group and interpersonal skills, teamwork skills include a shared understanding, or **team mental model,** of the team and its work (Cannon-Bowers et al., 1995; Klimoski & Mohammed, 1997). Essentially, this is the team's transactive memory system (see Chapter 11, Group Decision Making, for a discussion of this topic). On effective teams, team members share the same "big picture" of the team (Moreland, Argote, & Krishnan, 1998). They have a similar understanding of the group's norms, resources, and objectives. Members understand the roles of other team members and how they relate to one another and task accomplishment. They understand enough about the knowledge, skills, and abilities of other team members that they know what to expect from them and can coordinate their actions more easily. Tacit coordination is more effective because it is known who does what; less time can be spent talking about it and more time can be spent doing it.

This understanding of who knows what and does what also helps members know which team member to turn to for the different problems that may arise. The limo team began with a clear understanding of and respect for what each member brought to the team. Depending on the stage of the project, different members assumed the lead and were relied on to find a way around technical and resource challenges. For example, the group looked to the limo expert when they were taking the limo apart, and the master machinist when they could not find a part and had to make one.

Cannon-Bowers and her colleagues (1995) conducted an extensive review of the research literature on teamwork skills and concluded that these could be summarized into eight different dimensions. These were all apparent as the limo team scrambled to accomplish its mission in five days with a limited budget.

Adaptability refers to the team's ability to reallocate team resources when needed and compensate for less-than-ideal conditions. The limo team saw the limited time and resources as a challenge, and one member spent many hours on the phone and scouring junkyards for materials the group could use. When Plan A did not work, the group did not get discouraged. Instead, they created and implemented a Plan B, and sometimes a Plan C.

The term *shared situational awareness* describes the extent to which team members have a common understanding of the group, its task, and the situation facing the group. The limo group's leader, Jesse James (descendant of the famous outlaw), led the group in an all-day design which the group came to an understanding about the task and one another's potential contributions.

Performance monitoring and feedback has to do with the ability of team members to monitor the group's productivity and provide constructive feedback to one another to improve performance. Members of the limo group could be seen admiring one another's work and giving each other positive feedback and encouragement. Daily, Jesse James reminded the group of remaining tasks and the timetable of what had to be completed when if the group was to succeed.

The skill dimension of *leadership/team management* is represented by the ability to manage the team's resources and direct, coordinate, and motivate team members. Not only did team leader Jesse James keep the group on track by reminding them of deadlines and the tasks that still needed to be completed, he made sure members were available when their expertise and skill was needed and maintained an infectious belief in the group's ability to accomplish the task.

Skills such as conflict resolution, the ability to cooperate, assertiveness, and support for other members go under the heading of *interpersonal relations*. Some differences of opinion were evident on the limo team, but these were expressed respectfully, and the group was not sidetracked by disagreement and defensiveness. One member averted disaster when he insisted on checking a gasket installed by another member and found that it was lacking a crucial hole. It was all handled good-naturedly.

Apply It! ••• Recall Your Best Teamwork Experience

What was your best team experience? How did that team rate on the eight teamwork skills dimensions described here?

Coordination is the process by which the team's resources and activities are synchronized and completed by certain times. The tasks required for the limo conversion had to be done in a certain order and by a certain time if others were to complete their work. The team leader kept members aware of this, and members did their part to coordinate with other members. The dimension of *communication* refers to the accurate exchange of information within the group. No communication problems were apparent in the limo team. Last, *decision making* has to do with the team's ability to gather and integrate information and assess and solve problems. The limo group met this key challenge. They began with nothing but a white stretch limo and a mission to turn it into a firefighting machine. The group had to figure out what this would involve and make decisions about how to spend their budget, how to overcome technological hurdles, and how to order and pace their work.

Cohesion and Teamwork

Cohesion is another factor related to team effectiveness. On the highest-performing teams, members are committed not just to the group's goals but to one another (Katzenbach & Smith, 1993). One definition of cohesion given in Chapter 6, Group Development, is that cohesion is "a dynamic process that is reflected in the tendency for a group to stick together and remain united in pursuit of its goals and objectives" (Carron, 1988, p. 124). To be effective and productive, teams need the time and training to become cohesive (Banker, Field, Schroeder, & Sinha, 1996; Goldstein & Ford, 2002). Chapter 6 discusses ways to build group cohesion, such as fostering personal acquaintance among members and emphasizing a shared group identity. We also know that cohesiveness is greater when physical and psychological distance (such as that created by status differences) between team members is minimized (Paris et al., 2000).

Cohesion Increases Team Performance

Meta-analyses find that group cohesiveness is positively related to group performance (Evans & Dion, 1991; Mullen & Copper, 1994). Cohesiveness may advance performance because individuals in cohesive work groups are more directed toward group tasks (Stodgill, 1972) and may be more committed to achieving group goals (Mullen & Copper, 1994; Shaw, 1981). Cohesiveness may also promote performance because members of cohesive groups interact and communicate more, and this increases performance (Gully, Devine, & Whitney, 1995). Cohesiveness also implies a certain familiarity of members with one another; that is, they know other team members well enough that they can predict their behavior and match member interests and strengths to tasks (Druskat & Kayes, 2000). Intermember familiarity is positively linked to team performance (Druskat & Kayes, 2000; Goodman & Leyden, 1991).

Members of cohesive groups also appear more likely to do things for the group that go "beyond the call of duty" and enhance the group's performance. Several studies indicate that workgroup cohesiveness is associated such "extra-role performance behavior" (George & Bettenhausen, 1990; Kidwell, Mossholder, & Bennett, 1997). For instance, by the time the limo group finished the vehicle conversion, the group had become quite tight. One member stayed up all night to paint it fire-engine red and add hot-rod-like chrome, a nice touch but not one that was technically required for team success. But he wanted to do this for the group as the crowning touch of their project. One study with athletic teams also found that group cohesion was positively related to the strength of the group's resistance to disruptive events such as team defeat (Brawley, Carron, & Widmeyer, 1988). Despite setbacks, the limo team kept going, and this made them closer because they weathered the storms that came their way.

Team Performance Increases Cohesion

Although it makes sense that cohesiveness would affect performance, the relationship is actually a complicated one. While cohesiveness can increase group performance, it is also the case that group performance can influence cohesiveness (Mullen & Copper, 1994). This makes sense when you think about it. Sharing success with others does bring you closer together. Indeed, Mullen and Copper (1994) found that research on cohesiveness and performance indicates that performance affects cohesiveness more than vice versa. When the limo team members realized they had met their goal and their product could compete with a fire engine, they felt even more like a team. They all decided to arrive at the scene of the competition wearing tuxes in a show of team unity.

Further Complexities in the Cohesion–Performance Relationship

Whether cohesiveness increases performance also depends on whether the group's norms are congruent with the organization's (or the leader's, teacher's, or manager's) goals. A cohesive workgroup, for instance, may have counterproductive work norms, such as not working hard or treating customers with indifference. Langfred (1998) studied Danish army units and found that groups with high cohesiveness and task norms were most effective, whereas high cohesiveness and nontask norms were associated with poor performance. In the case of the limo team, success was clearly tied to the fact that the original source of the group's cohesion was that all members were committed to high performance goals.

Also, because cohesiveness increases conformity, it is likely to enhance performance in situations in which deviance and lack of coordination may endanger the group, but can hurt performance when creativity and new ideas are needed (Brehm, Kassin, & Fein, 1999). It is also true that the influence of group cohesion on performance is greater when completion of the task requires that group members interact, communicate, and cooperate (Gully et al., 1995). In

Figure 12-3
Factors Affecting Team Effectiveness

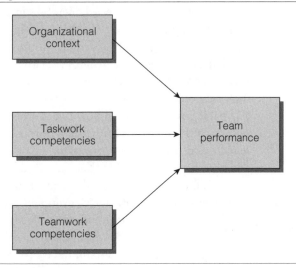

other words, cohesion is more important for interdependent tasks requiring teamwork. For instance, the lack of cohesion among faculty in many academic departments does not harm teaching performance, but it may harm the productivity of committees or group decision making in faculty meetings.

Team Effectiveness

Team-Related Attitudes

In contrast to "nominal" teams (teams in name only) or "pseudo" teams, "real" teams are teams in which morale is high and members agree on the group's mission and feel responsible for the group's results. In effective teams, members collaborate to achieve common goals and have attitudes supportive of teamwork.

Collective orientation

Having positive attitudes toward working as part of a team.

A number of attitudes affect teamwork. For instance, several studies find that positive attitudes toward teamwork, or a **collective orientation,** are positively associated with team effectiveness (Cannon-Bowers et al., 1995). As discussed in earlier chapters, compared to individuals from collectivistic cultures, people from individualistic cultures are more likely to have a competitive orientation that interferes with cooperation and positive teamwork attitudes. Turning a group into a team may be easier in some cultures than in others. Fortunately, all the members of the limo team were accustomed to working as part of a team and understood the importance of cooperation.

Shared vision

When team members are committed to a common purpose and common performance goals.

A **shared vision** is another important team attitude. The limo team members all agreed on their mission and were excited by the challenge and their role in making it happen. Effective teams are committed to a common purpose and common performance goals (Katzenbach & Smith, 1993). The importance of shared goals has been discussed throughout this book. Early in the history of group dynamics, theorists noted the importance of goals to group locomotion. For the group to move forward, members must agree on what forward is and how they are going to get there. As discussed in Chapter 9, Group Productivity, research clearly suggests that member commitment to group goals enhances productivity. Group goals contribute to team effectiveness especially when goals are specific and somewhat challenging and when team members are committed to the goals, receive feedback on progress toward their goals, believe the goals are attainable, and understand how to achieve the goals. On effective teams, members not only agree on a broad team purpose but transform broad directives into specific and measurable performance goals that help the team track its progress and hold itself accountable (Katzenbach & Smith, 1993).

Collective efficacy (group efficacy)

Members' beliefs that the team's efforts will lead to success.

Collective efficacy is another team attitude studied for its effect on team performance. **Collective efficacy,** or **group efficacy,** is the aggregation of group members' perceptions that the group can perform a particular task (Lindsley, Brass, & Thomas, 1995; Mulvey & Klein, 1998). In other words, do team members believe that the group's efforts will result in task success? If they do believe the group will be successful if it tries, they are more likely to make an effort. If they don't, they won't make the effort—after all, why bother? According to Bandura (2000), the higher the perceived collective efficacy, the higher will be group members' motivational investment in their undertakings, the stronger their staying power in the face of impediments and setbacks, and the greater their performance accomplishments (Bandura, 2000). Research findings support the idea that collective efficacy is related to group goals and performance (Earley, 1993; Little & Madigan, 1997; Prussia & Kiniki, 1996). In other words, it appears that when group members believe they will be successful, they are more likely to set higher goals and to achieve them.

Collective efficacy is influenced by a number of factors, including the group's past performance. High-efficacy groups are likely to have had high performance success in the past and, are likely to set goals that are equal to or higher than their own past performance or those of less efficacious groups (Mulvey & Klein, 1998; Prussia & Kiniki, 1996; Zander, 1994). Adequate resources and skills (training may be needed), assurances that other members are committed to the goal, and encouragement that they can perform complex tasks (verbal coaching) also increase collective efficacy. Providing the group with examples of similar groups who have achieved difficult goals also enhances collective efficacy

---

Apply It! ••• **Do You Have Attitudes Supportive of Teamwork?**

Fill out the questionnaire in **Box 12-3.** Based on your responses, would you say you have the attitudes supportive of teamwork? Where did your teamwork attitudes come from? Your culture? Your past team experiences? Your personality?

BOX 12-3 / ASSESSING YOUR TEAMWORK ATTITUDES

Directions: Indicate how strongly you agree with each of the following statements.

Strongly Disagree	Disagree	Disagree Somewhat	Neutral	Agree Somewhat	Agree	Strongly Agree
1	2	3	4	5	6	7

_____ 1. I prefer to work alone rather than as part of a group.

_____ 2. I am a competitive person, even with members of my own group.

_____ 3. In a group task situation, I try to take on tasks that I can do by myself without interacting much with other team members.

_____ 4. I would rather do most of the group's work myself than work with team members to reach agreement on what our goal is and how to achieve it.

_____ 5. In general, I am not confident in the ability of groups to do a quality job.

_____ 6. I really like working with other people to get a job done.

_____ 7. I do not have a problem with sharing power with other group members.

_____ 8. I do not mind sharing credit with other group members.

_____ 9. When on a team, I usually have confidence that we will accomplish our task efficiently.

_____ 10. In a group task situation, I do not avoid situations where I will have to coordinate my efforts with other team members.

Scoring: Agreement with the first five statements is indicative of attitudes contrary to teamwork. Agreement with the second five suggests a person with attitudes supportive of working on a team.

(Prussia & Kiniki, 1996). These features were all present for the limo team. For instance, knowing that other teams (such as the team that converted a Ford Explorer into a garbage truck) had succeeded, as well as their confidence in the skills of their fellow team members, increased the limo group members' confidence that they could meet the challenge.

Team Leadership

Leadership is obviously important to team effectiveness. It is usually the leader who secures the team's resources, runs interference with the organization, makes sure that members have the appropriate training, and creates the situations that will foster a positive team climate. Team leaders and managers make sure the team has organizational support, build and maintain the team as a performing unit, and coach and help the group (Hackman, 1990). Team leaders provide the group with the structure needed to develop healthy teamwork (Hackman, 1998). They provide the group with a well-designed task, make sure members know what their jobs are and how to do them, and specify the basic norms that support teamwork.

As discussed earlier in the chapter, teams vary in the extent to which they are self-run and range from those that are entirely self-managed to those that have relatively little say in what they are to do and how they are to do it. One message throughout this book is the importance of group member participation. In general, group members work harder and are more committed to groups when they are allowed a say in the decisions that affect them. Group effectiveness is also enhanced because group members are often a wealthy source of information about the task and how to improve efficiency and effectiveness. An autocratic leader who delivers all orders top-down without any consultation not only fails to obtain decision-relevant information, but also reduces the likelihood that members will engage in extra-role behavior and that the decision will be well implemented. The limo team would have failed had the members not been consulted. Of course, a laissez-faire leader who provides no guidance is equally problematic. A group with no leadership will flounder around, unsure of what to do and unclear on how the team and its tasks fit together. This means that team leadership is leading enough, but not too much.

Team leadership is clearly about balance. For instance, in Chapter 10, Leadership, it was clear that a balance of task and socioemotional leadership is best. A leader should provide directive or supportive leadership depending on the task's difficulty and stressfulness and depending on subordinates' personal needs and skills. Team leadership is also about finding this equilibrium. As Katzenbach and Smith (1993) note, the essence of a team leader's job is striking the right balance between providing guidance and giving up control, between making tough decisions and letting others make them, and between doing difficult things alone and letting others learn to do them. Too much command, or too little, will stifle the capability, initiative, and creativity of the team.

Team Training

It is rare for team members to have all the desired skills at the outset, and training is often needed in both taskwork and teamwork skills. In the United States, companies spend $30 billion to $100 billion annually on training (Thompson, 2000), but when training is provided, it is almost always designed for the individual worker and does not train people to work in groups (Moreland et al., 1998).

Team training
Training designed to improve members' taskwork and teamwork skills.

Ideally, **team training** is ongoing. Over the course of a project or team task, things may change so that new skills are needed. For example, hardware breakdowns and software updates may mean that members of a technological support team have to acquire new skills. Keeping member knowledge and skills current can be a constant challenge, especially if the task is one that regularly changes (Davis-Sacks, Denison, & Eisenstat, 1990). Fortunately, members often rise to the occasion by developing the skills the team is lacking. In this way, teams are powerful vehicles for individual learning and development (Katzenbach & Smith, 1993).

It is not enough to train team members in individual responsibilities and simply hope that they will figure out how to operate as a team (Paris et al., 2000).

BOX 12-4 / GROUP SKILLS RECOMMENDATIONS RELEVANT TO TEAMWORK

- Develop norms and roles compatible with team success.
- Build a group with norms of cooperation.
- Make status assignments based on specific-status characteristics.
- Minimize status differences.
- Engage in constructive controversy.
- Use constructive confrontation when group norms are violated.
- Establish a supportive communication climate.
- Recognize the benefits of member diversity.
- Create a superordinate (shared) group identity.
- Generate superordinate goals.
- Use group goal setting.
- Rely on explicit coordination and pre-planning.
- Persuade members that their contributions are needed, noticed, and valued.
- Tie valued individual outcomes to group outcomes.
- Balance task and socioemotional leadership.
- Choose discussion and decision-making procedures that prevent domination by a few members and ensure that all relevant information and perspectives are considered.

Indeed, training in teamwork skills is often needed so that members can better communicate and coordinate their work. Coaching in teamwork skills is especially important in cultures where individualism is a dominant value and members are unaccustomed to working as a team (Hackman, 1998).

The main vehicles for teamwork skills training are lectures, demonstrations, practice (such as role-playing and simulations), and feedback. Each chapter of this book offers suggestions for improving group skills relevant to teamwork. For example, one study found that constructively confronting team members who violate group norms contributes to team performance (Druskat & Kayes, 2000). Chapter 5, Communication in Groups, gives guidelines on constructive confrontation. **Box 12-4** summarizes some of the most important team skill recommendations from earlier chapters. Information found in this book can be used to develop instructional materials for teamwork skills training.

Many organizations try to encourage the development of teamwork skills by paying for their employees to be led through a series of challenging games or outdoor activities. Sometimes this is called **challenge education.** For instance, corporations will sometimes pay for a group to go on a whitewater rafting trip or some other sort of wilderness exploration trip such as rock climbing. The expectation is that team members will learn teamwork skills as they must cooperate and coordinate as part of the activity. Ropes courses—a set of team-oriented games that require the team to solve a series of structured problems under time pressure—are also popular. For instance, group members are given a limited number of materials and told they must construct a bridge over a river (often a

Challenge education

Games or outdoor activities intended to develop teamwork skills.

stream or an imagined one), cross it, and bring the bridge over to the other side so that enemies cannot use it. Afterwards, a ropes facilitator leads the group in a discussion of how they dealt with team-related issues such as coordination, communication, and conflict resolution. Unfortunately, the little research that has been done on the effectiveness of such activities for team building has yielded mixed results, some reporting positive effects on self-insight and group cohesion, and others finding no positive effects (Kemp, 1998; Kugath, 1997; Leenders & Henderson, 1991; Thiagarajan, 1999).

Thompson (2000) suggests that there are good reasons to believe that challenge education and teamwork games should be effective in team building. For instance, such activities can provide group members with metaphorical experiences for problems that they face as a group in their typical setting. If they are well led, the activities can give the team an opportunity to identity communication and coordination problems that are typical of the group and talk about how to remedy them. In my experience, though, too often facilitators are not very skilled and this potential goes unrealized, or the activities do not translate well to the group's regular work together. The experience may be fun, perhaps resulting in some group cohesion gains, but for the most part, little team-relevant learning actually occurs. Participants may even be resentful that they have been taken away from their work or that the organization has given money to consultants instead of to them.

It is also important to understand that these activities cannot be expected to solve serious team problems, especially ones caused by poor leadership, faulty reward systems, poor training, difficult members, and inadequate resources. As Katzenbach and Smith (1993) note, when teams have problems, managers often go for a "quick fix" instead of thinking carefully about the specifics of the team's problems.

For example, I remember one organization that had significant problems with morale and conflict because of competition for resources, puny raises, and poor team-management relations. There was also so much bureaucracy that the team's work was constantly slowed up. Anything they wanted to do had to receive approval from higher-ups that could only be obtained by filling out lots of paperwork and waiting several months. The leadership seemed reluctant to look deep enough to identify the problems' causes. Instead, their solution was to require that teams attend a conflict workshop. At this workshop, a consultant (paid $10,000) held up a stick and announced that whoever held the "talking stick" could say whatever he or she wanted before passing the stick on to another team member, who was to do likewise. While some took the opportunity to vent, most thought the whole thing stupid and were reluctant to speak honestly. Many were angered that management was doing nothing about the real source of the team's problems.

Context-driven team training

Training that is tailor-made for a specific team based on the team's context and task.

Many experts on teams recommend **context-driven team training.** This is training that is tailor-made for the team based on the context, the task, and the team (Stout, Salas, & Fowlkes, 1997). The idea is that team training developed specifically for the team's task is more likely to be useful to the team. Remember the eight different dimensions of teamwork skills discussed earlier in the chapter (adaptability, shared situational awareness, performance monitoring, leadership, interpersonal relations, coordination, communication, and decision making)? According to Cannon-Bowers and her fellow researchers (1995), each of these may require a different type of training or instruction, and some of these may be more relevant to a given team context than others.

Context-specific teamwork skills programs start by identifying the mission requirements and procedures and assessing the specific tasks requiring teamwork and coordination (Salas et al., 1999). This information is then used to create specific training objectives. From these, training procedures (lectures, videos, role-plays, and the like) are developed to increase trainees' competencies in the identified areas. Post-training evaluations are then conducted in which individuals and the team are given feedback. Because this framework for developing teamwork skills is used most often with military crews, it is called **crew resource management (CRM).**

Crew resource management (CRM)
Context-driven training in which specific training objectives are identified before training materials are developed.

Stout and her colleagues (1997) provide a good example of context-driven team training (and CRM) in a program tailored for naval pilot teams. The training emphasized the skills of communication, assertiveness, and situational awareness because these were deemed most important to team effectiveness in this setting. Before designing their training, they interviewed people knowledgeable in the crew dynamics required to fly the particular aircraft. They then developed lectures, demonstrations, role-plays, and simulator scenarios specific to the context. For instance, in the simulator exercise, trainees had to deal with a navigational problem, an electrical malfunction, and constant interruptions from controlling agencies. Events were built into the scenario to serve as cues for coordination or assertiveness behaviors. If trainees did not exhibit the expected and desired behavior, they received feedback on this. An evaluation of the context-driven training in comparison to traditional pilot training showed that the program was effective in creating better teamwork skills.

Other research also supports the effectiveness of context-specific team training (see, for example, Smith-Jentsch, Salas, & Baker, 1996; Salas, Fowlkes, Stout, Milanovich, & Prince, 1999). In sum, research to date suggests that team training is most effective when it focuses on required competencies and gives team members the opportunity to practice and receive feedback on specific, task-related team skills (Salas & Cannon-Bowers, 2000). This ensures that what is learned is readily transferred and useful to the team's real work.

Group training is often not conducted in groups, or at least not in the groups people will ultimately be working in. The assumption is that team skills learned in these training groups will be carried into the actual teams. Moreland and colleagues (1998) strongly recommend a different approach to group training, with people trained in the groups with which they will actually be working. They base this recommendation on research suggesting its importance for the development of transactive memory systems or team mental models (TMMs). As you learned earlier in the chapter, groups that have a shared understanding of the task and what each member knows and can do are better able to plan and coordinate their work.

Although TMMs often develop over time as the group works together, a shared team understanding develops more quickly when team members are trained together, rather than individually (Thompson, 2000). For instance, in one study (Moreland et al., 1998), participants were trained to assemble radios. Some were randomly assigned to be trained in groups of three and others to be trained individually. Both groups received identical information in the training phase and got to practice assembling the radios. One week later, all participants were placed in teams of three to assemble radios, relying solely on memory. Those trained in groups were placed in the same group they had trained with, and they performed significantly better than the groups comprised of people who had trained individually. They were able to rely on the team mental model that had evolved during their group training.

Training explicitly designed to promote a TMM is even better. For example, **interpositional training** is training designed to give members a working knowledge of their teammates' duties and tasks and the interrelationships among them (Volpe, Cannon-Bowers, Salas, & Spector, 1996). Interpositional training is important because it promotes a team mental model. Interpositional training can take three different forms (Blickensderfer, Cannon-Bowers, & Salas, 1998; Goldstein & Ford, 2002). *Positional clarification* is simply the provision of information, verbal or written, to team members about one another's jobs. *Positional modeling* adds observation and discussion of teammates' jobs. *Positional rotation* requires that members actually perform one another's jobs to get direct experience with each role's tasks and responsibilities. The type of interpositional training used should be based on the level of interdependence of the team. Positional clarification is often sufficient for teams low in interdependence, but positional rotation is believed to be appropriate when team interdependence is high (Blickensderfer et al., 1998). Several research studies have found interpositional training to be positively related to team effectiveness (Cannon-Bowers, Salas, Blickensderfer, & Bowers, 1998; Volpe et al., 1996).

> **Interpositional training**
> Training designed to promote a team mental model by giving members a working knowledge of teammate duties and tasks, and how they are related.

Improving Team Effectiveness

When it comes to teams, it's important to remember that old saying, "An ounce of prevention is worth a pound of cure." Teams that start on a good track tend to perform even better as time goes on, but those that get off to a bad start find their problems getting worse over time (Hackman, 1990). Taking the time to design the team well and to properly "launch" the team makes a big difference. A proper team launch includes introducing members, creating common team goals, developing specific objectives, creating healthy team norms, clarifying the chain of command and how decisions will be made, and talking about member skills (Bens, 1999).

Hackman (1998, p. 261) says that the conditions that foster effective teamwork are simple and seemingly straightforward to put into place: "A real team with work that lends itself to teamwork. A clear and engaging direction. A group structure—task, composition, and norms—that promotes competent teamwork. Team-friendly reward, educational, and information systems. And some coaching to help team members take advantage of their favorable performance circumstances." Like many things in this book, all of this is easier said than done. This section focuses on how you can put into practice what you have learned about teams so far.

One of the most important factors in increasing team effectiveness is to make sure that the team has the organizational supports it needs.

1. Make sure that the team has the human, informational, and material resources it needs to accomplish its mission.
2. Provide training or education to members on an as-needed basis.
3. Make it possible for the team to monitor its productivity. Give the team access to information about progress toward its goals.
4. Use a two-pronged reward system. Reward the team's performance with team incentives and team recognition, *and* reward team members based on their individual performance, expertise, or seniority.

It is also important to consider member skills when composing the group.

1. Select team members who have complementary taskwork skills (unique skills and expertise relevant to the various tasks the group must perform).
2. Choose members who are skilled and experienced in interpersonal and group skills, or provide them with the necessary training in teamwork skills.
3. Choose a team leader with the ability to manage the team's resources and direct, coordinate, and motivate team members. The team leader should have a clear understanding of the group's mission, know when consultation with team members is appropriate, and be good at balancing directive (task) and supportive (socioemotional) leadership.

Another important team enhancer is to develop the team's process.

1. Before beginning the task, use discussion and training to create a shared situational awareness and team mental model so that team members have a common understanding of the group, its task, and the situation facing the group.
2. Encourage team members to get to know one another. Knowledge of teammate strengths, tendencies, and preferences enables effective communication and allows the team to take advantage of member strengths (Cannon-Bowers, Tannenbaum, Salas, & Volpe, 1995; Druskat & Kayes, 2000).
3. Encourage members to provide constructive feedback to one another to improve performance.
4. Build team cohesiveness by emphasizing shared goals and team successes along the way.

5. Transform general goals into specific and measurable performance goals that help the team track its progress and hold itself accountable.

6. Increase collective efficacy by providing adequate resources, appropriate training, assurances that other members are committed to the goal, examples of similar groups that have succeeded, and encouragement that they can perform complex tasks.

Last, consider taking the time to train the team.

1. Use context-driven team training in which the training bears a direct relationship to the team's real tasks.

2. Design a context-specific teamwork skills program by identifying mission requirements and procedures and the specific tasks requiring teamwork and coordination. Use this information to create specific training objectives, and tailor training materials accordingly. Provide verbal instruction and demonstration, and have trainees practice the skills and receive feedback.

3. Train teams in the groups that they will be working in to promote the development of a team mental model.

4. Provide interpositional training if team members are highly interdependent.

Difficult Team Members

Does one "bad team apple" spoil the whole team experience? Although most team researchers emphasize other reasons for team failure, such as poor organizational supports, fuzzy goals, and skills gaps, there are times when the reason is that one or more team members make teamwork difficult. Keyton (1999) points out that although many group members feel trapped in teams in which member relations become strained because of a difficult or confusing group member, there is little research on the influence of dysfunctional team members on team dynamics.

Types of Difficult Team Members

Dysfunctional team members are of several types. One is the dominating group member who insists on controlling the group process and getting his or her way. Another is the independent team member who does not know how to work interdependently and therefore doesn't communicate or coordinate adequately with other team members and also interferes with the team's work. Then there's the competitive group member who competes with other team members and makes cooperation difficult. And of course, there's the uninvolved team member who contributes little to task accomplishment, and the quiet member who denies the group the benefits of his or her knowledge and abilities. These types of team members create problems for the team because all act in ways contrary to teamwork.

They also create problems because other team members spend too much energy thinking about and talking about difficult members instead of focusing on the task.

Keyton (1999) describes a difficult or dysfunctional group member called the "primary provoker." This person's demands on the group distract the team from its tasks. Other group members become enmeshed with the primary provoker and act as "secondary provokers," either by giving the primary provoker lots of attention or by avoiding him or her altogether. Borrowing from Stohl and Schell (1991), Keyton identifies three related conditions that foster the behavior of the primary provoker. First is *interpretive omnipotence*, in which the primary provoker insists that his or her understanding of the situation is the correct one. Much tension ensues as the group tries to understand what the primary provoker's "issue" is (usually the other group members don't see what the problem is). Once they think they understand, they spend more time trying to compromise or persuade the inflexible primary provoker. Second, the primary provoker usually exhibits a *heroic stance*, claiming to know what is best for the group and staking out a position of moral superiority. This is one reason why primary provokers command so much attention; the group wants to do the right thing and is horrified at the thought that they might be behaving immorally. Third is *undifferentiated passion*, in which the primary provoker appears far more emotionally invested and devotes considerably more time to the issue than is "normal" given the issue and the individual's role in the group (for instance, it is the leader's responsibility to manage the problem at hand).

In general, the team's energies become focused on the primary provoker and his or her concerns instead of on task accomplishment (Keyton, 1999). The team is usually caught off guard by the primary provoker's passion and does not feel that it can be ignored. If team members pride themselves on being caring and responsive, they have an especially strong desire to soothe and appease the primary provoker. They work to prove that this is a team in which all members are heard and consensus is reached. Unfortunately, the primary provoker is not easily satisfied by the group's reassurances or offers of compromise. These make him or her feel unheard and more passionate. More attention from the group is demanded. At this point, negative emotion and energy threaten to pollute the group as team members become frustrated and angry. The more dominant team members openly engage in conflict with the primary provoker. Less dominant members distance themselves from the team and especially from the primary provoker. If possible, some members may choose to leave and join a different team, or are turned off from the team experience altogether.

Suggestions for Dealing With Difficult Team Members

There is little question that difficult team members can waylay a team and interfere with goal accomplishment. The group may still accomplish its task, but it will be less efficient in doing so, and members will be dissatisfied with the team experience (Keyton, 1999). As suggested earlier, many undesirable team member behaviors can be averted by if the group develops norms supportive of teamwork early in the life of the team. For instance, teams that take the time to identify mutual goals and objectives, and the importance of each member to achieving them, are going to have fewer problems with social loafers. In reality, though, many teams plunge into the task without doing this work. Also, even when the group does what it can to create a healthy team, a difficult group member can mess things up.

Sometimes the simplest solution is to relocate the difficult team member, but this is not always possible. Constructive confrontation (see Chapter 5, Communication in Groups) is often useful in dealing with difficult members. In the case of primary provokers, after the group has made an honest attempt to deal with the provoker's concerns, a leader or senior group member may have to privately inform the provoker that it's time for the team to move on.

You can ignore or tolerate the difficult group member. Especially for temporary team assignments, the benefits of working through the problem may not outweigh the costs of lost time (Druskat & Kayes, 2000). In the long-term team, however, it is usually worth the effort to come up with a better solution than just ignoring and tolerating. If difficult members continue in their disruptive behavior, team member commitment may be harmed to the point that important members leave and coordination and communication become strained as members avoid the difficult member and distance from the group because of its unpleasantness.

There is a particular risk in ignoring primary provokers. Because they are convinced of their moral superiority and have a very strong need to be heard, ignoring them usually causes them to become even more passionate. They may threaten to "blow the whistle" by going to the top leadership with their concerns (which of course only makes the secondary provokers angry because they have tried to be sensitive to the primary provoker's concerns). If that threat doesn't work, the primary provoker may very well take his or concerns to leadership outside of the team. Even if the team is ultimately vindicated, defending against charges of incompetence, poor leadership, and unethical behavior will consume even more of the team's energy and time.

Keyton (1999) recommends outside intervention to help the group discuss the tension and become "unstuck." Katzenbach and Smith (1993) agree that outside help may be useful for dealing with problems created by difficult group members, but they caution against focusing too much on the conflict itself. Instead, they say that reemphasizing "team basics" is more likely to get the team back on task. What is the team's mission, what are the deadlines for its accomplishment, and how is the team going to get done what it needs to get done? Even when interpersonal difficulties linger as a result of conflict or drama, they suggest the best thing is for the involved parties is to identify specific actions that each will take so that they can move on and cooperate enough that tasks can be accomplished efficiently and effectively.

Concept Review

Teams vs. Groups

- Not all groups are teams. **Teams** are composed of people with the right balance of skills who cooperate to do a job within a larger organization. Teams range in size from two to twenty-five members, and team members' tasks are highly interdependent.

Ways to Classify Teams

- Some classifications categorize teams on the basis of the type of task they perform. Temporal duration (whether the team is short term or long term) is also used to classify teams. Other systems categorize a team according to who determines the team's objectives and how these are to be accomplished.

Teams and the Organizational Context

- The organizational context determines the team's resources, how much freedom the team is given, how the team will be rewarded, how it obtains information, and how it monitors its work. Teams need a supportive organizational context if they are to be successful.
- Four main **organizational team supports** are: (1) a reward system that recognizes and reinforces excellent team performance; (2) an educational system that provides any training or technical consultations that are needed; (3) an information system that helps the team manage its work; and (4) a resource system that supplies the material resources that the work requires.
- The two most common practices for rewarding and motivating team performance are **team incentives** and **team recognition.** Because rewarding only team success can create social loafing and free rider effects, it is best to reward both the team's performance and individual performance.

Group Composition

- **Group composition** refers to the types of individuals that comprise the team.
- The transformation of a group of individuals into an effective team requires **team competencies**—the knowledge, skills, and attitudes (KSAs) necessary for the performance of the group's tasks.
- Members should have complementary **taskwork skills.** Each should bring to the team unique skills and expertise relevant to the various tasks the group must perform.
- **Teamwork skills**—the ability to work together as a team—are as important as technical skills and task-specific knowledge. In addition to group and interpersonal skills, teamwork skills include a shared understanding, or **team mental model,** of the team, its work, and abilities of other team members.

- Eight teamwork skills dimensions are adaptability, shared situational awareness, performance monitoring and feedback, leadership/team management, interpersonal relations, coordination, communication, and decision making.

Cohesion and Teamwork

- Meta-analyses find that group cohesiveness is positively related to group performance.
- Cohesive work groups are more directed toward group tasks and more committed to achieving group goals. Members of cohesive groups interact and communicate more, and this increases performance. In cohesive groups, members know one another well enough that they can predict their behavior and match member interests and strengths to tasks. Cohesiveness is also associated with "extra-role performance behavior."
- Although cohesiveness influences performance, performance also increases cohesiveness.
- Cohesiveness does not always increase performance; it depends on whether the group has norms consistent with high performance.

Team Effectiveness

- Team-related attitudes are related to team effectiveness. A **collective orientation, shared vision,** and **collective efficacy** are positively related to team performance.
- Good team leaders secure team resources, run interference with the organization, make sure that members have the appropriate training, and foster a positive team climate.
- Ongoing training in is often needed in both taskwork and teamwork skills. The main vehicles for teamwork skills training are lectures, demonstrations, practice (such as role-playing and simulations), and feedback.
- Team-oriented games and **challenge education** are sometimes used to encourage the development of teamwork skills. Research on the effectiveness of such activities has yielded mixed results.
- Research supports the effectiveness of **context-driven team training**— training that is tailor-made for the team based on the context, the task, and the team.
- A shared team mental model develops more quickly when team members are trained together. **Interpositional training** is designed to give members a working knowledge of their teammates' duties and tasks and the interrelationships among them.

Difficult Team Members

- Difficult team members can waylay a team and interfere with goal accomplishment. The group may still accomplish its task, but it will be less efficient in doing so, and members will be dissatisfied with the team experience.
- Dysfunctional team members are of several types. These include dominating group members, overly independent or competitive members, and uninvolved team members. The "primary provoker" is a difficult group member who makes many demands on the team and distracts the team from its tasks.

Skill Review

Create a Supportive Organizational Context

- Give the team the human, informational, and material resources it needs to accomplish its mission.
- Provide training or education to members on an as-needed basis.
- Give the team feedback about progress toward its goals.
- Reward the team's performance with team incentives and team recognition, *and* reward team members based on their individual performance, expertise, or seniority.

Consider Member Skills When Composing the Group

- Select team members who have complementary taskwork skills.
- Choose members who are skilled and experienced in interpersonal and group skills, or provide them with the necessary training in teamwork skills.
- Choose a team leader with the ability to manage the team's resources and direct, coordinate, and motivate team members.

Enhance Team Process

- Before beginning the task, create a shared situational awareness and team mental model.
- Encourage team members to get to know one another.
- Encourage members to provide constructive feedback to one another to improve performance.
- Build team cohesiveness by emphasizing shared goals and team successes along the way.
- Transform general goals into specific and measurable performance goals.

- Increase collective efficacy by providing adequate resources, appropriate training, assurances that other members are committed to the goal, examples of similar groups that have succeeded, and encouragement that they can perform complex tasks.

Implement Context-Specific Team Training

- Design a context-specific teamwork skills program by identifying mission requirements and procedures and the specific tasks requiring teamwork and coordination. Use this information to create specific training objectives and tailor training materials. Provide verbal instruction and demonstration, and have trainees practice the skills and receive feedback.
- Train teams in the groups that they will be working in.
- Provide interpositional training to give members a working knowledge of their teammates' duties and tasks and the interrelationships among them.

Deal With Difficult Team Members

- To avert some negative behaviors, develop norms supportive of teamwork early in the life of the team.
- Consider relocating a difficult group member.
- Use constructive confrontation to deal with difficult members.
- For temporary team assignments, ignore or tolerate difficult team members. However, in the long-term team, ignoring primary provokers can be risky.
- Obtain help from outside the group to help the group discuss the tension and become "unstuck."

Study Questions

1. What distinguishes a "team" from a "group"?
2. What size should a team be?
3. What are the different ways in which teams can be classified?
4. How does the organizational context affect team success? What are the four key supports an organization can offer? What are the two most common practices for rewarding and motivating team performance?
5. When composing a team, what team competencies should be taken into consideration?
6. What different types of teamwork skills are described in the chapter?
7. Why is a "team mental model" important to team success?
8. How does cohesion relate to team performance?

9. What "team-related attitudes" were discussed in the chapter, and how do they affect teamwork?
10. What do we mean when we say that "team leadership is leading enough but not too much" and that "team leadership is about balance"?
11. What recommendations are given in the chapter to increase team effectiveness?
12. Why is context-driven team training recommended over challenge education and team-oriented games? What are the different types? Why should team members be trained together?
13. How do difficult team members affect the group? What is a "primary provoker"? What recommendations are given for dealing with difficult group members?

Group Activities

Activity 1: Do a Proper Team Launch

Pretend that your six-person group has one month to raise funds for the local women's shelter, an organization that provides assistance to battered women. Before jumping into the task, take the time to do a proper "team launch." Begin with member introductions (think of good questions ahead of time). Talk about members' knowledge, skills, and abilities relevant to the project. Create common team goals, and develop specific objectives (what needs to be done, who will do it, by what date). Create a team policy on lateness, missed meetings, and social loafing. Your instructor may or may not want you to actually complete the fundraising project.

Activity 2: Experience Challenge Education

Most communities offer some challenge education-like experiences. For instance, many universities have ropes courses or offer instruction in kayaking, and some cities have climbing gyms. With your small group (five to ten members), have a challenge education experience. Afterwards, evaluate the experience. Was it helpful in team building?

Activity 3: Design a Team Support System

Activity 1 describes a group project in which students are expected to work as a team. Review the chapter section on organizational context. With your five-person group, create a written set of specific recommendations for your teacher that would help him/her create an organizational context supportive of teamwork for students undertaking the project described in Activity 1.

InfoTrac College Edition Search Terms

To do research for your papers and assignments, use InfoTrac that's provided free with new copies of this book. Go to http://infotrac.thomsonlearning.com and enter the following search terms:

- Team Effectiveness
- Leadership of Teams
- Collective Efficacy

- Crew Resource Management
- 360-degree Feedback

References

Abramis, D. J. (1994). Work role ambiguity, job satisfaction, and job performance: Meta-analyses and review. *Psychological Reports, 75,* 1411–1433.

Abrams, D., Wetherell, M., Cochrane, S., Hogg, M. A., & Turner, J. C. (1990). Knowing what to think by knowing who you are: Self-categorization and the nature of norm formation, conformity, and group polarization. *British Journal of Social Psychology, 29,* 97–119.

Adams, J. S. (1965). Inequity in social exchange. In L. Berkowitz (Ed.), *Advances in experimental social psychology* (Vol. 2, pp. 267–299). New York: Academic Press.

Adams, R. A., Piercy, F. P., Jurdich, J. A., & Lewis, R. A. (2001). Components of a model adolescent AIDS/drug abuse prevention program: A Delphi study. *Family Relations, 41,* 312–317.

Adler, P. A., & Adler, P. (1995). Dynamics of inclusion and exclusion in preadolescent cliques. *Social Psychology Quarterly, 58,* 145–162.

Albert, A. A., & Porter, J. R. (1988). *Women in management worldwide.* Armonk, NY: M. E. Sharpe.

Albert, R. D. (1996). A framework and model for understanding Latin American and Latino/Hispanic cultural patterns. In D. Landis & R. S. Bhagat (Eds.), *Handbook of intercultural training* (pp. 327–348). Thousand Oaks, CA: Sage.

Alberti, R., & Emmons, M. (1995). *Your perfect right: A guide to assertive living* (7th ed.). San Luis Obispo, CA: Impact Press.

Aldag, R. J., & Fuller, S. R. (1993). Beyond fiasco: A reappraisal of the groupthink phenomenon and a new model of group decision processes. *Psychological Bulletin, 113,* 533–552.

Allen, R. W., Madison, D. L., Porter, L. W., Renwick, P. A., & Mayes, B. T. (1979). Organizational politics: Tactics and characteristics of its actors. *California Management Review, 22,* 77–83.

Allen, V. L., & Levine, J. M. (1969). Consensus and conformity. *Journal of Experimental Social Psychology, 5,* 389–399.

Allen, V. L., & Levine, J. M. (1971). Social support and conformity: The role of independent assessment of reality. *Journal of Experimental Social Psychology, 7,* 4–58.

Allison, S. (2002). Videos are weapons in surf city feud. *Los Angeles Times,* Sept. 1, B1.

Allport, F. H. (1924). The group fallacy in relation to social science. *Journal of Abnormal and Social Psychology, 19,* 60–73.

Allport, G. W. (1954). *The nature of prejudice.* Cambridge, MA: Addison-Wesley.

Allport, G. W. (1997). Foreword to the 1948 edition. In K. Lewin (Ed.), *Resolving social conflicts: Selected papers on group dynamics* (pp. 5–9). Washington, DC: American Psychological Association. (Original work published 1948)

Altman, I. & Taylor, D. A. (1973). *Social penetration: The development of interpersonal relationships.* New York: Holt, Rinehart, & Winston.

Altman, I., Vinsel, A., & Brown, B. A. (1981). Dialectic conceptions in social psychology: An appreciation to social penetration and privacy regulation. In L. Berkowitz (Ed.), *Advances in Experimental Social Psychology* (Vol. 14, pp. 107–160). New York: Academic Press.

Anderson, C., John, O. P., Keltner, D., & Kring, A. M. (2001). Who attains social status? Effects of personality and physical attractiveness in social groups. *Journal of Personality and Social Psychology, 81,* 116–132.

Anderson, C. M., & Martin, M. M. (1999). The relationship of argumentativeness and verbal aggressiveness to cohesion, consensus, and satisfaction in small groups. *Communication Reports, 12,* 21–32.

Ansari, M. A., & Kapoor, A. (1987). Organizational context and upward influence tactics. *Organizational Behavior and Human Decision Processes, 40,* 39–49.

Antonioni, D. (1996). Two strategies for responding to stressors: Managing conflict and clarifying work expectations. *Journal of Business and Psychology, 11,* 287–295.

Aron, A., Dutton, D. G., Aron, E. N., & Iverson, A. (1989). Experiences of falling in love. *Journal of Social and Personal Relationships, 6,* 243–257.

Aronson, E., & Bridgeman, D. (1979). Jigsaw groups and the desegregated classroom: In pursuit of common goals. *Personality and Social Psychology Bulletin, 5,* 438–446.

Aronson, E., & Gonzalez, A. (1988). Desegregation, jigsaw, and the Mexican-American experience. In P. A. Katz & D. Taylor (Eds.), *Eliminating racism: Profiles in controversy* (pp. 301–314). New York: Plenum.

Aronson, E., & Patnoe, S. (1997). *Cooperation in the classroom: The jigsaw method.* New York: Longman.

Aronson, E., Wilson, T. D., & Akert, R. M. (1999). *Social psychology* (3rd ed.). New York: Longman.

Arrow, H., & McGrath, J. E. (1993). Membership matters: How member change and continuity affect small group structure, process, and performance. *Small Group Research, 24,* 334–361.

Arrow, H., & McGrath, J. E. (1995). Membership dynamics in groups at work: A theoretical framework. In L. L. Cummings & B. M. Staw (Eds.), *Research in Organizational Behavior,* (Vol.17, pp. 373–412). Middlesex, England: JAI Press.

Asch, S. E. (1951). Effects of group pressure upon the modification and distortion of judgement. In H.

Guetzkow (Ed.), *Groups, leadership, and men* (pp. 177–190). Pittsburgh: Carnegie Press.

Asch, S. E. (1955). Opinions and social pressure. *Scientific American, 193,* 31–35.

Asch, S. E. (1956). Studies of independence and conformity: A minority of one against a unanimous majority. *Psychological Monographs, 70* (9, whole no. 416).

Asch, S. E. (1957). An experimental investigation of group influence. In Walter Reed Army Institute of Research, *Symposium on preventive and social psychiatry* (pp. 15–17). Washington, DC: U.S. Government Printing Office.

Aspinwall, L. G. & Taylor, S. E. (1993). Effects of social comparison direction, threat, and self-esteem on affect, evaluation, and expected success. *Journal of Personality and Social Psychology, 64,* 708–722.

Atwater, L. E., Carey, J. A., & Waldman, D. A. (2001). Gender and discipline in the workplace: Wait until your father gets home. *Journal of Management, 27,* 537–566.

Ayman, R., & Chemers, M. M. (1983). Relationship of supervisory behavior ratings to work group effectiveness and subordinate satisfaction among Iranian managers. *Journal of Applied Psychology, 68,* 338–341.

Babad, E. Y., & Amir, L. (1978). Bennis and Shepard's theory of group development: An empirical examination. *Small Group Behavior, 9,* 47–49.

Bakeman, R. (2000). Behavioral observation and coding. In H. T. Reis & C. M. Judd (Ed.), *Handbook of research methods in social and personality psychology* (pp. 138–159). Cambridge: Cambridge University Press.

Bales, R. F. (1950). *Interaction Process Analysis: A method for the study of small groups.* Chicago: University of Chicago Press.

Bales, R. F. (1953). The equilibrium problem in small groups. In T. Parsons, R. F. Bales, & E. A. Shils (Eds.), *Working papers in the theory of action* (pp. 111–162). New York: Free Press.

Bales, R. F. (1955). How people interact in conferences. *Scientific American, 192,* 31–35.

Bales, R. F. (1970). *Personality and interpersonal behavior.* New York: Holt, Rinehart, & Winston.

Bales, R. F. (1980). *SYMLOG case study kit.* New York: Free Press.

Bales, R. F. (1988). A new overview of the SYMLOG system: Measuring and changing behavior in groups. In R. B. Polley, A. P. Hare, & P. J. Stone (Eds.), *The SYMLOG practitioner: Applications of small group research* (pp. 319–344). New York: Praeger.

Bales, R. F., & Slater, P. E. (1955). Role differentiation in small decision making groups. In T. Parsons & R. F. Bales (Eds.), *Family, socialization, and interaction processes* (pp. 259–306). New York: Free Press.

Bales, R. F., Strodtbeck, F. L., Mills, T. M., & Roseborough, M. E. (1951). Channels of communication in small groups. *American Sociological Review, 16,* 461–468.

Banaji, M. R., Hardin, C., & Rothman, A. J. (1993). Implicit stereotyping in person judgment. *Journal of Personality and Social Psychology, 65,* 272–281.

Bandura, A. (2000). Exercise of human agency through collective efficacy. *Current Directions in Psychological Science, 9,* 17–20.

Banker, R. D., Field, J. M., Schroeder, R. G., & Sinha, K. K. (1996). Impact of work teams on manufacturing performance: A longitudinal field study. *Academy of Management Journal, 39,* 867–890.

Barchas, P. (1986). A sociophysiological orientation to small groups. In E. Lawler (Ed.), *Advances in group processes* (Vol. 3, pp. 209–246). Greenwich, CT: JAI Press.

Barchas, P. R., & Fisek, M. H. (1984). Hierarchical differentiation in newly formed groups of rhesus and humans. In P. R. Barchas (Ed.), *Essays toward a sociophysiological perspective* (pp. 23–33). Westport, CT: Greenwood Press.

Bargal, D., Gold, M., & Lewin, M. (1992). Introduction: The heritage of Kurt Lewin. *Journal of Social Issues, 48,* 3–14.

Barley, S. R., & Bechky, B. A. (1994). In the backrooms of science: The work of technicians in science labs. *Work and Occupations, 21,* 85–126.

Barnlund, D., & Harland, C. (1963). Propinquity and prestige as deterimants of communication networks. *Sociometry, 26,* 464–479.

Baron, J. N., Davis-Blake, A., & Bielby, W. T. (1986). The structure of opportunity: How promotion ladders vary within and among organizations. *Administrative Science Quarterly, 31,* 248–273.

Baron, R. S., Vandello, J. A., & Brunsman, B. (1996). The forgotten variable in conformity research: Impact of task importance on social influence. *Journal of Personality and Social Psychology, 71,* 915–927.

Barrick, M. R., & Mount, M. K. (1991). The Big Five personality dimensions and job performance: A meta-analysis. *Personnel Psychology, 44,* 1–26.

Bass, B. M. (1990). *Bass and Stogdill's handbook of leadership: A survey of theory and research.* New York: Free Press.

Bass, B. M. (1997). Does the transactional-transformational paradigm transcend organizational and national boundaries? *American Psychologist, 52,* 130–139.

Bass, B. M., & Avolio, B. J. (1990). *The Multifactor Leadership Questionnaire.* Palo Alto, CA: Consulting Psychologists Press.

Bass, B. M. & Avolio, B. J. (1993). Transformational leadership: A response to critiques. In M. M. Chemers & R. Ayman (Eds.), *Leadership Theory & Research: Perspectives and Directions.* San Diego, CA: Academic Press.

Bass, B. M., & Avolio, B. J. (1994). Transformational leadership and organizational culture. *International Journal of Public Administration, 17,* 541–554.

Bastien, D., & Hostiger, T. (1988). Jazz as a process of organizational innovation. *Communication Research, 15,* 582–602.

Baumeister, R. F., & Leary, M. R. (1995). The need to belong: Desire for interpersonal attachments as a fundamental human motivation. *Psychological Bulletin, 117,* 497–529.

Bavelas, A. (1950). Communication patterns in task-oriented groups. *Journal of the Acoustical Society of America, 22,* 725–730.

Baxter, L. (1986). Gender differences in the heterosexual relationship rules embedded in break-up accounts. *Journal of Social and Personal Relationships, 3,* 289–306.

Baxter, L. (1988). A dialectical perspective in communication strategies in relationship development. In S. W. Duck, D. F. Hayt, S. E. Hobfoll, W. Ickes, & B. M. Montgomery (Eds.), *Handbook of personal relationships: Theory, research, and interventions* (pp. 257–273). New York: Wiley.

Baxter, L. (1990). Dialectical contradictions in relationship development. *Journal of Social and Personal Relationships, 7,* 69–88.

Baxter, L. (1993). The social side of personal relationships: A dialectical perspective. In S. W. Duck (Ed.), *Social contexts of relationships* (Vol. 3, pp. 139–165). Newbury Park, CA: Sage.

Baxter, L. (1994). A dialogic approach to relationship maintenance. In D. J. Canary & L. Stafford (Eds.), *Communication and relational maintenance* (pp. 233–254). New York: Academic Press.

Beebe, S. A., & Masterson, J. T. (1994). *Communication in small groups: Principles and practices* (4th ed.). New York: Harper Collins.

Beemon, D. R., & Sharkey, T. W. (1987). The use and abuse of corporate politics. *Business Horizons,* March–April, 26–30.

Benne, K. D., & Sheats, P. (1949). Functional roles of group members. *Journal of Social Issues, 4,* 41–49.

Bennis, W., & Nanus, B. (1985). *Leaders: The strategies for taking charge.* New York: Harper & Row.

Bennis, W., & Shepard, H. (1956). A theory of group development. *Human Relations, 9,* 415–437.

Bens, I. (1999). Keeping your team out of trouble. *Journal for Quality and Participation, 22,* 45–47.

Berg, B. L. (1998). *Qualitative research methods for the social sciences* (3rd ed.). Boston: Allyn & Bacon.

Berger, J., & Conner, T. L. (1974). Performance expectations and behavior in small groups: A revised formulation. In J. Berger, T. L. Conner, & M. H. Fisek (Eds.), *Expectation states theory: A theoretical research program* (pp. 85–110). Cambridge, MA: Winthrop.

Berger, J., Rosenholtz, S. J., & Zelditch, M. (1980). Status organizing processes. *Annual Review of Sociology, 6,* 479–508.

Berger, J., Webster, M. Jr., Ridgeway, C. L., & Rosenholtz, S. J. (1986). Status cues, expectations, and behavior. In E. J. Lawler (Ed.), *Advances in group processes* (pp. 1–22). Greenwich, CT: JAI Press.

Bergmann, B. (1986). *The economic emergence of women.* New York: Basic Books.

Berman-Rossi, T. (1997). Empowering groups through understanding stages of group development. *Social Work with Groups, 15,* 239–255.

Berry, J. W. (1997). Individual and group relations in plural societies. In C. S. Granrose & S. Oskamp (Eds.), *Cross-cultural work groups* (pp. 17–35). Thousand Oaks, CA: Sage.

Bersheid, E., & Reis, H. T. (1998). Attraction and close relationships. In D. Gilbert, S. Fiske, & G. Lindzey (Eds.), *Handbook of social psychology* (4th ed.). New York: McGraw-Hill.

Bersheid, E., & Walster, E. (1978). *Interpersonal attraction.* Reading, MA: Addison-Wesley.

Bettencourt, H. (1990). Attribution in intergroup and international conflict. In S. Graham & V. S. Folkes (Eds.), *Attribution theory: Applications to achievement, mental and interpersonal conflict* (pp. 208–216). Hillsdale, NJ: Erlbaum.

Bettenhausen, K., & Murnighan, J. K. (1985). The emergence of norms in competitive decision-making groups. *Administrative Science Quarterly, 30,* 350–372.

Bhagat, R. S., & Prien, K. O. (1996). Cross-cultural training in organizational contexts. In D. Landis & R. S. Bhagat (Eds.), *Handbook of intercultural Training* (2nd ed.), pp. 216–230.

Biernat, M., & Kobrynowicz, D. (1997). Gender- and-race based standards of competence: Lower minimum standards but higher ability standards for devalued groups. *Journal of Personality and Social Psychology, 72,* 544–557.

Bion, W. (1961). *Experiences in groups.* New York: Basic Books.

Blake, R. R., & McCanse, A. A. (1991). *Leadership dilemmas: Grid solutions.* Houston: Gulf Publishing.

Blake, R. R., & Mouton, J. S. (1964). *The managerial grid.* Houston: Gulf Publishing.

Blake, R. R., & Mouton, J. S. (1985). *The managerial grid III.* Houston: Gulf Publishing.

Blanchard, K., Zigarmi, P., & Nelson, R. (1993). Situational leadership after 25 years: A retrospective. *Journal of Leadership Studies, 1,* 22–36.

Blanchard, K., Zigarmi, P., & Zigarmi, D. (1985). *Leadership and the one-minute manager: Increasing effectiveness through situational leadership.* New York: William Morrow.

Blascovich, J., Wyer, N. A., Swart, L. A., & Kibler, J. L. (1997). Racism and racial categorization. *Journal of Personality and Social Psychology, 72,* 1364–1372.

Blau, P. (1977). *Inequality and heterogeneity.* New York: Free Press.

Blickensderfer, E., Cannon-Bowers, J. A., & Salas, E. (1998). Cross-training and team performance. In J. A. Cannon-Bowers & E. Salas (Eds.), *Making decisions under stress: Implications for individual and team training* (pp. 299–311). Washington, DC: American Psychological Association.

Bock, J. D. (2000). Doing the right thing: Single mothers by choice and the struggle for legitimacy. *Gender and Society, 14,* 62–86.

Bodine, R. J., & Crawford, D. K. (1998). *The handbook of conflict resolution education: A guide to building quality programs in schools.* San Francisco: Jossey-Bass.

Bollen, K. A., & Hoyle, R. H. (1990). Perceived cohesion: A conceptual and empirical examination. *Social Forces, 69,* 479–504.

Bond, M. H., & Hwang, K. K. (1986). The social psychology of the Chinese people. In M. H. Bond (Ed.), *The psychology of the Chinese people.* Hong Kong: Oxford University Press.

Bond, M. H., & Smith, P. B. (1996). Culture and conformity: A meta-analysis of studies using Asch's

(1952, 1956) line judgement task. *Psychological Bulletin, 119,* 111–137.

Bons, P. M., & Fiedler, F. E. (1976). Changes in organizational leadership and the behavior of relationship-and-task-motivated leaders. *Administrative Science Quarterly, 21,* 433–472.

Bormann, E. G. (1990). *Small group communication: Theory and practice* (3rd ed.). New York: Harper & Row.

Bornstein, R. F. (1989). Exposure and affect: Overview and meta-analysis of resarch, 1968–1987. *Psychological Bulletin, 106,* 265–289.

Bornstein, R. F., & D'Agostino, P. R. (1992). Stimulus recognition and the mere exposure effect. *Journal of Personality and Social Psychology, 63,* 545–552.

Bottger, P. C., & Yetton, P. W. (1987). Improving group performance by training in individual problem solving. *Journal of Applied Psychology, 72,* 651–657.

Bottorff, J. L. (1994). Using videotape recordings in qualitative research. In J. M. Morse (Ed.), *Critical thinking in qualitative research methods* (pp. 149–162). Thousand Oaks, CA: Sage.

Bowers, C. A., Pharmer, J. A., & Salas, E. (2000). When member homogeneity is needed in work teams: A meta-analysis. *Small Group Research, 31,* 305–327.

Braaten, L. J. (1974–1975). Developmental phases of encounter groups and related intensive groups: A critical review of models and a new proposal. *Interpersonal Development, 5,* 112–129.

Braithewaite, D. O., & Baxter, L. A. (1995). "I do" again: The relational dialectics of renewing marriage vows. *Journal of Social and Personal Relationships, 12,* 177–198.

Brauer, M., Judd, C. M., & Gliner, M. D. (1995). The effects of repeated expressions on attitude polarization during group discussions. *Journal of Personality and Social Psychology, 68,* 1014–1029.

Brawley, L. R., Carron, A. V., & Widmeyer, W. N. (1988). Exploring the relationship between cohesion and group resistance to disruption. *Journal of Sport and Exercise Psychology, 10,* 199–213.

Bray, R. M., Johnson, D., & Chilstrom, J. T., Jr. (1982). Social influence by group members with minority opinions: A comparison of Hollander and Moscovici. *Journal of Personality and Social Psychology, 43,* 78–88.

Brehm, S. S. (1992). *Intimate relationships.* New York: McGraw-Hill.

Brehm, S. S., Kassin, S. M., & Fein, S. (1999). *Social psychology.* (4th ed.). Boston: Houghton Mifflin.

Brewer, M. B. (1979). In-group bias in the minimal intergroup situation: A cognitive-motivational analysis. *Psychological Bulletin, 86,* 307–324.

Brewer, M. B. (1991). The social self: On being the same and different at the same time. *Personality and Social Psychology Bulletin, 17,* 475–482.

Brewer, M. B., & Miller, N. (1996). *Intergroup relations.* Pacific Grove, CA: Brooks/Cole.

Bronfenbrenner, U. (1961). The mirror image in Soviet-American relations: A social psychologist's report. *Journal of Social Issues, 17,* 45–56.

Brown, B. B., Clasen, D. R., & Eicher, S. A. (1986). Perceptions of peer pressure, peer conformity, dispositions, and self-reported behavior among adolescents. *Developmental Psychology, 22,* 521–530.

Brown, R. (1988). *Group processes: Dynamics within and between groups.* Oxford: Basil Blackwell.

Brown, T. M., & Miller, C. E. (2000). Communication networks in task performance groups. *Small Group Research, 31,* 131–158.

Brown, V., Tumeo, M., Larey, T. S., & Paulus, P. B. (1998). Modeling cognitive interactions during group brainstorming. *Small Group Research, 29,* 495–527.

Bruins, J. (1999). Social power and influence tactics: A theoretical introduction. *Journal of Social Issues, 55,* 7–14.

Bugental, D. B., & Lewis, J. C. (1999). The paradoxical misuse of power by those who see themselves as powerless: How does it happen? *Journal of Social Issues, 55,* 51–64.

Bui, K. T., Raven, B. H., & Schwarzwald, J. (1994). Influence strategies in dating relationships: The effects of relationship satisfaction, gender, and perspective. *Journal of Social Behavior and Personality, 9,* 429–442.

Buller, P. F., & Bell, C. H. (1986). Effects of team building and goal setting on productivity: A field experiment. *Academy of Management Journal, 29,* 305–328.

Burke, R. J., & McKeen, C. A. (1996). Do women at the top make a difference? Gender proportions and the experiences of managerial and professional women. *Human Relations, 49,* 1093–1104.

Burn, S. M. (1991). Social psychology and the stimulation of recycling behaviors: The block leader approach. *Journal of Applied Social Psychology, 21,* 629–661.

Burn, S. M. (1996). *The Social Psychology of Gender.* New York: McGraw-Hill.

Burn, S. M. (2000). *Women across cultures: A global perspective.* New York: McGraw-Hill.

Burn, S. M., Aboud, R., & Moyles, C. (2000). The relationship between gender social identity and support for feminism. *Sex Roles, 42,* 1081–1089.

Burn, S. M., & Oskamp, S. (1989). Ingroup biases and the U.S.-Soviet conflict. *Journal of Social Issues, 45,* 73–89.

Burns, J. M. (1978). *Leadership.* New York: Harper & Row.

Burrow, T. L. (1924). The group method of analysis. *Psychoanalytic Review, 16,* 268–280.

Buss, D. M. (1990). The evolution of anxiety and social exclusion. *Journal of Social and Clinical Psychology, 9,* 196–210.

Buss, D. M. (1991). Evolutionary personality psychology. *Annual Review of Psychology, 42,* 459–491.

Butler, D., & Geis, F. L. (1990). Nonverbal affect responses to male and female leaders: Implications for leadership evaluations. *Journal of Personality and Social Psychology, 58,* 48–59.

Buttner, E. H., & McEnally, M. (1996). The interactive effect of influence tactic, applicant gender, and type of job on hiring recommendations. *Sex Roles, 34,* 581–591.

Byrne, D., Clore, G. L., & Smeaton, G. (1986). The attraction hypothesis: Do similar attitudes affect anything? *Journal of Personality and Social Psychology, 51,* 1167–1170.

Cady, S. H., & Valentine, J. (1999). Team innovation and perceptions of consideration: What difference does diversity make? *Small Group Research, 30,* 730–750.

Canary, D. J., & Stafford, L. (1994). Maintaining relationships through strategic and routine interaction. In D. J. Canary & L. Stafford (Eds.), *Communication and relational maintenance* (pp. 3–22). New York: Academic Press.

Cann, A., & Siegfried, W. D. (1990). Gender stereotypes and dimensions of effective leader behavior. *Sex Roles, 23,* 413–419.

Cannon-Bowers, J. A., Salas, E., Blickensderfer, E., & Bowers, C. A. (1998). The impact of cross-training and workload on team functioning: A replication and extension of initial findings. *Human Factors, 40,* 92–101.

Cannon-Bowers, J. A., Tannenbaum, S. I., Salas, E., & Volpe, C. E. (1995). Defining competencies and establishing team training requirements. In R. A. Guzzo & E. Salas (Eds.), *Team effectiveness and decision making in organizations* (pp. 333–380). San Francisco: Jossey-Bass.

Cantor, N., & Mischel, W. (1977). Traits as prototypes: Effects on recognition memory. *Journal of Personality and Social Psychology, 35,* 38–48.

Caple, R. (1978). The sequential stages of group development. *Small Group Behavior, 9,* 470–476.

Carli, L. L. (1991). Gender, status, and influence. In E. J. Lawler, B. Markovsky, C. Ridgeway, & H. A. Walker (Eds.), *Advances in group processes* (Vol. 8, pp. 89–113). Greenwich, CT: JAI Press.

Carli, L. L. (1999). Gender, interpersonal power, and social influence. *Journal of Social Issues, 55,* 81–99.

Carli, L. L. (2001). Gender and social influence. *Journal of Social Issues, 57,* 725–742.

Carli, L. L., & Eagly, A. H. (1999). Gender effects on social influence and emergent leadership. In G. N. Powell (Ed.), *Handbook of gender and work* (pp. 203–222). Thousand Oaks, CA: Sage.

Carnevale, P. J., Conlon, D. E., Hanisch, K. A., & Harris, K. L. (1989). Experimental research on the strategic-choice model of mediation. In K. Kressel, D. G. Pruitt, & Associates (Eds.), *Mediation research* (pp. 344–367). San Francisco: Jossey-Bass.

Carnevale, P. J., & Leung, K. (2001). Cultural dimensions of negotiation. In M. A. Hogg & S. Tindale (Eds.), *Blackwell Handbook of Social Psychology: group processes* (pp. 482–496). Oxford UK: Blackwell.

Carron, A. V. (1988). *Group Dynamics in Sport: Theoretical and Practical Issues.* London, ONT: Spodym Publishers.

Carr-Ruffino, N. (1996). *Managing diversity: People skills for a multicultural workplace.* Cincinnati: Southwestern.

Carron, A. V. (1982). Cohesiveness in sports groups: Interpretations and considerations. *Journal of Sport Psychology, 4,* 123–128.

Carron, A. V., Widmeyer, W. N., & Brawley, L. R. (1985). The development of an instrument to assess cohesion in sport teams: The Group Environment Questionnaire. *Journal of Sports Psychology, 7,* 244–266.

Cartwright, D., & Zander, A. (1968). *Group dynamics: Research and theory* (3rd ed.). New York: Harper & Row.

Cejka, M. A., & Eagly, A. H. (1999). Gender-stereotypic images of occupations correspond to the sex segregation of employment. *Personality and Social Psychology Bulletin, 25,* 413–423.

Chataway, C. J., & Kolb, D. M. (1994). Informal contributions to the conflict management process. In A. Taylor & J. B. Miller (Eds.), *Conflict and gender* (pp. 259–280). Cresskill, NJ: Hampton Press.

Cheek, D. K. (1976). *Assertive black . . . puzzled white: A black perspective on assertive behavior.* San Luis Obispo, CA: Impact.

Chemers, M. M. (1983). Leadership theory and research: A systems-process integration. In P. B. Paulus (Ed.), *Basic group processes* (pp. 9–40). New York: Springer-Verlag.

Chemers, M. M., Hays, R. B., Rhodewalt, F., & Wysocki, J. (1985). A person-environment analysis of job stress: A contingency model explanation.

Journal of Personality and Social Psychology, 49, 628–635.

Chesney, A. A., & Locke, E. A. (1991). Relationship among goal difficulty, business strategies, and performance on a complex management simulation activity. *Academy of Management Journal, 34,* 400–424.

Chusmir, L. H., & Mills, J. (1989). Gender differences in conflict resolution styles of managers: At work and at home. *Sex Roles, 20,* 149–163.

Cialdini, R. B. (2001). *Influence: Science and practice* (4th edition). Boston: Allyn & Bacon.

Cianni, M., & Romberger, B. (1995). Perceived racial, ethnic, and gender differences in access to developmental experiences. *Group and Organization Management, 20,* 440–459.

Clark, N. K., Stephenson, G. M., & Kniveton, B. (1990). Social remembering: Quantitative aspects of individual and collaborative remembering by police officers and students. *British Journal of Psychology, 81,* 73–94.

Clark, R. D., III, & Maas, A. (1988). The role of social categorization and perceived source credibility in minority influence. *European Journal of Social Psychology, 18,* 347–364.

Clayton, M. J. (1997). Delphi: A technique to harness expert opinion for critical decision-making tasks in education. *Educational Psychology, 17,* 373–387.

Coch, L., & French, J. R. P., Jr. (1948). Overcoming resistance to change. *Human Relations, 1,* 512–532.

Cohen, C. E. (1981). Person categories and social perception: Testing some boundaries of the processing effects of prior knowledge. *Journal of Personality and Social Psychology, 40,* 441–452.

Cohen, J. (1969). *Statistical power analysis for the behavioral sciences.* New York: Academic Press.

Cohen, S., & Bailey, D. (1997). What makes teams work. *Journal of Management, 23,* 239–290.

Cohn, D., & Fears, D. (2001, March 13). Multiracial growth seen in census: Numbers show diversity, complexity of U.S. count. *Washington Post,* p. A1.

Colligan, M. J., & Murphy L. R., (1979). Mass psychogenic illness in organization: An overview. *Journal of Occupational Psychology, 52,* 77–90.

Colligan, M. J., Pennebaker, J. W., & Murphy, L. R. (Eds.). (1982). *Mass psychogenic illness: A social psychological analysis.* Hillsdale, NJ: Erlbaum.

Collins, S. (1993). Blacks on the bubble: The vulnerability of black executives in white corporations. *Sociological Quarterly, 34,* 29–47.

Comas-Diaz, L., & Duncan, J. W. (1985). The cultural context: A factor in assertiveness training with mainland Puerto Rican women. *Psychology of Women Quarterly, 9,* 463–476.

Condon, J. W., & Crano, W. D. (1988). Inferred evaluation and the relation between attitude similarity and interpersonal attraction. *Journal of Personality and Social Psychology, 54,* 789–797.

Conger, J. A. (1989). *The charismatic leader: Behind the mystique of exceptional leadership.* San Francisco: Jossey-Bass.

Conrad, C. (1991). Communication in conflict: Style-strategy relationships. *Communication Monographs, 58,* 135–155.

Cook, S. W. (1985). Experimenting on social issues: The case of school desegregation. *American Psychologist, 40,* 452–460.

Cooley, C. H. (1998). Social organization: A study of the larger mind. In H. J. Schubert (Ed.), *Charles Horton Cooley: On self and social organization* (pp. 179–184). Chicago: University of Chicago Press. (Original work published 1909)

Corey, G., Corey, M. S., Callanan, P., & Russell, J. M. (1992). *Group techniques* (2nd ed.). Pacific Grove, CA: Brooks/Cole.

Corey, M. S., & Corey, G. (1997). *Groups: Process and practice* (5th ed.). Pacific Grove, CA: Brooks/Cole.

Cox, T. (1993). *Cultural diversity in organizations: Theory, research, and practice.* San Francisco: Berrett-Koehler.

Cox, T., Lobel, S., & McLeod, P. (1991). Effects of ethnic group cultural differences on cooperative and competitive behavior on a group task. *Academy of Management Journal, 34,* 827–847.

Cox, T. H., & Blake, S. (1991). Managing cultural diversity: Implications for organizational competitiveness. *Academy of Management Executive, 5,* 45–56.

Crandall, C. S. (1988). Social contagion of binge eating. *Journal of Personality and Social Psychology, 55,* 588–598.

Crocker, J., & Luhtanen, R. (1990). Collective self-esteem and ingroup bias. *Journal of Personality and Social Psychology, 58,* 60–67.

Crocker, J., & McGraw, K. M. (1984). What's good for the goose is not good for the gander: Solo status as an obstacle to occupational achievement for males and females. *American Behavioral Scientist, 27,* 357–369.

Crosby, F. *Relative deprivation and working women.* New York: Oxford University Press.

Crouch, A., & Yetton, P. (1987). Manager behavior, leadership style, and subordinate performance: An empirical extension of the Vroom-Yetton conflict rule. *Organizational Behavior and Human Decision Processes, 39,* 384–396.

Cunningham, R., & Olshfski, D. (1985). Objectifying assessment centers. *Review of Public Personnel Administration, 5,* 42–49.

Curtis, R. C., & Miller, K. (1986). Believing that another likes or dislikes you: Behaviors making the beliefs come true. *Journal of Personality and Social Psychology, 51,* 284–290.

Cushner, K., & Landis, D. (1996). The intercultural sensitizer. In D. Landis & R. S. Bhagat (Eds.), *Handbook of intercultural training* (pp. 185–202). Thousand Oaks, CA: Sage.

Dalkey, N. (1969). *The Delphi method: An experimental study of group decisions.* Santa Monica, CA: Rand Corporation.

Damanpour, F. (1991). Organizational innovation: A meta-analysis of effects of determinants and moderators. *Academy of Management Journal, 34,* 555–590.

Darley, J. M., & Latane, B. (1968). Bystander intervention in emergencies: Diffusion of responsibility. *Journal of Personality and Social Psychology, 8,* 377–383.

Davies, M. F. (1996). Social interaction. In A. P. Hare, H. H. Blumberg, M. F. Davies, & M. V. Kent (Eds.), *Small groups: An introduction* (pp. 115–134). Westport, CT: Praeger.

Davis-Sacks, M. L., Denison, D. R., & Eisenstat, R. A. (1990). Summary: Professional support teams. In J. R. Hackman (Ed.), *Groups that work (and those that don't): Creating conditions for effective teamwork* (pp. 195–202). San Francisco: Jossey-Bass.

Delbecq, A., Van de Van, A., & Gustafson, D. (1975). *Group techniques: A guide to nominal and Delphi processes.* Glenview, IL: Scott Foresman.

DeMatteo, J. S., Eby, L. T., & Sundstrom, E. (1998). Team-based rewards: Current empirical evidence and directions for future research. *Research on Organization Behavior, 20,* 141–183.

Den Hartog, D. N., House, R. J., Hanges, P. J., Ruiz-Quintanilla, S. A., & Dorfman, P. W. (1999). Culture specific and cross-culturally generalizable implicit leadership theories: Are attributes of charismatic/transformational leadership universally endorsed? *Leadership Quarterly, 10,* 219–257.

Dennis, A. R. (1996). Information exchange and use in small group decision making. *Small Group Research, 27,* 532–551.

Deutsch, M. (1949a). An experimental study of the effects of cooperation and competition upon group processes. *Human Relations, 2,* 199–234.

Deutsch, M. (1949b). A theory of cooperation and competition. *Human Relations, 2,* 129–152.

Deutsch, M. (1973). *Conflicts: Constructive and destructive processes.* New Haven, CT: Yale University Press.

Deutsch, M. (1992). Kurt Lewin: The tough-minded and tender-hearted scientist. *Journal of Social Issues, 48,* 31–44.

Deutsch, M. (1994). Constructive conflict resolution: Principles, training, and research. *Journal of Social Issues, 50,* 13–32.

Deutsch, M. (2000a). Cooperation and competition. In M. Deutsch & P. T. Coleman (Eds.), *The handbook of conflict resolution* (pp. 21–40). San Francisco: Jossey-Bass.

Deutsch, M. (2000b). Introduction. In M. Deutsch & P. T. Coleman (Eds.), *The handbook of conflict resolution* (pp. 1–18). San Francisco: Jossey-Bass.

Devine, D. J., Clayton, L. D., Philips, J. L., Dunford, B. B., & Melner, S. B. (1999). Teams in organizations: Prevalence, characteristics, and effectiveness. *Small Group Research, 30,* 678–712.

Devine, P. G. (1995). Prejudice and out-group perception. In A. Tesser (Ed.), *Advanced social psychology* (pp. 467–524). New York: McGraw-Hill.

Dewhurst, M. L., & Wall, V. D., Jr. (1994). Gender and mediation of conflict: Communication differences. In A. Taylor & J. B. Miller (Eds.), *Conflict and gender* (pp. 281–302). Cresskill, NJ: Hampton Press.

Diamant, N. J. (2000). Conflict and conflict resolution in China: Beyond mediation-centered approaches. *Journal of Conflict Resolution, 44,* 523–547.

Diehl, M., & Stroebe, W. (1989). Productivity loss in brainstorming groups: Toward the solution of a riddle. *Journal of Personality and Social Psychology, 535,* 497–509.

Dion, K. L. (1986). Responses to perceived discrimination and relative deprivation. In J. M. Olson, C. P. Herman, & M. P. Zanna (Eds.), *Relative deprivation and social comparison* (pp. 159–179). Hillsdale, NJ: Erlbaum.

Dion, K. L. (1990). Group morale. In R. Brown (Ed.), *The Marshall Caendish encyclopedia of personal relationships* (Vol. 15, pp. 1854–1861). Oxford: Cavendish.

Dion, K. L., & Evans, C. R. (1992). On cohesiveness: Reply to Keyton and other critics of the construct. *Small Group Research, 23,* 242–251.

Dion, K. L., & Schuller, R. A. (1990). Ms. and the manager: A tale of two stereotypes. *Sex Roles, 22,* 569–577.

Donnell, S. M., & Hall, J. (1980). Men and women as managers: A significant case of no significant difference. *Organizational Dynamics, 8,* 60–76.

Donohue, W. A., & Kolt, R. (1992). *Managing interpersonal conflict.* Newbury Park, CA: Sage.

Dorfman, P. W., Howell, J. P., Hibino, S., Lee, J. K., Tate, U., & Bautista, A. (1997). Leadership in Western and Asian countries: Commonalities and differences in effective leadership processes across cultures. *Leadership Quarterly, 8,* 233–274.

Dovidio, J. F., Brown, C. E., Heltman, K., Ellyson, S. L., & Keating, C. F. (1988). Power displays between women and men in discussions of gender-linked tasks: A multichannel study. *Journal of Personality and Social Psychology, 55,* 580–587.

Dovidio, J. F., Ellyson, S. L., Keating, C. F., Heltman, K., & Brown, C. E. (1988). The relationship of social power to visual displays of social dominance between men and women. *Journal of Personality and Social Psychology, 54,* 233–242.

Driskell, J. E., & Mullen, B. (1990). Status, expectations, and behavior: A meta-analytic review and test of the theory. *Personality and Social Psychology Bulletin, 16,* 541–543.

Drury, J., & Reicher, S. (2000). Collective action and psychological change: The emergence of new social identities. *British Journal of Social Psychology, 39,* 579–604.

Drury, J., & Stott, C. (2001). Bias as a research strategy in participant observation: The case of intergroup conflict. *Field Methods, 13,* 47–67.

Druskat, V. U., & Kayes, D. C. (2000). Learning versus performance in short-term project teams. *Small Group Research, 31,* 328–362.

Duane, M. J. (1989). Sex differences in styles of conflict management. *Psychological Reports, 65,* 1033–1034.

Dugger, K. (1996). Social location and gender-role attitudes: A comparison of black and white women. In E. N. Chow, D. Wilkinson, & M. B. Zinn (Eds.), *Race, class, & gender: Common bonds, different voices* (pp.32–51). Thousand Oaks, CA: Sage.

Dunphy, D. (1964). *Social changes in analytic groups.* Unpublished doctoral dissertation, Harvard University, Cambridge, MA.

Durham, C. C., Knight, D., & Locke, E. A. (1997). Effects of leader role, team-set goal difficulty, efficacy, and tactics on team effectiveness. *Organizational Behavior and Human Decision Processes, 72,* 203–231.

Durkheim, E. (1895). *Les reles de la méthode sociolgique.* Paris: F. Alcan.

Eagly, A. H. (1983). Gender and social influence: A social psychological analysis. *American Psychologist, 38,* 971–995.

Eagly, A. H. (1987). *Sex differences in social behavior: A social-role interpretation.* Hillsdale, NJ: Erlbaum.

Eagly, A. H. (1995). The science and politics of comparing women and men. *American Psychologist, 50,* 145–158.

Eagly, A. H., & Carli, L. L. (1981). Sex of researchers and sex typed communications as determinants of sex differences in influencability: A meta-analysis of social influence studies. *Psychological Bulletin, 90,* 1–20.

Eagly, A. H., & Johnson, B. T. (1990). Gender and leadership style: A meta-analysis. *Journal of Personality and Social Psychology, 60,* 685–710.

Eagly, A. H., & Karau, S. J. (1991). Gender and the emergence of leaders: A meta-analysis. *Journal of Personality and Social Psychology, 60,* 685–710.

Eagly, A. H., Karau, S. J., & Makhijani, M. G. (1995). Gender and the effectiveness of leaders: A meta-analysis. *Journal of Personality and Social Psychology, 60,* 685–710.

Eagly, A. H., Makhijani, M. G., & Klonsky, B. G. (1992). Gender and the evaluation of leaders: A meta-analysis. *Psychological Bulletin, 111,* 3–22.

Eagly, A. H., & Wood, W. (1982). Inferred sex differences in status as a determinant of gender stereotypes about social influence. *Journal of Personality and Social Psychology, 43,* 915–928.

Eagly, A. H., & Wood, W. (1985). Gender and influence ability: Stereotype versus behavior, In V. E. O'Leary, R. K. Unger, & B. S. Wallston (Eds.), *Women, gender, and social psychology* (pp. 225–256). Hillsdale, NJ: Erlbaum.

Eagly, A. H., Wood, W., & Fishbaugh, L. (1981). Sex differences in conformity: Surveillance by the group as a determinant male nonconformity. *Journal of Personality and Social Psychology, 40,* 384–394.

Earley, P. C. (1989). Social loafing and collectivism: A comparison of the United States and the People's Republic of China. *Administrative Science Quarterly, 34,* 565–581.

Earley, P. C. (1993). East meets West meets Mideast: Further explorations of collectivistic and individualistic work groups. *Academy of Management Journal, 36,* 319–348.

Ellemers, N. (1993). The influence of socio-structural variables on identity management strategies. In W. Stroebe & M. Hewstone (Eds.), *European review of social psychology* (Vol. 4, pp. 27–57). Chichester, England: Wiley.

El Nasser, E., & Overberg, P. (2001, March 15). Index charts growth in diversity. *USA Today,* p. 3A.

Ely, R. (1994). The effects of organizational demographics and social identity on relationships among professional women. *Administrative Science Quarterly, 39,* 203–238.

Ennett, S. T., & Bauman, K. E. (1993). Peer group structure and adolescent cigarette smoking: A social network analysis. *Journal of Health and Social Behavior, 34,* 226–236.

Erez, M. R., Earley, R. C., & Hulin, C. L. (1985). The impact of participation on goal acceptance and performance: A two-step model. *Academy of Management Journal, 28,* 50–56.

Erez, M. R., & Kanfer, F. H. (1983). The role of goal acceptance in goal setting and task performance. *Academy of Management Review, 8,* 454–463.

Evans, C. R., & Dion, K. L. (1991). Group cohesion and performance: A meta-analysis. *Small Group Research, 22,* 175–186.

Evans, R. (2001). Examining the informal sanctioning of deviance in a chat room culture. *Deviant Behavior, 22,* 195–210.

Ezekiel, R. S. (1995). *The racist mind: Portraits of American neo-Nazis and Klansmen.* New York: Viking.

Falicov, C. J. (1998). The cultural meaning of family triangles. In M. McGoldrick (Ed.), *Re-visioning family therapy* (pp. 37–48). New York: Guilford Press.

Farrell, M. (1976). Patterns in the development of self-analytic groups. *Journal of Applied Behavioral Science, 12,* 523–542.

Federal Glass Ceiling Commission. (1995). *A solid investment: Making full use of the nation's human capital: Recommendations of the Federal Glass Ceiling Commission.* Washington, DC: U.S. Department of Labor, Glass Ceiling Commission.

Feldman, D. C. (1984). The development and enforcement of group norms. *Academy of Management Review, 9,* 47–53.

Ferdman, B. (1995). Cultural identity and diversity in organizations: Bridging the gap between group differences and individual uniqueness. In M. M. Chemers, S. Oskamp, & M. A. Constanzo (Eds.), *Diversity in organizations* (pp. 37–60). Thousand Oaks, CA: Sage.

Ferdman, B., & Brody, S. E. (1996). Models of diversity training. In D. Landis & R. S. Bhagat (Eds.), *Handbook of intercultural training* (pp. 282–306). Thousand Oaks, CA: Sage.

Fernandez, J. P. (1991). *Managing a diverse workforce: Regaining the competitive edge.* Lexington, MA: Lexington Books.

Festinger, L. (1950). Informal social communication. *Psychological Review, 57,* 271–282.

Festinger, L. (1954). A theory of social comparison processes. *Human Relations, 7,* 117–140.

Festinger, L., Rieken, H. W., & Schacter, S. (1956). *When prophecy fails.* Minneapolis: Minnesota Press.

Festinger, L., Schacter, S., & Back, K. (1950). *Social pressures in informal groups: A study of a housing project.* New York: Harper.

Fiedler, F. F. (1967). *A theory of leadership effectiveness.* New York: Harper.

Fiedler, F. F. (1993). The leadership situation and the black box in contingency theories. In M. M. Chemers & R. Ayman (Eds.), *Leadership, theory, and researcher: Perspectives and directions* (pp. 1–28). New York: Academic Press.

Fiedler, F. F., & Chemers, M. M. (1984). *Improving leadership effectiveness: The leader match concept* (2nd ed.). New York: Wiley.

Field, H. G., & Andrews, J. P. (1998). Testing the incremental validity of the Vroom-Jago versus Vroom-Yetton models of participation in decision making. *Journal of Behavioral Decision Making, 11,* 251–261.

Filardo, E.K. (1996). Gender patterns in African American and white adolescents' social interaction in same-race, mixed-gender groups. *Journal of Personality and Social Psychology, 71,* 71–82.

Fine, G. A., & Holyfield, L. (1996). Secrecy, trust, and dangerous leisure: Generating group cohesion in voluntary organizations. *Social Psychology Quarterly, 59,* 22–38.

Fiol, C. M., Harris, D., & House, R. J. (1999). Charismatic leadership: Strategies for effecting social change. *Leadership Quarterly, 10,* 449–482.

Fisher, R., & Brown, S. (1988). *Getting together: Building a relationship that gets to yes.* Boston: Houghton Mifflin.

Fisher, R., Ury, W., & Patton, B. (1991). *Getting to yes: Negotiating agreement without giving in* (2nd ed.). New York: Penguin.

Fiske, S. T., & Taylor, S. E. (1984). *Social cognition.* New York: Random House.

Foels, R., Driskell, J. E., Mullen, B., & Salas, E. (2000). The effects of democratic leadership on group member satisfaction: An integration. *Small Group Research, 31,* 676–701.

Forsyth, D. R. (1999). *Group dynamics* (3rd ed.). Pacific Grove, CA: Brooks/Cole.

Foschi, M. (1992). Gender and double standards for competence. In C. L. Ridgeway (Ed.), *Gender, interaction and inequality* (pp. 181–207). New York: Springer-Verlag.

Foschi, M. (1996). Double standards in the evaluation of men and women. *Social Psychology Quarterly, 57,* 326–339.

Foschi, M., Lai, L., & Sigerson, K. (1994). Gender and double standards in the assessment of job applicants. *Social Psychology Quarterly, 57,* 326–339.

Foti, R. J., & Luch, C. H. (1992). The influence of individual differences on the perception and categorization of leaders. *Leadership Quarterly, 3,* 55–66.

Foushee, H. C. (1984). Dyads and triads at 35,000 feet. *American Psychologist, 39,* 885–893.

Freedman, S. M., & Phillips, J. S. (1988). The changing nature of research on women at work. *Journal of Management, 14,* 231–251.

French, J. R. P., & Raven, B. (1959). The bases of social power. In D. Cartwright (Ed.), *Studies in social power* (pp. 150–167). Ann Arbor: University of Michigan, Institute for Social Research.

Friend, R., Rafferty, Y., & Bramel, D. (1990). A puzzling misinterpretation of the Asch "conformity" study. *European Journal of Social Psychology, 20,* 29–44.

Fulkerson, J. R., & Schuler, R. S. (1992). Managing worldwide diversity at Pepsi-Cola International. In S. E. Jackson & Associates, *Diversity in the workplace: Human resources initiatives* (pp. 248–276). New York: Guilford Press.

Gabrenya, W. K., Wang, Y. E., & Latane, B. (1985). Social loafing on an optimising task: Cross-cultural differences among Chinese and Americans. *Journal of Cross-Cultural Psychology, 16,* 223–242.

Gabrielidis, C., Stephan, W. G., Ybarra, O., Dos Santos Pearson, V. M., & Villareal, L. (1997). Preferred styles of conflict resolution. *Journal of Conflict Resolution, 28,* 661–678.

Gaertner, S., & Dovidio, J. (1986). The aversive form of racism. In J. Dovidio & S. Gaertner (Eds.), *Prejudice, discrimination, and racism* (pp. 61–89). New York: Academic Press.

Gandz, J., & Murray V. V. (1980). The experience of workplace politics. *Academy of Management Journal, 23,* 237–251.

Gavin, L., & Furman, W. (1989). Age difference in adolescents' perceptions of their peer groups. *Developmental Psychology, 25,* 827–834.

George, J. M. (1992). Extrinsic and intrinsic origins of perceived social loafing in organizations. *Academy of Management Journal, 35,* 191–202.

George, J. M. (1995). Asymmetrical effects of rewards and punishments: The case of social loafing. *Journal of Occupational and Organizational Psychology, 68,* 327–339.

George, J. M., & Bettenhausen, K. (1990). Understanding prosocial behavior, sales performance, and turnover: A group-level analysis in a service context. *Journal of Applied Psychology, 75,* 698–709.

Gersick, C. J. G. (1988). Time and transition in work teams: Toward a new model of group development. *Academy of Management Journal, 31,* 9–41.

Gersick, C. J. G. (1989). Marking time: Predictable transitions in task groups. *Academy of Management Journal, 32,* 274–309.

Gibb, J. R. (1961). Defensive communication. *Journal of Communication, 11,* 141–148.

Gibbard, G., & Hartman, J. (1973). The Oedipal paradigm in group development: A clinical and empirical study. *Small Group Behavior, 4,* 305–354.

Gigone, D., & Hastie, R. (1993). The common knowledge effect: Information sharing and group judgment. *Journal of Personality and Social Psychology, 65,* 959–974.

Gilbert, D. T., & Hixon, J. G. (1991). The trouble of thinking: Activation and application of stereotypic beliefs. *Journal of Personality and Social Psychology, 60,* 509–517.

Giordano, P. C. (1983). Sanctioning the high-status deviant: An attributional analysis. *Social Psychology Quarterly, 46,* 329–342.

Gire, J. T., & Carment, D. W. (1992). Dealing with disputes: The influence of individualism-collectivism. *Journal of Social Psychology, 133,* 81–95.

Glick, P. (1991). Trait-based and sex-based discrimination in occupational prestige, occupational salary, and hiring. *Sex Roles, 25,* 351–378.

Gluckman, M. (1963). Gossip and scandal. *Current Anthropology, 4,* 307–316.

Godfrey, D. K., Jones, E. E., & Lord, C. G. (1986). Self-promotion is not ingratiating. *Journal of Personality and Social Psychology, 50,* 106–115.

Goethals, G. R., & Darley, J. M. (1977). Social comparison theory: An attributional approach. In J. M. Suls & R. L. Miller (Eds.), *Social comparison processes: Theoretical and empirical perspectives* (pp. 259–278). Washington, DC: Hemisphere/Halsted.

Gold, J. A., Ryckman, R. M., & Mosely, N. R. (1984). Romantic mood induction and attraction to a dissimilar other: Is love blind? *Personality and Social Psychology Bulletin, 10,* 358–368.

Goldstein, I. L., & Ford, J. K. (2002). *Training in organizations* (4th ed.). Pacific Grove, CA: Brooks/Cole.

Goodman, P. S. (1977). Social comparison processes in organizations. In B. M. Staw & G. R. Salancik (Eds.), *New directions in organizational behavior* (pp. 97–132). Chicago: St. Clair Press.

Goodman, P. S., & Leyden, D. P. (1991). Familiarity and group productivity. *Journal of Applied Psychology, 76,* 578–586.

Gottman, J. (1994). *Why marriages succeed or fail.* New York: Simon & Schuster.

Gouran, D. S., & Hirokawa, R. Y. (1996). Functional theory and communication in decision-making and problem-solving groups: An expanded view. In M. S. Poole & R. Y. Hirokawa (Eds.), *Communication and group decision making* (2nd ed.), (pp. 55–80). Thousand Oaks, CA: Sage.

Granrose, C. S., & Oskamp, S. (1997). Cross-cultural work groups: An overview. In C. S. Granrose & S. Oskamp (Eds.), *Cross-cultural work groups* (pp. 1–16). Thousand Oaks, CA: Sage.

Gross, S. E. (1995). *Compensation for teams: How to design and implement team-based reward programs.* New York: AMACOM.

Guetzkow, H., & Gyr, J. (1954). An analysis of conflict in decision-making groups. *Human Relations, 7,* 367–382.

Gully, S. M., Devine, D. J., & Whitney, D. J. (1995). A meta-analysis of cohesion and performance: Effects of level of analysis and task interdependence. *Small Group Research, 26,* 497–520.

Gurin, P., Miller, A. H., & Gurin, G. (1980). Stratum identification and consciousness. *Social Psychology Quarterly, 43,* 30–47.

Guzzo, R. A. (1995). Introduction: At the intersection of team effectiveness and decision making. In R. A. Guzzo, E. Salas, & Associates, *Team effectiveness and decision making in organizations* (pp. 1–8). San Francisco: Jossey-Bass.

Guzzo, R. A., & Dickson, M. W. (1996). Teams in organizations: Recent research on performance and effectiveness. *Annual Review of Psychology, 47,* 307–308.

Guzzo, R. A., Yost, P. R., Campbell, R. J., & Shea, G. P. (1993). Potency in groups: Articulating a construct. *British Journal of Social Psychology, 32,* 87–106.

Hackman, J. R. (1987). The design of work teams. In J. W. Lorsch (Ed.), *Handbook of organizational behavior* (pp. 315–342). Upper Saddle River, NJ: Prentice Hall.

Hackman, J. R. (1990). *Groups that work (and those that don't).* San Francisco: Jossey-Bass.

Hackman, J. R. (1998). Why teams don't work. In R. S. Tindale, L. Heath, J. Edwards, E. J. Posavac, F. B. Bryant, Y. Suarez-Balcazr, E. Henderson-King, & J. Myers (Eds.), *Theory and research on small groups* (pp. 248–266). New York: Plenum.

Hall, J. A. (1998). How big are nonverbal sex differences? The case of smiling and sensitivity to nonverbal cues. In O. J. Canary & K. Dindia (Eds.), *Sex differences and similarities in communication* (pp. 155–177). Mahwah, NJ: Erlbaum.

Halpin, A. W., & Winer, B. J. (1957). A factorial study of the leader behavior descriptions. In R. M. Stogdill & A. E. Coons (Eds.), *Leader behavior: Its description and measurement.* Columbus: Ohio State University, Bureau of Business Research.

Hamilton, D. L. (1981). Illusory correlation as a basis for stereotyping. In D. L. Hamilton (Ed.), *Cognitive processes in stereotyping and intergroup behavior.* Hillsdale, NJ: Erlbaum.

Hamilton, D. L., & Rose, T. (1980). Illusory correlation and the maintenance of stereotypic beliefs. *Journal of Personality and Social Psychology, 39,* 832–845.

Hardy, C. J., & Latane, B. (1988). Social loafing in cheerleaders: Effects of team membership and competition. *Journal of Sport and Exercise Psychology, 10,* 109–114.

Hare, A. P. (1973). Theories of group development and categories for interaction analysis. *Small Group Behavior, 4,* 259–304.

Hare, A. P. (1992). *Groups, teams, and social interaction.* New York: Praeger.

Hare, A. P. (1996a). A brief history of SYMLOG: In headlines and footnotes. In S. E. Hare & A. P. Hare (Eds.), *SYMLOG field theory: Organizational consultation, value differences, personality and social perception* (pp. 193–200). Westport, CT: Praeger.

Hare, A. P. (1996b). SYMLOG field theory. In S. E. Hare & A. P. Hare (Eds.), *SYMLOG field theory: Organizational consultation, value differences, personality and social perception* (pp. 1–8). Westport, CT: Praeger.

Hare, A. P., Koenigs, R. J., & Hare, S. E. (1997). Perceptions of observed and model values of male and female managers. *Journal of Organizational Behavior, 18,* 437–447.

Hare, S. E., & Hare, A. P. (Eds.), (1996). *SYMLOG field theory: Organizational consultation, value differences, personality and social perception.* Westport, CT: Praeger.

Harkins, S. G., & Jackson, J. (1985). The role of evaluation in eliminating social loafing. *Personality and Social Psychology Bulletin, 11,* 457–465.

Harkins, S. G., & Petty, R. E. (1982). Effects of task difficulty and task uniqueness on social loafing. *Journal of Personality and Social Psychology, 43,* 1214–1229.

Harkins, S. G., & Syzmanski, K. (1988). Social loafing and self-evaluation with an objective standard. *Journal of Experimental Social Psychology, 24,* 354–365.

Harkins, S. G., & Syzmanski, K. (1989). Social loafing and group evaluation. *Journal of Personality and Social Psychology, 56,* 934–941.

Harper, R. G. (1985). Power, dominance, and nonverbal behavior: An overview. In S. L. Ellyson & J. F. Dovidio (Eds.), *Power, dominance, and nonverbal behavior* (pp. 29–48). New York: Springer-Verlag.

Harrington, C. L., & Bielby, D. D. (1995). Where did you hear that? *Sociological Quarterly, 36,* 607–629.

Harrison, D. A., Price, K. H., & Bell, M. P. (1998). Beyond relational demography: Time and the effects of surface and deep-level diversity on work group cohesion. *Academy of Management Journal, 41,* 96–107.

Harvey, J. (1988). *The Abilene Paradox and other meditations on management.* Lexington, MA: Lexington Books.

Hater, J. J., & Bass, B. M. (1988). Superiors' evaluations and subordinates' perceptions of transformational and transactional leadership. *Journal of Applied Psychology, 73,* 695–702.

Heilman, M. E., & Martell, R. F. (1986). Exposure to successful women: Antidote to sex discrimination in applicant screening decisions? *Organizational Behavior and Human Decision Processes, 37,* 376–390.

Hendricks, G., & Hendricks, K. (1990). *Conscious loving: The journey to co-commitment.* New York: Bantam.

Henry, K. B., Arrow, H., & Carini, B. (1998). A tripartite model of group identification: Theory and measurement. *Small Group Research, 30,* 558–581.

Herek, G. M., Janis, I. L., & Huth, P. (1987). Decision-making during international crises: Is quality of process related to outcome? *Journal of Conflict Resolution, 31,* 203–226.

Hershey, P., & Blanchard, K. (1982). *Management of organizational behavior: Utilizing human resources* (4th ed.). Englewood Cliffs, NJ: Prentice Hall.

Hershey, P., & Blanchard, K. (1988). *Management of organizational behavior: Utilizing human resources* (5th ed.). Englewood Cliffs, NJ: Prentice Hall.

Higham, P. A., & Carment, D. W. (1992). The rise and fall of politicians. *Canadian Journal of Behavioral Science,* 404–409.

Hill, W. F. (1974). Systematic group development: SGD therapy. In A. Jacobs & W. Spradlin (Eds.), *The group as an agent of change* (pp. 111–121). New York: Behavioral Publications.

Hilton, J. L., & Darley, J. M. (1991). The effects of interaction goals on person perception. *Advances in Experimental Social Psychology, 24,* 235–267.

Hilton, J. L., & Fein, S. (1989). The role of typical diagnosticity in stereotype-based judgments. *Journal of Personality and Social Psychology, 57,* 201–211.

Hinsz, V. B., Tindale, R. S., & Volrath, D. A. (1997). The emerging conceptualization of groups as information processors. *Psychological Bulletin, 121,* 43–64.

Hirokawa, R. Y. (1985). Discussion procedures and decision-making performance: A test of a functional perspective. *Human Communication Research, 12,* 203–224.

Hirokawa, R. Y. (1990). The role of communication in group decision-making efficacy. *Small Group Research, 21,* 190–204.

Hirokawa, R. Y., DeGooyer, D., & Valde, K. (2000). Using narratives to study task group effectiveness. *Small Group Research, 31,* 573–591.

Hirokawa, R. Y., Erbert, L., & Hurst, A. (1996). Communication and group decision-making effectiveness. In M. S. Poole & R. Y. Hirokawa (Eds.), *Communication and group decision making* (2nd ed.), (pp. 269–300). Thousand Oaks, CA: Sage.

Hirokawa, R. Y., Kodama, R. A., & Harper, N. L. (1990). Impact of managerial power on persuasive strategy selection by male and female managers. *Management Communication Quarterly, 34,* 250–265.

Hirokawa, R. Y., & Miyahara, A. (1986). A comparison of influence strategies used by managers in American and Japanese organizations. *Communications Quarterly, 34,* 260–265.

Hirokawa, R. Y., & Scheerhorn, D. R. (1986). Communication in faulty group decision-making. In R. Y. Hirokawa & M. S. Poole (Eds.), *Communication and group decision making* (pp. 63–80). Beverly Hills, CA: Sage.

Hoffman, C. C., Wilcom, L., Gomez, E., & Hollander, C. (1992). Sociometric applications in a corporate environment. *Journal of Group Psychotherapy, Psychodrama, and Sociometry, 45,* 3–16.

Hofstede, G. (1980). Motivation, leadership, and organization: Do American theories apply? *Organizational Dynamics, 3,* 27–33.

Hofstede, G. (1991). *Cultures and organizations: Software of the mind.* New York: McGraw-Hill.

Hogan, R., Curphy, G. J., & Hogan, J. (1994). What we know about leadership: Effectiveness and personality. *American Psychologist, 49,* 493–504.

Hollander, E. P. (1958). Conformity, status, and idiosyncrasy credit. *Psychological Review, 65,* 117–127.

Hollander, E. P. (1960). Competence and conformity in the acceptance of influence. *Journal of Abnormal and Social Psychology, 61,* 361–365.

Hollander, E. P., & Offermann, L.R. (1990). Power and leadership in organizations: Relationships in transition. *American Psychologist, 45,* 179–189.

Hollenbeck, J. R., & Klein, H. J. (1987). Goal commitment and the goal-setting process: Problems, prospects, and proposals for the future. *Journal of Applied Psychology, 72,* 212–220.

Homans, G. C. (1950). *The human group.* New York: Harcourt Brace.

Hooijberg, R., & DiTomaso, N. (1996). Leadership in and of demographically diverse organizations. *Leadership Quarterly, 7,* 1–19.

House, R. J. (1971). A path-goal theory of leaders' effectiveness. *Administrative Science Quarterly, 16,* 321–339.

House, R. J. (1977). A 1976 theory of charismatic leadersip. In J. G. Hunt & L. L. Larson (Eds.), *Leadership: The cutting edge* (pp. 189–207). Carbondale: Southern Illinois University Press.

House, R. J., & Dessler, G. (1974). The path-goal theory of leadership: Some post hoc and a priori tests. In J. G. Hunt & L. L. Larson (Eds.), *Contingency approaches to leadership* (pp. 29–55). Carbondale: Southern Illinois University Press.

House, R. J., & Mitchell, T. R. (1974). Path-goal theory of leadership. *Contemporary Business, 3*(Fall), 81–98.

House, R. J., Woycke, J., & Fodor, E. M. (1991). Charismatic and noncharismatic leaders: Differences in behavior and effectiveness. In B. M. Staw (Ed.), *Psychological dimensions of organizational behavior* (pp. 437–450). New York: MacMillan.

Howard, J., & Rothbart, M. (1980). Social categorization and memory for ingroup and outgroup behavior. *Journal of Personality and Social Psychology, 38,* 301–310.

Howell, J. M., & Avolio, B. J. (1992). The ethics of charismatic leadership: Submission or liberation. *Academy of Management Executive, 6,* 43–54.

Howell, J. M., & Frost, P. J. (1989). A laboratory study of charismatic leadership. *Organizational Behavior and Human Decision Processes, 43,* 243–269.

Howell, J. P., Dorfman, P. W., Hibino, S., Lee, J. K., & Tate, U. (1997). Leadership in Western and Asian countries: Commonalities and differences in effective leadership processes across cultures. *Leadership Quarterly, 8,* 233–274.

Huang, W., Raman, K. S., & Wei, K. K. (1993). A process study of the effects of GSS and task type on informational and normative influence in small groups. In J. I. DeGross, R. P. Bostrom, & D. Robey (Eds.), *Proceedings of the 14th International Conference on Information Systems* (pp. 77–87). Orlando, FLA: ACM.

Humphrey, R. (1985). How work roles influence perception: Structural-cognitive processes and organizational behavior. *American Sociological Review, 50,* 242–252.

Hurtado, A., Rodriguez, J., Gurin, P., & Beals, J. (1993). The impact of Mexican descendants' social identity on the ethnic socialization of children. In M. E. Bernal & G. F. Knight (Eds.), *Ethnic identity: Formation and transmission among Hispanics and other minorities* (pp. 131–162). Albany: State University of New York Press.

Hutson-Comeaux, S. L., & Kelly, J. R. (1996). Sex differences in interaction style and group task performance: The process-performance relationship. *Journal of Social Behavior and Personality, 11,* 255–275.

Ilgen, D. R., & Youtz, M. A. (1986). Factors affecting the evaluation and development of minorities in organizations. *Personnel and Human Resources Management, 4,* 307–337.

Ingham, A. G., Levinger, G., Graves, J., & Peckham, V. (1974). The Ringelmann effect: Studies of group size and group performance. *Journal of Experimental Social Psychology, 10,* 371–384.

International Labour Organization. (1998). *Will the glass ceiling ever be broken? Women in management: It's still lonely at the top.* (http://www.ilo.org/public/english/235press/magazine/23/glass.htm)

Jackson, J. M., & Harkins, S. G. (1985). Equity in effort: An explanation of the social loafing effect. *Journal of Personality and Social Psychology, 49,* 1199–1206.

Jackson, S. (1992). Team composition in organizational settings: Issues in managing a diverse work force. In S. Worchel, W. Wood, & J. Simpson (Eds.), *Group process and productivity* (pp. 138–176). Beverly Hills, CA: Sage.

Jackson, S., & Schuler, R. S. (1985). A meta-analysis and conceptual critique of research on role ambiguity and role conflict in work settings. *Organizational Behavior, 36,* 16–78.

Jackson, S., Stone, V., & Alvarez, E. (1993). Socialization amidst diversity: Impact of demographics on work team oldtimers and newcomers. In L. Cummings & B. Staw (Eds.), *Research in organizational behavior* (Vol. 15), (pp. 45–110). Greenwich, CT: JAI Press.

Janis, L. L. (1982). *Groupthink: Psychological studies of policy decisions and fiascoes* (2nd ed.). Boston: Houghton Mifflin.

Janis, L. L. (1989). *Crucial decisions: Leadership in policy making and crisis management.* New York: Free Press.

Janis, L. L., & Mann, L. (1977). *Decision making: A psychological analysis of conflict, choice, and commitment.* New York: Free Press.

Jehn, K. A., Chadwick, C., & Thatcher, S. (1997). To agree or not to agree: Diversity, conflict, and group outcomes. *International Journal of Conflict Management, 8,* 287–306.

Jehn, K. A., Northcraft, G. B., & Neale, M. A. (1999). Why differences make a difference: A field study of diversity, conflict, and performance in workgroups. *Administrative Science Quarterly, 44,* 741–763.

Jessup, L. M., & Valacich, J. S. (Eds.). (1993). *Group support systems: New perspectives.* New York: Macmillan.

Johnson, B. T., & Eagly, A. H. (2000). Quantitative synthesis of social psychological research. In H. T. Reis & C. M. Judd (Eds.), *Handbook of research methods in social and personality psychology* (pp. 496–528). Cambridge: Cambridge University Press.

Johnson, D. M. (1945). The phantom anesthetist of Matton: A field study of mass hysteria. *Journal of Abnormal and Social Psychology, 40,* 175–186.

Johnson, D. W. (2000). *Reaching out: Interpersonal effectiveness and self-actualization* (7th ed.). Boston: Allyn & Bacon.

Johnson, D. W., & Johnson, F. P. (2000). *Joining together: Group theory and group skills* (7th ed.). Boston: Allyn & Bacon.

Johnson, D. W., & Johnson, R. T. (1989). *Cooperation and competition: Theory and research.* Edina, MN: Interaction.

Johnson, D. W., Johnson, R. T., & Tjosvold, D. (2000). Constructive controversy: The value of intellectual opposition. In M. Deutsch & P. T. Coleman (Eds.), *The handbook of conflict resolution* (pp. 65–85). San Francisco: Jossey-Bass.

Johnson, H. L. (1985). Bribery in international markets: Diagnosis, clarification, and remedy. *Journal of Business Ethics, 4,* 447–455.

Johnson, P. (1976). Women and power: Toward a theory of effectiveness. *Journal of Social Issues, 32,* 99–110.

Johnson, S. (1994). A game of two halves? On men, football, and gossip. *Journal of Gender Studies, 3,* 145–155.

Jones, E. E. (1985). Major developments in social psychology during the past five decades. In G. Lindzey & E. Aronson (Eds.), *Handbook of Social Psychology,* (Vol. 1, pp. 47–108). New York: Random House.

Jones, E. W. (1986). Black managers: The dream deferred. *Harvard Business Review, 64,* 84–93.

Kacen, L., & Rozovski, U. (1998). Assessing group processes: A comparison among group participants', direct observers', and indirect observers' assessment. *Small Group Research, 29,* 179–197.

Kahn, R. L., & Katz, D. (1953). Leadership practices in relation to productivity and morale. In D. Cartwright & A. Zander (Eds.), *Group dynamics.* New York: Harper & Row.

Kane, E. W. (1992). Race, gender, and attitudes toward gender stratification. *Social Psychology Quarterly, 55,* 311–320.

Kanter, R. (1977). Some effects of proportions on group life: Skewed sex ratios and responses to token women. *American Journal of Sociology, 82,* 965–990.

Karau, S. J., & Williams, K. D. (1993). Social loafing: A meta-analytic review and theoretical integration. *Journal of Personality and Social Psychology, 65,* 681–706.

Katzenbach, J. R., & Smith, D. K. (1993). *The wisdom of teams: Creating the high-performance organization.* Boston: Harvard Business School.

Kelman, H. C. (1992). Informal mediation by the scholar/practitioner. In J. Bercovitch & J. Z. Rubin (Eds.), *Mediation in international relations: Multiple approaches to conflict management* (pp. 64–96). New York: St. Martin's Press.

Kelman, H. C. (1997). Group processes in the resolution of international conflicts: The Israeli-Palestinian case. *American Psychologist, 52,* 212–220.

Kemmelmeier, M., & Winter, D. G. (2000). Putting threat into perspective: Experimental studies on perceptual distortion in international conflict. *Personality and Social Psychology Bulletin, 26,* 795–810.

Kemp, T. (1998, July). Panacea or poison? Building self-esteem through adventure experiences. *Proceedings of the International Adventure Therapy Conference,* Perth, Australia.

Kemper, T. D. (1991). Predicting emotions from social relations. *Social Psychology Quarterly, 54,* 330–342.

Kenny, D. A. (1994). Using the social relations model to understand relationships. In R. Erber & R. Gilmour (Eds.), *Theoretical frameworks for personal relationships* (pp. 111–127). Hillsdale, NJ: Erlbaum.

Kerr, N. L. (1983). Motivation losses in small groups: A social dilemma analysis. *Journal of Personality and Social Psychology, 45,* 819–828.

Kerr, N. L., Aronoff, J., & Messe, L. A. (2000). Methods of small group research. In H. T. Reis & C. M. Judd (Eds.), *Handbook of research methods in social and personality psychology* (pp. 160–189). Cambridge: Cambridge University Press.

Kerr, N. L., & Bruun, S. E. (1981). Ringelmann revisited: Alternative explanations for the social loafing effect. *Personality and Social Psychology Bulletin, 7,* 224–231.

Kerr, N. L., & Bruun, S. E. (1983). Dispensability of member effort and group motivation losses: Free-rider effects. *Journal of Personality and Social Psychology, 44,* 78–94.

Kerr, N. L., MacCoun, R. J., & Kramer, G. P. (1996). Bias in judgment: Comparing individuals and groups. *Psychological Review, 103,* 687–719.

Keyton, J. (1993). Group termination: Completing the study of group development. *Small Group Research, 24,* 84–100.

Keyton, J. (1999). Analyzing interaction patterns in dysfunctional teams. *Small Group Research, 30,* 491–519.

Kidwell, R. E., Mossholder, K. W., & Bennett, N. (1997). Cohesiveness and organizational citizenship behavior: A multi-level analysis using work groups and individuals. *Journal of Management, 23,* 775–793.

Kimmel, P. R. (1994). Cultural perspectives on inter-national negotiations. *Journal of Social Issues, 50,* 179–196.

Kimmel, P. R. (2000). Culture and conflict. In M. Deutsch & P. T. Coleman (Eds.), *The handbook of conflict resolution* (pp. 453–474). San Francisco: Jossey-Bass.

Kipnis, D., Schmidt, S., & Wilkinson, I. (1980). Intraorganizational influence tactics: Explorations in getting one's way. *Journal of Applied Psychology, 65,* 440–452.

Kirchmeyer, C., & Cohen, A. (1992). Multicultural groups: Their performance and reactions with con-structive conflict. *Group and Organization Management, 17,* 153–170.

Kirkpatrick, S. A., & Locke, E. A. (1991). Leadership: Do traits matter? *Academy of Management Executive, 5,* 48–60.

Klein, W. M. (1997). Objective standards are not enough: Affective, self-evaluative, and behavioral responses to social comparison information. *Journal of Personality and Social Psychology, 72,* 763–774.

Klein, W. M., & Mulvey, P. W. (1989, August). *Performance goals in group settings: An investigation of group and goal setting processes.* Paper presented at the meeting of the National Academy of Management, Washington, DC.

Klein, W. M., & Mulvey, P. W. (1995). The setting of goals in groups: An examination of processes and performance. *Organizational Behavior and Human Decision Processes, 61,* 44–53.

Klimoski, R., & Jones, R. G. (1995). Staffing issues for effective group decision making: Key issues in matching people and teams. In R. A. Guzzo & E. Salas (Eds.), *Team effectiveness and decision making in organizations* (pp. 291–332). San Francisco: Jossey-Bass.

Klimoski, R., & Mohammed, S. (1997). Team mental model: Construct or metaphor? *Journal of Management, 20,* 403–437.

Knight, D., Pearce, C. L., Smith, K. G., Olian, J. D., Sims, H. P., Smith, K. A., & Flood, P. (1999). Top management team diversity, group process, and strategic consensus. *Strategic Management Journal, 20,* 445–465.

Knottnerus, J. D. (1997). Social structural analysis and status generalization: The contributions and poten-tial of expectation states theory. In J. Szmatka, J. Skvoretz, & J. Berger, (Eds.), *Status, network, and structure* (pp. 119–136). Stanford, CA: Stanford University Press.

Knouse, S. B., & Chretien, D. (1996). Workforce diversity and TQM. In S. B. Knouse (Ed.), *Human resources management perspectives on TQM: Concepts and practices* (pp. 261–274). Milwaukee: American Society for Quality Control Press.

Knouse, S. B., & Dansby, M. R. (1999). Percentage of work-group diversity and work-group effectiveness. *Journal of Psychology: Interdisciplinary and Applied, 133,* 486–495.

Kolb, J. A. (1999). The effect of gender role, attitude toward leadership, and self-confidence on leader emergence: Implications for leadership develop-ment. *Human Resource Development Quarterly, 10,* 305–320.

Komaki, J., Heinzmann, A. T., & Lawson, L. (1980). Effect of training and feedback: Component analysis of a behavioral safety program. *Journal of Applied Psychology, 65,* 261–270.

Konrad, A. M., Winter, S., & Gutek, B. A. (1992). Diversity in work group sex composition: Implications for majority and minority members. In I. P. Tolbert & S. B. Bacharach (Eds.), *Research in the sociology of organizations* (Vol. 10, pp. 115–140). Greenwich, CT: JAI Press.

Koomen, W. (1988). The relationship between participation rate and liking ratings in groups. *British Journal of Social Psychology, 27,* 127–132.

Koslowsky, M., & Schwarzwald, J. (1993). The use of power strategies to gain compliance. *Journal of Social Behavior and Personality, 21,* 135–144.

Koslowsky, M., & Schwarzwald, J. (1999). Gender, self-esteem, and focus of interest in the use of power strategies by adolescents in conflict situations. *Journal of Social Issues, 55,* 15–32.

Kotter, J. P. (1990). *A force for change: How leadership differs from management.* New York: Free Press.

Kramer, M. W., & Kuo, C. L. (1997). The impact of brainstorming techniques on subsequent group processes. *Small Group Research, 28,* 218–241.

Kravitz, D. A., & Martin, B. (1986). Ringelmann rediscovered: The original article. *Journal of Personality and Social Psychology, 50,* 936–941.

Krichevskii, R. L. (1983). The phenomenon of the differentiation of the leadership role in small groups. In H. H. Blumberg, A. P. Hare, V. Kent, & M. Davies (Eds.), *Small groups and social interaction* (Vol. 1). Chichester: Wiley.

Krone, K. J., Ling, C., & Xia, H. (1997). Approaches to managerial influence in the People's Republic of China. *Journal of Business Communication, 34,* 289–318.

Kroon, M. B., van Kreveld, D., & Rabbie, J. (1992). Group versus individual decision making: Effects of accountability and gender on groupthink. *Small Group Research, 23,* 427–459.

Kugath, S. D. (1997). The effects of family participation in an outdoor adventure program. *Proceedings of the International Conference on Outdoor Recreation.* ERRIC Documentation Reproduction Service (ED417050). (http://ericae.net/ericdb/ED417050.htm).

Kyl-Heku, L. M., & Buss, D. M. (1996). Tactics as units of analysis in personality psychology: An illustration using tactics of hierarchy negotiation. *Personality and Individual Differences, 21,* 497–517.

Lambert, A. J., Khan, S. R., Lickel, B. A., & Fricke, K. (1997). Mood and the correction of positive versus negative stereotypes. *Journal of Personality and Social Psychology, 72,* 1002–1016.

Lamm, H. (1988). A review of our research on group polarization: Eleven experiments on the effects of group discussion on risk acceptance, probability estimation, and negotiation positions. *Psychological Reports, 62,* 807–813.

Landau, J. (1995). The relationship of race and gender to managers' ratings of promotion potential. *Journal of Organizational Behavior, 16,* 391–400.

Langfred, C. W. (1998). Is group cohesiveness a double-edged sword? *Small Group Research, 29,* 124–144.

Larkey, L. K. (1996). Toward a theory of communicative interactions in culturally diverse workgroups. *Academy of Management Review, 21,* 463–491.

Larsen, K. S. (1990). The Asch conformity experiment: Replication and transhistorical comparisons. *Journal of Social Behavior and Personality, 5,* 163–168.

Larson, C. E., & LaFasto, F. M. (1989). *Teamwork: What must go right/what can go wrong.* Newbury Park, CA: Sage.

Latane, B. (1981). The psychology of social impact. *American Psychologist, 36,* 343–356.

Latane, B., & Darley, J. M. (1970). *The unresponsive bystander: Why doesn't he help?* Englewood Cliffs, NJ: Prentice Hall.

Latane, B., Williams, K., & Harkins, S. (1979). Many hands make light the work: The causes and consequences of social loafing. *Journal of Personality and Social Psychology, 37,* 822–832.

Latham, G. P., & Locke, E. A. (1975). Increasing productivity with decreasing time limits: A field replication of Parkinson's law. *Journal of Applied Psychology, 60,* 524–526.

Latham, G. P., Winters, D. C., & Locke, E. A. (1994). Cognitive and motivational effects of participation: A mediator study. *Journal of Organizational Behavior, 15,* 49–63.

Lau, D. C., & Murnighan, J. K. (1998). Demographic diversity and faultlines: The compositional dynamics of organizational groups. *Academy of Management Review, 23,* 325–340.

Lawler, E. E. (1992). *The ultimate advantage: Creating the high-involvement organization.* San Francisco: Jossey-Bass.

Lawler, E. E., & Hackman, J. R. (1969). Impact of employee participation in the development of pay incentive plans: A field experiment. *Journal of Applied Psychology, 53,* 467–471.

Lawrence, H. V., & Wiswell, A. K. (1993). Using the work group as a laboratory for learning: Increasing leadership and team effectiveness through feedback. *Human Resource Development Quarterly, 4,* 135–148.

Leary, M. R., & Forsyth, D. R. (1987). Attributions of responsibility for collective endeavors. In C. Hendrick (Ed.), *Group processes* (pp. 167–188). Newbury Park, CA: Sage.

Leavitt, H. J. (1951). Some effects of certain communication patterns on group performance. *Journal of Abnormal and Social Psychology, 46,* 38–50.

LeBon, G. (1968). *The crowd.* Dunwoody, GA: Berg. (Original work published 1895)

Lee, M. T., & Ofshe, R. (1981). The impact of behavioral style and status characteristics on social influence: A test of two competing theories. *Social Psychology Quarterly, 44,* 73–82.

Leenders, G., & Henderson, B. (1991). Dialogue of new directions: The spiritual heart of adventure learning. *Journal of Experiential Education, 14,* 32–38.

Leffler, A., Gilespie, D. L., & Conaty, J. C. (1982). The effects of status differentiation on non-verbal behavior. *Social Psychology Quarterly, 45,* 153–161.

Lepore, L., & Brown, R. (1997). Category and stereotype activation: Is prejudice inevitable? *Journal of Personality and Social Psychology, 72,* 275–287.

Lerner, H. G. (1989). *The dance of intimacy: A woman's guide to courageous acts of change in key relationships.* New York: Harper & Row.

Leung, K., Au, Y., Fernandez-Dol, J. M., & Iwawaki, S. (1992). Preference for methods of conflict processing in two collectivist cultures. *International Journal of Psychology, 27,* 195–209.

Levi, D. (2001). *Group dynamics for teams.* Newbury Park, CA: Sage.

Levine, J. M. (1989). Reaction to opinion deviance in small groups. In P. B. Paulus (Ed.), *Psychology of group influence,* (2nd ed.) (pp. 187–232). Hillsdale, NJ: Erlbaum.

Levine, J. M., & Moreland, R. L. (1990). Progress in small group research. In M. R. Rosenweig & L. W. Porter (Eds.), *Annual Review of Psychology, 41,* 585–634.

Levine, J. M., & Moreland, R. L. (1995). *Group processes.* In A. Tesser (Ed.), *Advanced social psychology* (pp. 419–466). New York: McGraw-Hill.

Lewicki, R. J., & Wiethoff, C. (2000). Trust, trust development, and trust repair. In M. Deutsch & P. T. Coleman (Eds.), *The handbook of conflict resolution* (pp. 21–40). San Francisco: Jossey-Bass.

Lewin, K. (1935). *A dynamic theory of personality.* New York: McGraw-Hill.

Lewin, K. (1941). Analysis of the concepts whole, differentiation, and unity. *University of Iowa Studies in Child Welfare, 18,* 226–261.

Lewin, K. (1943). Forces behind food habits and methods of change. *Bulletin of the National Research Council, 108,* 35–65.

Lewin, K. (1947). *The Research Center for Group Dynamics.* New York: Beacon House.

Lewin, K. (1948). *Resolving social conflicts.* New York: Harper & Row.

Lewin, K. (1951a). *Field theory in social science.* New York: Harper & Row.

Lewin, K. (1951b). Problems of research in social psychology. In D. Cartwright (Ed.), *Field theory in social science: Selected theoretical papers* (pp. 130–154). Westport, CT: Greenwood.

Lewin, K. (1997a). Behavior and development as a function of the total situation. In G. W. Lewin (Ed.), *Resolving social conflicts,* (3rd ed.), (pp. 337–382). Washington, DC: American Psychological Association. (Original work published 1946)

Lewin, K. (1997b). Frontiers in group dynamics. In G. W. Lewin (Ed.), *Resolving social conflicts,* (3rd ed.), (pp. 301–336). Washington, DC: American Psychological Association. (Original work published 1947)

Lewin, K., Lippit, R., & White, R. K. (1939). Patterns of aggressive behavior in experimentally created social climates. *Journal of Social Psychology, 10,* 271–299.

Lewis, C. M., & Beck, A. P. (1983). Experiencing level in the process of group development. *Group, 7,* 18–26.

Li, J., Karakowsky, L., & Siegel, J.P. (1999). The effects of proportional representation on intragroup behavior in mixed-race decision-making groups. *Small Group Research, 30,* 259–280.

Libby, R., Trotman, K. T., & Zimmer, I. (1987). Member variation, recognition of expertise, and group performance. *Journal of Applied Psychology, 72,* 81–87.

Lindsley, D. H., Brass, D. J., & Thomas, J. (1995). Efficacy-performance spirals: A multilevel perspective. *Academy of Management Review, 20,* 645–678.

Linnehan, F., & Konrad, A. M. (1999). Diluting diversity: Implications for intergroup inequality in organizations. *Journal of Management Inquiry, 8,* 399–414.

Lippit, R., & White, R. K. (1958). An experimental study of leadership and group life. In E. E. Maccoby, T. M. Newcomb, & E. L. Hartley (Eds.), *Reading in social psychology* (3rd ed.), (pp. 496–511). New York: Holt, Rinehart, & Winston.

Lipsey, M. W., & Wilson, D. B. (1993). The efficacy of psychological, educational, and behavioral treatment. *American Psychologist, 48,* 1181–1209.

Little, B. L., & Madigan, R. M. (1997). The relationship between collective efficacy and performance in manufacturing work teams. *Small Group Research, 28,* 517–535.

Littlepage, G. E., Robison, W., & Reddington, K. (1997). Effects of task experience and group experience on group performance, member ability, and recognition of expertise. *Organizational Behavior and Human Decision Processes, 69,* 133–147.

Locke, E. A., & Latham, G. P. (1988). The determinants of goal commitment. *Academy of Management Review, 13,* 23–39.

Locke, E. A., Latham, G. P., & Erez, M. (1988). The determinants of goal commitment. *Academy of Management Review, 13,* 23–39.

Locke, E. A., Latham, G. P., & Erez, M. (1990). *A theory of goal setting and task performance.* Englewood Cliffs, NJ: Prentice Hall.

London, M. (1997). Job feedback: Giving, seeking, and using feedback for performance improvement. Mahwah, NJ: Erlbaum.

Lord, C. G., Desforges, D. M., Fein, S., Pugh, M., & Lepper, M. R. (1994). Typicality effects in attitudes toward social policies: A concept-mapping approach. *Journal of Personality and Social Psychology, 66,* 658–673.

Lord, C. G., & Maher, K. J. (1991). *Leadership and information processing.* London: Routledge.

Lord, C. G., & Saenz, D. S. (1985). Memory deficits and memory surfeits: Differential cognitive consequences of tokenism for tokens and observers. *Journal of Personality & Social Psychology, 49,* 918–926.

Lortie-Lussier, M. (1987). Minority influence and idiosyncracy credit: A new comparison of the Moscovici and Hollander theories of innovation. *European Journal of Social Psychology, 17,* 431–446.

Lott, A. J., & Lott, B. E. (1965). Group cohesiveness as interpersonal attraction: A review of relationships with antecedent and consequent variables. *Psychological Bulletin, 64,* 259–309.

Lovaglia, M. J., & Houser, J. A. (1996). Emotional reactions and status in groups. *American Sociological Review, 61,* 867–883.

Lundgren, D., & Knight, D. (1978). Sequential stages of development in sensitivity training groups. *Journal of Applied Behavioral Science, 14,* 204–222.

Mackie, D. M. (1986). Social identification effects in group polarization. *Journal of Personality and Social Psychology, 50,* 720–728.

Mackie, D. M., Allison, S. T., Worth, L. T., & Asuncion, A.G. (1992a). The generalization of outcome-biased counter-stereotypic inferences. *Journal of Experimental Social Psychology, 28,* 43–64.

Mackie, D. M., Allison, S. T., Worth, L. T., & Asuncion, A. G. (1992b). The impact of outcome biases on counterstereotypic inferences about groups. *Personality and Social Psychology Bulletin, 18,* 44–51.

Macrae, C. N., Bodenhausen, G. V., Milne, A. B. (1998). Saying no to unwanted thoughts: Self-focus and the regulation of mental life. *Journal of Personality and Social Psychology, 74,* 578–589.

Macrae, C. N., Bodenhausen, G. V., Milne, A. B., & Jetten, J. (1994). Out of mind but back in sight: Stereotypes on the rebound. *Journal of Personality and Social Psychology, 67,* 808–817.

Macrae, C. N., Milne, A. B., & Bodenhausen, G. V. (1994). Stereotypes as energy-saving devices: A peek inside the cognitive toolbox. *Journal of Personality and Social Psychology, 66,* 37–47.

Manias, E., & Street, A. (2001). The interplay of knowledge and decision making between nurses and doctors in critical care. *International Journal of Nursing Studies, 38,* 129–140.

Mann, R., Gibbard, G., & Hartman, J. (1967). *Interpersonal style and group development.* New York: Wiley.

Markus, H., & Zajonc, R. B. (1985). The cognitive perspective in social psychology. In G. Lindzey & E. Aronson (Eds.), *Handbook of social psychology,* (3rd ed.),(Vol. 1, pp. 137–230). New York: Random House.

Martel, E. (2001). From mensch to macho? The social construction of a Jewish masculinity. *Men and Masculinities, 3,* 347–369.

Martin, C. L. (1987). A ratio measure of sex stereotyping. *Journal of Personality and Social Psychology, 52,* 489–499.

Martin, R., & Davids, K. (1995). The effects of group development techniques on a professional athletic team. *Journal of Social Psychology, 135,* 533–535.

Maslow, A. H. (1970). *Motivation and personality* (2nd ed.). New York: Harper & Row.

Maslow, A. H. (1971). *The farther reaches of human nature.* New York: Viking Press.

Matsui, T., Kakuyama, T., & Onglato, M. U. (1987). Effects of goals and feedback on performance in groups. *Journal of Applied Psychology, 72,* 407–415.

Maupin, H. E., & Fisher, R. J. (1989). The effects of superior female performance and sex role orientation on gender infirmity. *Canadian Journal of Behavioral Science, 21,* 55–69.

Mayer, B. (2000). *The dynamics of conflict resolution: A practitioner's guide.* San Francisco: Jossey-Bass.

Mayo, E. (1933). *The human problems of an industrial civilization.* New York: Macmillan.

Mazur, A. (1985). A biosocial model of status in face-to-face groups. *Social Forces, 64,* 377–402.

McCauley, C. (1989). The nature of social influences in groupthink: Compliance and internalization. *Journal of Personality and Social Psychology, 57,* 250–260.

McCauley, C. (1998). Group dynamics in Janis's theory of groupthink: Backward and forward. *Organizational Behavior and Human Decision Processes, 73,* 142–162.

McClelland, D. C. (1985). *Human motivation.* Glenview, IL: Scott Foresman.

McEwen, C. A., & Milburn, T. W. (1993). Explaining a paradox of mediation. *Negotiation Journal, 9,* 23–36.

McGarty, C., Turner, J. C., Hogg, M. A., David, B., & Wetherell, M. S. (1992). Group polarization as conformity to the prototypical group member. *British Journal of Social Psychology, 31,* 1–20.

McGoldrick, M. (1998). *Re-visioning family therapy.* New York: Guilford.

McGrath, J. E. (1984). *Groups: Interaction and performance.* Englewood Cliffs, NJ: Prentice Hall.

McGrath, J. E. (1990). Time, interaction, and performance (TIP): A theory of groups. *Small Group Research, 22,* 147–194.

McGrath, J.E. (1993). The GEMCO Workshop: Description of a longitudinal study. *Small Group Research, 24,* 285–306.

McGrath, J. E. (1997). Small group research, that once and future field: An interpretation of the past with an eye to the future. *Group Dynamics, 1,* 7–27.

McGuire, W. (1973). The yin and yang of progress in social psychology. *Journal of Personality and Social Psychology, 26,* 446–456.

McLeod, P. L., Lobel., S. A., & Cox, T. H. J. (1996). Racioethnic diversity and creativity in small groups. *Small Group Research, 27,* 248–264.

Mead, G. H. (1934). *Mind, self, and society.* Chicago: University of Chicago Press.

Meeker, B. F. (1994). Performance evaluation. In M. Foschi & E. J. Lawler (Eds.), *Group processes: Sociological analyses* (pp. 95–118). Chicago: Nelson-Hall.

Mehrabian, A. (1972). *Nonverbal communication.* Chicago: Aldine Atherton.

Mennecke, B. E., Hoffer, J. A., & Wynne, B. E. (1992). The implications of group development and history for group support system theory and practice. *Small Group Research, 23,* 524–572.

Merry, S. E. (1984). Rethinking gossip and scandal. In D. Black (Ed.), *Toward a general theory of social control* (Vol. 1). Orlando, FL: Academic Press.

Miles, J. A., & Greenberg, J. (1993). Using punishment threats to attenuate social loafing effects among swimmers. *Organizational Behavior and Human Decision Processes, 56,* 246–265.

Miles, M. (1971). *Learning to work in groups.* New York: Teachers College Press.

Miller, C. T. (1982). The role of performance-related similarity in social comparison of abilities: A test of the related attributes hypothesis. *Journal of Experimental Social Psychology, 18,* 513–523.

Milliken, F. J., & Martins, L. L. (1996). Search for common threads: Understanding the multiple effects of diversity in organizational groups. *Academy of Management Review, 21,* 402–433.

Mills, T. M. (1964). *Group transformations: An analysis of a learning group.* Englewood Cliffs, NJ: Prentice Hall.

Mills, T. M. (1967). *The sociology of small groups.* Englewood Cliffs, NJ: Prentice Hall.

Milstein, M. M. (1983). Toward more effective meetings. *1983 Annual for Facilitators, Trainers, and Consultants.* San Francisco: Jossey-Bass.

Mintzberg, H. (1983). *Power in and around organizations.* Englewood Cliffs, NJ: Prentice Hall.

Miranda, S. M. (1994). Avoidance of groupthink: Meeting management using group support systems. *Small Group Research, 25,* 105–137.

Misumi, J. (1985). *The behavioral science of leadership: An interdisciplinary Japanese research program.* Ann Arbor: University of Michigan Press.

Misumi, J., & Peterson, M. (1985). The performance-maintenance (PM) theory of leadership: Review of a Japanese research program. *Administrative Science Quarterly, 30,* 198–223.

Monteith, M. J., Devine, P. G., & Zuwerink, J. R. (1993). Self-directed versus other-directed affect as a consequence of prejudice-related discrepancies. *Journal of Personality and Social Psychology, 64,* 198–210.

Montgomery, B. M. (1993). Relationship maintenance versus relationship change: A dialectical dilemma. *Journal of Social and Personal Relationships, 10,* 205–224.

Moreland, R. L., Argote, L., & Krishnan, R. (1996). Social shared cognition at work: Transactive memory and group performance. In J. L. Nye & A. M. Brower (Eds.), *What's social about social cognition? Social cognition research in small groups* (pp. 57–84). Newbury Park, CA: Sage.

Moreland, R. L., Argote, L., & Krishnan, R. (1998). Training people to work in groups. In R. S. Tindale,

L. Heath, J. Edwards, E. J. Posavac, F. B. Bryant, Y. Suarez-Balcazar, E. Henderson-King, & J. Myers (Eds.), *Theory and research on small groups* (pp. 37–56). New York: Plenum.

Moreland, R. L., & Levine, J. M. (1988). Group dynamics over time: Development and socialization in small groups. In J. E. McGrath (Ed.), *The social psychology of time: New perspectives* (pp. 151–181). Newbury Park, CA: Sage.

Moreland, R. L., & Levine J. M. (1995). *Group processes.* In A. Tesser (Ed.), *Advanced social psychology* (pp. 419–466). New York: McGraw-Hill.

Moreno, J. L. (1934). *Who shall survive?* Beacon, NY: Beacon House.

Moreno, J. L. (1943). Sociometry and the social order. *Sociometry, 6,* 299–344.

Moreno, J. L. (1953). *Who shall survive?* (Rev. ed.). Beacon, NY: Beacon House.

Morrison, A. M., & Von Glinow, M. A. (1990). Women and minorities in management. *American Psychologist, 45,* 200–208.

Morrison, J. G., Kelly, R. T., Moore, R. A., & Hutchins, S. G. (1998). Implications of decision-making research for decision support and displays. In J. A. Cannon-Bowers & E. Salas (Eds.), *Making decisions under stress: Implications for individual and team training* (pp. 375–406). Washington, DC: American Psychological Association.

Moscovici, S. (1985). Social influence and conformity. In G. Lindzey & E. Aronson (Eds.), *Handbook of social psychology* (Vol. 2, pp. 347–412). New York: Random House.

Moscovici, S. (1994). Three concepts: Minority, conflict, and behavioral style. In S. Moscovici, A. Mucchi-Faina, & A. Maass (Eds.), *Minority influence* (pp. 233–251). Chicago: Nelson-Hall.

Moscovici, S., Lage, E., & Naffrechoux, M. (1969). Influence of a consistent minority on the responses of a majority in a color perception task. *Sociometry, 32,* 365–380.

Moscovici, S., & Zavalloni, M. (1969). The group as a polarizer of attitudes. *Journal of Personality and Social Psychology, 12,* 125–135.

Moscowitz, G. B. (1996). The mediational effects of attributions and information processing in minority social influence. *British Journal of Social Psychology, 35,* 47–66.

Mosvick, R. K., & Nelson, R. B. (1987). *We've got to start meeting like this!* Glenview, IL: Scott Foresman, & Co.

Mullen, B. (1989). *Advanced BASIC meta-analysis.* Hillsdale, NJ: Erlbaum.

Mullen, B. (1991). Group composition, salience, and cognitive representations: The phenomenology of being in a group. *Journal of Experimental Social Psychology, 27,* 297–323.

Mullen, B., Anthony, T., Salas, E., & Driskell, J. E. (1994). Group cohesiveness and quality of decision making: An integration of tests of the groupthink hypothesis. *Small Group Research, 25,* 189–204.

Mullen, B., Brown, R., & Smith, C. (1992). Ingroup bias as a function of salience, relevance, and status: An integration. *European Journal of Social Psychology, 22,* 103–122.

Mullen, B., & Copper, C. (1994). The relation between group cohesiveness and performance: An integration. *Psychological Bulletin, 115,* 210–227.

Mullen, B., & Driskell, J. E. (1998). Meta-analysis and the study of group dynamics. *Group Dynamics: Theory, Research, and Practice, 2,* 213–229.

Mullen, B., Johnson, C., & Salas, E. (1991). Productivity loss in brainstorming groups: A meta-analytic integration. *Basic and Applied Social Psychology, 12,* 3–23.

Mullen, B., Salas, E., & Driskell, J. E. (1989). Salience, motivation, and artifact as contributions to the relation between participation and leadership. *Journal of Experimental Social Psychology, 25,* 545–559.

Mulvey, P. W., & Klein, H. J. (1998). The impact of perceived loafing and collective efficacy on group goal performance and group performance. *Organizational Behavior and Human Decision Processes, 74,* 62–87.

Nemeth, C. J. (1994). The value of minority dissent. In S. Moscovici, A. Mucchi-Faina, & A. Maas

(Eds.), *Minority influence* (pp. 3–16). Chicago: Nelson-Hall.

Nemeth, C. J., & Chiles, C. (1988). Modeling courage: The role of dissent in fostering independence. *European Journal of Social Psychology, 18,* 275–280.

Nemeth, C. J., & Wachtler, J. (1983). Creative problem solving as a result of majority versus minority influence. *European Journal of Social Psychology, 13,* 45–55.

Nevo, O., & Nevo, B. (1993). Gossip and counseling. *Counseling Psychology Quarterly, 6,* 229–239.

Northouse, P. G. (1997). *Leadership: Theory and practice.* Thousand Oaks, CA: Sage.

Nowack, A., Szamrej, J., & Latane, B. (1990). From private attitude to public opinion: A dynamic theory of social impact. *Psychological Review, 97,* 363–376.

Offermann, L. R., Kennedy, J. K., & Wirtz, P. W. (1994). Implicit leadership theories: Content, structure, and generalizability. *Leadership Quarterly, 5,* 43–55.

Ohbuchi, K., Fukushima, O., & Tedeschi, J. T. (1999). Cultural values in conflict management. *Journal of Cross-Cultural Psychology, 30,* 51–72.

Ohbuchi, K., & Takahashi, Y. (1994). Cultural styles of conflict. *Journal of Applied Social Psychology, 24,* 1345–1366.

Ohlott, P. J., Ruderman, M. N., & McCauley, C. D. (1994). Gender differences in managers' developmental job experiences. *Academy of Management Journal, 37,* 46–67.

O'Leary, A. M., Ilgen, D. R., Whitener, E. M., Salas, E., DeGregorio, M. B., & Shapiro, J. (1989, August). *Group goal setting: Generalizations from and extensions of goal setting theory.* Paper presented at the meeting of the National Academy of Management, Washington, DC.

O'Leary-Kelly, A. M., Martocchio, J. J., & Frink, D. D. (1994). A review of the influence of group goals on group performance. *Academy of Management Journal, 37,* 1285–1301.

Ones, D. S., Mount, M. K., Barrick, M. R., & Hunter, J. E. (1994). Personality and job performance: A

critique of the Tett, Jackson, and Rothsteing (1991) meta-analysis. *Personnel Psychology, 47,* 147–156.

Opp, K. D. (1982). The evolutionary emergence of norms. *British Journal of Social Psychology, 21,* 139–149.

Orasanu, J., Fischer, U., & Davison, J. (1997). Cross-cultural barriers to effective communication in aviation. In C. S. Granrose & S. Oskamp (Eds.), *Cross-cultural work groups* (pp. 134–162). Thousand Oaks, CA: Sage.

O'Reilly, C. A., III, Williams, K. Y., & Barsade, S. (1997). Group demography and innovation: Does diversity help? In M. A. Neale & E. A. Mannix (Eds.), *Research in the management of groups and teams* (Vol. 1, pp. 183–207). Greenwich, CT: JAI Press.

Osborn, A. F. (1957). *Applied imagination* New York: Scribner.

Osborn, A. F. (1963). *Applied imagination.* (2nd ed.). New York: Scribner.

Osgood, C. E. (1962). *An alternative to war or surrender.* Urbana: University of Illinois Press.

Ouchi, W. G. (1981). *Theory Z: How American business can meet the Japanese challenge.* Reading, MA: Addison-Wesley.

Owens, D. A., & Sutton, R. I. (2001). Status contests in meetings: Negotiating the informal order. In M. E. Turner (Ed.), *Groups at work: Theory and research* (pp. 299–316). Mahwah, NJ: Erlbaum.

Pandey, J. (1986). Sociocultural perspectives on ingratiation. In B. A. Maher & W. B. Maher (Eds.), *Progress in experimental personality research (14).* Orlando, FL: Academic Press.

Paris, C. R., Salas, E., & Cannon-Bowers, J. A. (2000). Teamwork in multi-person systems: A review and analysis. *Ergonomics, 43,* 1052–1075.

Parks, C. D., & Sanna, L. J. (1999). *Group performance and interaction.* Boulder, CO: Westview.

Parks, C. D., & Vu, A. D. (1994). Social dilemma behavior of individuals from highly individualist and collectivist cultures. *Journal of Conflict Resolution, 38,* 708–718.

Pelled, L. H. (1996). Demographic diversity, conflict, and work group outcomes: An intervening process theory. *Organization Science, 7,* 615–631.

Pelled, L. H. (1997). Relational demography and perceptions of group conflict and performance: A field investigation. *International Journal of Conflict Resolution, 7,* 230–246.

Pelled, L. H., Eisenhardt, K. M., & Xin, K. R. (1999). Exploring the black box: An analysis of work group diversity, conflict, and performance. *Administrative Science Quarterly, 44,* 1–28.

Peters, L. H., Hartke, D. D., & Pohlman, J. T. (1985). Fiedler's contingency theory of leadership: An application of the meta-analysis procedures of Schmidt and Hunter. *Psychological Bulletin, 97,* 274–285.

Peterson, R. S. (1997). A directive leadership style in group decision making can be both virtue and vice: Evidence from elite and experimental groups. *Journal of Personality and Social Psychology, 72,* 1107–1121.

Peterson, R. S., Owens, P. D., Tetlock, P. E., Fan, E. T., & Martorana, P. (1998). *Organizational Behavior and Human Decision Processes, 73,* 272–305.

Pettigrew, T. F. (1979). The ultimate attribution error: Extending Allport's cognitive analysis of prejudice. *Personality and Social Psychology Bulletin, 5,* 461–476.

Petty, R. E., Harkins, S. G., Williams, K., & Latane, B. (1977). The effects of group size on cognitive effort and evaluation. *Personality and Social Psychology Bulletin, 3,* 579–582.

Pfeffer, J. (1992). *Managing with power: Politics and influence in organizations.* Boston: Harvard Business School Press.

Podsakoff, P. M., Ahearne, M., & MacKenzie, S. B. (1997). Organizational citizenship behavior and the quantity and quality of work group performance. *Journal of Applied Psychology, 82,* 262–270.

Podsakoff, P. M., MacKenzie, S. B., Ahearne, M., & Bommer, W. H. (1995). Searching for a needle in a haystack: Trying to identify the elusive moderators of leadership behaviors. *Journal of Management, 21,* 423–470.

Podsakoff, P. M., Todor, W. D., Grover, R. A., & Huber, V. L. (1984). Situational moderators of leader reward and punishment behavior: Fact or fiction? *Organizational Behavior and Human Performance, 34,* 21–63.

Polley, R. B., Hare, A. P., & Stone, P. J. (1988). *The SYMLOG practitioner: Applications of small group research.* New York: Praeger.

Poole, M. S., & Hirokawa, R. Y. (1996). Introduction: Communication and group decision making. In M. S. Poole & R. Y. Hirokawa (Eds.), *Communication and group decision making,* (2nd ed.), (pp. 3–18). Thousand Oaks, CA: Sage.

Popielarz, P., & McPherson, M. (1995). On the edge or in between: Niche position, niche overlap, and the duration of voluntary association memberships. *American Journal of Sociology, 101,* 698–720.

Porter, L. W., & Lawler, E. E. (1968). *Managerial attitudes and performance.* Homewood, IL: Dorsey.

Powell, G. N. (1990). One more time: Do female and male managers differ? *Academy of Management Executive, 4,* 68–75.

Powell, G. N. (1999). Reflections on the glass ceiling: Recent trends and future prospects. In G. N. Powell (Ed.), *Handbook of gender and work* (pp. 325–346). Thousand Oaks, CA: Sage.

Pratto, F., & Bargh, J. A. (1991). Stereotyping based on apparently individuating information: Trait and global components of sex stereotypes under attention overload. *Journal of Experimental Social Psychology, 27,* 26–47.

Prentice, D. A., & Miller, D. T. (1996). Pluralistic ignorance and the perpetuation of social norms by unwitting actors. *Advances in Experimental Social Psychology, 28,* 161–209.

Pritchard, R. D., Jones, S. D., Roth, P. L., Struebing, K. K., & Ekeberg, S. E. (1988). Effects of group feedback, goal setting, and incentives on organizational productivity. *Journal of Applied Psychology, 73,* 139–145.

Pritchard, R. D., & Watson, M. D. (1992). Understanding and measuring group productivity. In S. Worchel, W. Wood, & J. A. Simpson (Eds.), *Group process and productivity* (pp. 251–276). Newbury Park, CA: Sage.

Propp, K. M. (1995). An experimental examination of biological sex as a status cue in decision making groups and its influence on information utilization. *Small Group Research, 26,* 451–474.

Propp, K. M. (1997). Information utilization in small group decision making. *Small Group Research, 28,* 424–454.

Pruitt, D. G., & Carnevale, P. J. (1993). *Negotiation in social conflict.* Pacific Grove, CA: Brooks/Cole.

Pruitt, D. G., Welton, G. L., Fry, W. R., McGillicuddy, N. B., Castrianno, L., & Zubek, J. M. (1989). The process of mediation: Caucusing, control, and problem solving. In M. A. Rahim (Ed.), *Managing conflict: An interdisciplinary approach.* New York: Praeger.

Prussia, G. E., & Kiniki, A. J. (1996). A motivational investigation of group effectiveness using social-cognitive theory. *Journal of Applied Psychology, 81,* 187–198.

Ragins, B. R. (1989). Barriers to mentoring: The female manager's dilemma. *Human Relations, 42,* 1–22.

Ragins, B. R. (1999). Gender and mentoring relationships: A review and research agenda for the next decade. In G. N. Powell (Ed.), *Handbook of gender and work* (pp. 203–222). Thousand Oaks, CA: Sage.

Ragins, B. R., & Sundstrom, E. (1989). Gender and power in organizations: A longitudinal perspective. *Psychological Bulletin, 105,* 51–88.

Ragins, B. R., Townsend, B., & Mattis, M. (1998). Gender gap in the executive suite: CEOs and female executives report on breaking the glass ceiling. *Academy of Management Executive, 12,* 28–42.

Rahim, M. A. (1983). A measure of styles of handling interpersonal conflict. *Academy of Management Journal, 26,* 368–376.

Raider, E., Coleman, S., & Gerson, J. (2000). Teaching conflict resolution skills in a workshop. In M. Deutsch & P. T. Coleman (Eds.), *The handbook of conflict resolution* (pp. 499–521). San Francisco: Jossey-Bass.

Rao, A., & Hashimoto, K. (1996). Intercultural influence: A study of Japanese expatriate managers in Canada. *Journal of International Business Studies, 27,* 443–467.

Rao, A., & Schmidt, S. M. (1995). Influence strategies in intercultural interaction: The view from Asia. *Advances in International Comparative Management, 10,* 79–98.

Rashotte, L. S., & Smith-Lovin, L. (1997). Who benefits from being bold? The interactive effects of task cues and status characteristics on influence in mock jury groups. In B. Markovsky, M. J. Lovaglia, & L. Troyer (Eds.), *Advances in group processes* (Vol. 14, pp. 235–246). London: Praeger.

Raven, B. (1993). Bases of power: Origins and recent developments. *Journal of Social Issues, 49,* 227–251.

Reber, G., Jago, A. G., & Bohnisch, W. (1993). Intercultural differences in leadership behavior. In M. Haller, K. Bleicher, E. Brauchlin, H.J. Pleitner, R. Wunderer, & A. Zund (Eds.), *Globalisierung der Wirtschaft: Einwirkungen auf die Betriebswirtschafslehre* (pp. 217–241). Bern, Switzerland: Verlag Paul Haupt.

Richardson, D. R., Green, L. R., & Lago, T. (1998). The relationship between perspective taking and nonaggressive responding in the face of an attack. *Journal of Personality, 66,* 235–254.

Ridgeway, C. L. (1982). Status in groups: The importance of motivation. *American Sociological Review, 47,* 76–88.

Ridgeway, C. L. (1987). Nonveral behavior, dominance, and the basis of status in task groups. *American Sociological Review, 52,* 683–694.

Ridgeway, C. L. (2001a). Gender, status, and leadership. *Journal of Social Issues, 57,* 637–656.

Ridgeway, C. L. (2001b). Social status and group structure. In M. A. Hogg & S. Tinsdale (Eds.), *Group processes* (pp. 352–375). Oxford, UK: Blackwell.

Ridgeway, C. L., & Balkwell, J. W. (1997). Group processes and the diffusion of status beliefs. *Social Psychology Quarterly, 60,* 14–31.

Ridgeway, C. L., & Berger, J. (1988). The legitimation of power and prestige orders in task groups. In M. Webster, Jr. & M. Foschi (Eds.), *Status Generalization: New Theory and Research* (pp. 207–31 and 497–501). Standford, CA: Stanford University Press.

Ridgeway, C. L., & Johnson, C. (1990). What is the relationship between socioemotional behavior and status in task groups? *American Journal of Sociology, 95,* 1189–1212.

Riordan, C., & Shore, L. (1997). Demographic diversity and employee attitudes: Examination of relational demography within work units. *Journal of Applied Psychology, 82,* 342–358.

Roan, S. (2001, October 27). Feel sick? Diagnosis: Hysteria. *Los Angeles Times,* p. A1.

Robert, H. M. Major (1876/1989). *Robert's rules of order.* New York: Berkeley Publishing Group.

Rodriguez, R. A. (1998). Challenging demographic reductionism: A pilot study investigating diversity, conflict, and performance. *Administrative Science Quarterly, 44,* 1–28.

Roethisberger, F. J., & Dickson, W. J. (1939). *Management and the worker.* Cambridge, MA: Harvard University Press.

Rogelberg, S. G., Barnes-Farrell, J. L., & Lowe, C. A. (1992). The stepladder technique: An alternative group structure facilitating effective group decision making. *Journal of Applied Psychology, 77,* 730–737.

Rogelberg, S. G., & Rumery, S. M. (1996). Gender diversity, team decision quality, time on task, and interpersonal cohesion. *Small Group Research, 27,* 79–90.

Rogers, C. (1970). *Carl Rogers on encounter groups.* New York: Harper & Row.

Rosenbaum, M. E. (1986). The repulsion hypothesis: On the nondevelopment of relationships. *Journal of Personality and Social Psychology, 51,* 1156–1166.

Rosenblatt, R. A. (2001, March 13). Census illustrates diversity from sea to shining sea. *Los Angeles Times,* p. A16.

Rosnow, R. L., & Fine, G. A. (1976). *Rumor and gossip: The social psychology of hearsay.* New York: Elsevier.

Roth, P. L. (1994). Group approaches to the Schmidt-Hunter global estimation procedure. *Organizational Behavior and Human Decision Processes, 59,* 428–451.

Rothman, J. (1997). *Resolving identity-based conflict.* San Francisco: Jossey-Bass.

Rouhana, N. N., & Kelman, H. C. (1994). Promoting joint thinking in international conflicts: An Israeli-Palestinian continuing workshop. *Journal of Social Issues, 50,* 157–178.

Rouse, W. B., Cannon-Bowers, J. A., & Salas, E. (1992). The role of mental models in team performance in complex systems. *IEEE Transactions on Systems, Man, and Cybernetics, 22,* 1296–1308.

Rowe, A. J., Boulgaides, J. D., & McGrath, M. R. (1984). *Managerial decision making.* Chicago: Science Research Associates.

Rubin, J. Z. (1989). Some wise and mistaken assumptions about conflict resolution. *Journal of Social Issues, 45,* 195–209.

Rubin, J. Z., Pruitt, D. G., & Kim, S. H. (1994). *Social conflict: Escalation, stalemate, and settlement* (2nd ed.). New York: McGraw-Hill.

Ruble, T. L., & Scheer, J. A. (1994). Gender differences in conflict-handling styles: Less than meets the eye? In A. Taylor & J. B. Miller (Eds.), *Conflict and gender* (pp. 155–166). Cresskill, NJ: Hampton Press.

Rudman, L., & Kilianski, S. (2000). Implicit and explicit attitudes toward female authority. *Prsonality and Social Psychology Bulletin, 26,* 1315–1328.

Rudman, L. A., & Glick, P. (2001). Prescriptive gender stereotypes and backlash toward agentic women. *Journal of Social Issues, 57,* 743–762.

Runnion, A., Johnson, T., & McWhorter, J. (1978). The effects of feedback and reinforcement on truck turnaround time in materials transportation. *Journal of Organizational Behavior Management, 1,* 110–117.

Salas, E., & Cannon-Bowers, J. A. (2000). The science of training: A decade of progress. *Annual Review of Psychology, 52,* 471–499.

Salas, E., Fowlkes, J., Stout, R. J., Milanovich, D. M., & Prince, C. (1999). Does CRM training improve teamwork skills in the cockpit? Two evaluation studies. *Human Factors, 41,* 326–343.

Salas, E., Prince, C., Bowers, C. A., Stout, R. J., Oser, R. L., & Cannon-Bowers, J. A. (1999). A methodology for enhancing crew resource management training. *Human Factors, 41,* 161–172.

Sande, G. N., Ellard, J. W., & Ross, M. (1986). Effect of arbitrarily assigned status labels on self perceptions and social perceptions: The mere position effect. *Journal of Personality and Social Psychology, 50,* 684–689.

Sapp, S. G., Harrod, W. J., & Zhao, L. (1996). Leadership emergence in task groups with egalitarian gender-role expectations. *Sex Roles, 34,* 65–80.

Satir, V., Banmen, J., Gerber, J., & Gormori, M. (1991). *The Satir model: Family therapy and beyond.* Palo Alto, CA: Science and Behavior Books, Inc.

Schacter, S. (1951). Deviation, rejection, and communication. *Journal of Abnormal and Social Psychology, 46,* 190–207.

Schafer, M., & Crichlow, S. (1996). Antecedents of groupthink: A quantitative study. *Journal of Conflict Resolution, 40,* 415–436.

Schaller, M. (1991). Social categorization and the formation of social stereotypes: Further evidence for biased information processing in the perception of group-behavior correlations. *European Journal of Social Psychology, 21,* 25–35.

Schmidt, S. M. (1992). The structure of leader influence: A cross-national comparison. *Journal of Cross-Cultural Psychology, 23,* 251–262.

Schriesheim, C. A., Tepper, B. J., & Tetrault, L. A. (1994). Least preferred co-worker score, situational control, and leadership effectiveness: A meta-analysis of contingency model performance predictions. *Journal of Applied Psychology, 79,* 561–573.

Scully, J. A., Kirkpatrick, S. A., & Locke, E. A. (1995). Locus of knowledge as a determinant of the effect of participation on performance, affect, and perceptions. *Organizational Behavior and Human Decision Processes, 61,* 276–288.

Shackleford, S., Wood, W., & Worchel, S. (1996). Behavioral styles and the influence of women in mixed sex groups. *Social Psychology Quarterly, 59,* 284–293.

Shaw, M. E. (1964). Communication networks. In L. Berkowitz (Ed.), *Advances in experimental social psy-chology* (Vol. 1, pp. 111–147). New York: Academic Press.

Shaw, M. E. (1971). *Group dynamics: The psychology of small group behavior.* New York: McGraw-Hill.

Shaw, M. E. (1978). Communication networks fourteen years later. In L. Berkowitz (Ed.), *Group processes: Papers from advances in experimental social psychology* (pp. 351–361). New York: Academic Press.

Shaw, M. E. (1981). *Group dynamics: The psychology of small group behavior* (3rd ed.). New York: McGraw-Hill.

Shaw, M. E., & Penrod, W. T. (1962). Does more information available to a group always improve group performance? *Sociometry, 25,* 377–390.

Shepperd, J. A. (1993). Productivity loss in performance groups: A motivational analysis. *Psychological Bulletin, 113,* 67–81.

Shepperd, J. A., & Taylor, K. (1999). Social loafing and expectancy-valence theory. *Personality and Social Psychology Bulletin, 25,* 1147–1159.

Sherif, M. (1936). *The Psychology of Social Norms.* New York: Harper & Row.

Sherif, M., Harvey, O. J., White, J., Hood, W., & Sherif, C. (1961). *Intergroup conflict and cooperation: The Robber's Cave experiment.* Norman: University of Oklahoma, Institute of Intergroup Relations.

Sherif, M., & Sherif, C. (1956). *An outline of social psychology* (rev. ed.). New York: Harper & Row.

Shimanoff, S. B. (1988). Group interaction via communication rules. In R. S. Cathcart & L. A. Samovar (Eds.), *Small group communication: A reader,* (5th ed.), (pp. 50–62). Dubuque, Iowa: W. C. Brown.

Sidanius, J., & Prado, F. (1999). *Social dominance.* New York: Cambridge University Press.

Sieberg, E., & Larson, C. (1971, April). Dimensions of interpersonal response. Paper presented to the annual conference of the International Communication Association, Phoenix.

Singer, J. E., Baum, C. S., Baum, A., & Thew, B. D. (1982). Mass psychogenic illness: The case for social comparison. In M. J. Colligan, J. W. Pennebaker, & L. R. Murphy (Eds.), *Mass psychogenic illness: A social psychological analysis* (pp. 155–169). Hillsdale, NJ: Erlbaum.

Singh, R., & Tan, L. S. C. (1992). Attitudes and attraction: A test of the similarity-attraction and dissimilarity-repulsion hypotheses. *British Journal of Social Psychology, 31,* 227–238.

Sinha, J. B. P. (1995). *The cultural context of leadership and power.* New Delhi: Sage.

Skevington, S., & Baker, D. (1989). Introduction. In S. Skevington & D. Baker (Eds.), *The social identity of women* (pp. 1–14). London: Sage.

Skvoretz, J. (1988). Models of participation in status-differentiated groups. *Social Psychology Quarterly, 51,* 43–57.

Slater, P. (1966). *Microcosm.* New York: Wiley.

Slavin, R. E., & Cooper, R. (1999). Improving intergroup relations: Lessons learned from cooperative education programs. *Journal of Social Issues, 55,* 647–665.

Slusher, M. P., & Anderson, C. A. (1987). When reality monitoring fails: The role of imagination in stereotype maintenance. *Journal of Personality and Social Psychology, 52,* 653–662.

Smith, H. J., & Tyler, T. R. (1997). Choosing the right pond: The impact of group membership on self-esteem and group-oriented behavior. *Journal of Experimental Social Psychology, 33,* 146–170.

Smith, K. G., Smith, K. A., O'Bannon, D. P., Olian, J. D., Sims, H. P., & Scully, J. (1994). Top management team demography and process: The role of social integration and communication. *Administrative Science Quarterly, 39,* 412–438.

Smith, P. B. (1963). Differentiation between sociometric rankings: A test of four theories. *Human Relations, 16,* 335–350.

Smith, P. B., & Bond, M. H. (1999). *Social psychology across cultures* (2nd ed). Boston: Allyn & Bacon.

Smith, P. B., & Tayeb, M. (1988). Organizational structure and processes. In M. H. Bond (Ed.), *The cross-cultural challenge to social psychology.* Newbury Park, CA: Sage.

Smith-Jentsch, K. A., Salas, E., & Baker, D. P. (1996). Training team performance-related assertiveness. *Personnel Psychology, 49,* 110–116.

Snyder, M. (1992). Motivational foundations of behavioral confirmation. In M. P. Zanna (Ed.), *Advances in experimental social psychology* (Vol. 25, pp. 67–114). San Diego: Academic Press.

Snyder, M., & Uranowitz, S. W. (1978). Reconstructing the past: Some cognitive consequences of person perception. *Journal of Personality and Social Psychology, 36,* 941–950.

Sorenson, P. S., Hawkins, K., & Sorenson, R. L. (1995). Gender, psychological type and conflict style preference. *Management Communication Quarterly, 9,* 115–127.

Spears, R., Lea, M., & Lee, S. (1990). De-individuation and group polarization in computer-mediated communication. *British Journal of Social Psychology, 29,* 121–134.

Spencer, S. J., Steele, C. M., & Quinn, D. (1999). Stereotype threat and women's math performance. *Journal of Experimental Social Psychology, 3,* 4–28.

Stahelski, A., Frost, D., & Patch, M. (1989). Use of Raveus socially dependent bases of power: French and Raveus theory applied to work group leadership. *Journal of Applied Social Psychology, 19,* 283–297.

Stahelski, A. J., & Paynton, C. F. (1995). The effects of status cues on choices of social power and influence strategies. *Journal of Social Psychology, 135,* 553–561.

Stasser, G., & Stewart, D. (1992). Discovery of hidden profiles by decision making groups: Solving a problem versus making a judgment. *Journal of Personality and Social Psychology, 53,* 81–93.

Steele, C. M. (1997). A threat is in the air: How stereotypes can shape intellectual ability and performance. *American Psychologist, 52,* 613–629.

Steele, C. M., & Aronson, J. (1995). Stereotype-threat and the intellectual test performance of African-Americans. *Journal of Personality and Social Psychology, 69,* 797–811.

Steele, C. M., Spencer, S. J., & Aronson, J. (1999). Stereotype threat, intellectual identification and the academic performance of women and minorities. In

M. Zanna (Ed.), *Advances in Experimental Psychology.*

Steil, J. M., & Weltman, K. (1992). Influence strategies at home and work: A study of six dual career couples. *Journal of Social and Personal Relationships, 9,* 65–88.

Steiner, I. D. (1972). *Group process and productivity.* New York: Academic Press.

Steiner, I. D. (1986). Paradigms and groups. *Advances in Experimental Social Psychology, 19,* 251–286.

Stephan, W. G. (1994, October). *Intergroup anxiety.* Paper presented at the meeting of the Society of Experimental Social Psychology, Lake Tahoe, CA.

Stiles, W. B., Lyall, L. M., Knight, D. P., Ickes, W., Waung, M., Hall, C. L., & Primeau, B. E. (1997). Gender differences in verbal presumptuousness and attentiveness. *Personality and Social Psychology Bulletin, 23,* 759–772.

Stodgill, R. M. (1948). Personal factors associated with leadership: A survey of the literature. *Journal of Psychology, 25,* 35–71.

Stodgill, R. M. (1972). Group productivity, drive and cohesiveness. *Organizational Behavior and Human Performance, 8,* 26–43.

Stodgill, R. M. (1974). *Handbook of leadership: A survey of the literature.* New York: Free Press.

Stohl, C., & Schell, S. E. (1991). A communication-based model of a small-group dysfunction. *Management Communication Quarterly, 5,* 90–110.

Stout, R. J., Salas, E., & Fowlkes, J. E. (1997). Enhancing teamwork in complex environments through team training. *Journal of Group Psychotherapy, Psychodrama, and Sociometry, 49,* 163–187.

Street, M. D. (1997). Groupthink: An examination of theoretical issues, implications, and future research suggestions. *Small Group Research, 28,* 72–92.

Suedfeld, P., & Tetlock, P. E. (1992). Psychological advice about political decision making: Heuristics, biases, and cognitive defects. In P. Suedfeld & P. E. Tetlock (Eds.), *Psychology and social policy* (pp. 51–70). Washington, DC: Hemisphere.

Suls, J., & Fletcher, B. (1983). Social comparison in the social and physical sciences: An archival study. *Journal of Personality and Social Psychology, 44,* 575–580.

Suls, J. M. (1977). Gossip as social comparison. *Journal of Communication, 27,* 164–167.

Sundstrom, E., DeMeuse, K. P., & Putrell, D. (1990). Work teams: Applications and effectiveness. *American Psychologist, 45,* 120–133.

Tajfel, H. (1981). *Human groups and social categories: Studies in social psychology.* Cambridge, England: Cambridge University Press.

Tajfel, H., Billig, M., Bundy, R., & Flament, C. (1971). Social categorization and intergroup behaviour. *European Journal of Social Psychology, 1,* 149–178.

Tang, J. (1997). The Model Minority thesis revisited: (Counter) evidence from the science and engineering fields. *Journal of Applied Behavioral Science, 33,* 291–314.

Tannen, D. (1995, September). The power of talk: Who gets heard and why. *Harvard Business Review,* pp. 138–148.

Taps, J., & Martin, P. Y. (1990). Gender composition, attributional accounts, and women's influence and likeability in task groups. *Small Group Research, 21,* 471–491.

Tavris, C. (1992). *The mismeasure of woman.* New York: Simon & Schuster.

Taylor, S. E. (1981). A categorization approach to stereotyping. In D. L. Hamilton (Ed.), *Cognitive processes in stereotyping and intergroup behavior* (pp. 358–369). Hillsdale, NJ: Erlbaum.

Taylor, S. E., Fiske, S. T., Etocoff, N. L., & Ruderman, A. J. (1978). Categorical and contextual bases of person memory and stereotyping. *Journal of Personality and Social Psychology, 36,* 778–793.

Tepper, B., Brown, S., & Hunt, M. D. (1993). Strength of subordinates' upward influence tactics and gender congruency effects. *Journal of Applied Social Psychology, 23,* 1903–1919.

Terry-Azios, D. A. (1999). Diversifying corporate America. *Hispanic, 12,* 82.

Tesser, A. (1988). Toward a self-evaluation maintenance model of social behavior. In L. Berkowitz (Ed.), *Advances in experimental social psychology* (Vol. 21, pp. 181–227). New York: Academic Press.

Tetlock, P., Peterson, R., McGuire, C., Chang, S., & Feld, P. (1992). Assessing political group dynamics: A test of the groupthink model. *Journal of Personality and Social Psychology, 63,* 403–425.

Thiagarajan, S. (1999). Challenge education. In D. G. Landon, K. S. Whiteside, & M. M. McKenna (Eds.), *Intervention resource guide: 50 performance improvement tools.* San Francisco: Jossey-Bass.

Thomas, D. A. (1990). The impact of race on managers' experiences of developmental relationship (mentoring and sponsorship): An intra-organizational study. *Journal of Organizational Behavior, 11,* 479–491.

Thomas, D. A, & Higgins, M. (1996). Mentoring and the boundaryless career: Lessons from the minority experience. In M. B. Arthur & D. M. Rousseau (Eds.), *The boundaryless career: A new employment principle for a new organizational era* (pp. 268–281). New York: Oxford University Press.

Thompson, L. (2000). *Making the team: A guide for managers.* Upper Saddle River, NJ: Prentice Hall.

Thorne, B. (1993). *Gender play.* New Brunswick, NJ: Rutgers University Press.

Timmerman, T. A. (2000). Racial diversity, age diversity, interdependence, and team performance. *Small Group Research, 31,* 592–606.

Tindale, R. S., & Anderson, E. M. (1998). Small group research and applied social psychology: An introduction in R. S. Tindale, L. Heath, J. Edwards, E. J. Posavac, R. B. Bryant, Y. Suarez-Bakazav, E. Henderson-King, & J. Myers (Eds.), *Theory and Research on Small Groups* (pp. 1–8). New York: Plenum.

Ting-Toomey, S. (1994). Managing conflict in intimate intercultural relationships. In D. D. Cahn (Ed.), *Conflict in personal relationships* (pp. 47–78). Hillsdale, NJ: Erlbaum.

Todd-Mancillas, W. R., & Rossi, A. (1985). Gender differences in the management of personnel disputes. *Women's Studies in Communication, 8,* 25–33.

Tolbert, P. S., Graham, M. E., & Andrews, A. O. (1999). Group gender composition and work group relations: Theories, evidence, and issues. In G. N. Powell (Ed.), *Handbook of gender and work* (pp. 179–202). Thousand Oaks, CA: Sage.

Tolbert, P. S., Simons, T., Andrews, A. O., & Rhee, J. (1995). The effects of gender composition in academic departments on faculty turnover. *Industrial and Labor Relations Review, 48,* 562–579.

Triandis, H. (1960). Cognitive similarity and communication in a dyad. *Human Relations, 13,* 279–287.

Triandis, H. (1994). *Culture and social behavior.* New York: McGraw-Hill.

Triandis, H., Hall, E., & Ewen, R. (1965). Member heterogeneity and dyadic creativity. *Human Relations, 18,* 33–55.

Triplett, N. (1898). The dynamogenic factors in pace making and competition. *American Journal of Psychology, 9,* 507–533.

Trubisky, P., Ting-Toomey, S., & Lin, S. L. (1991). The influence of individualism-collectivism and self-monitoring on conflict styles. *International Journal of Intercultural Relation, 15,* 65–84.

Tsui, A. S., Egan, T. D., & O'Reilly, C. A., III (1992). Being different: Relational demography and organizational attachment. *Administrative Science Quarterly, 37,* 549–579.

Tsui, A. S., & O'Reilly, C. A., III (1989). Beyond simple demographic effects: The importance of relational demography in superior-subordinate dyads. *Academy of Management Journal, 32,* 402–423.

Tuckman, B. W. (1965). Developmental sequence in small groups. *Psychological Bulletin, 63,* 384–399.

Tuckman, B. W., & Jensen, M. A. (1977). Stages of small-group development revisited. *Group and Organization Studies, 2,* 419–427.

Tung, R. L. (1997). International and intranational diversity. In C. S. Granrose & S. Oskamp (Eds.), *Cross-cultural work groups* (pp. 163–185). Thousand Oaks, CA: Sage.

Turner, J. C. (1981). The experimental social psychology of intergroup behaviour. In J. Turner & H. Giles (Eds.), *Intergroup behaviour* (pp. 66–101). Oxford: Blackwell.

Turner, J. C. (1982). Towards a cognitive redefinition of the social group. In H. Tajfel (Ed.), *Social identity and intergroup relations.* Cambridge: Cambridge University Press.

Turner, J. C., & Haslam, S. A. (2001). Social identity, organizations, and leadership. In M. E. Turner (Ed.), *Groups at work: Theory and research* (pp. 25–65). Mahwah, NJ: Erlbaum.

Turner, J. C., Wetherell, M. S., & Hogg, M. A. (1989). Referent informational influence and group polarization. *British Journal of Social Psychology, 28,* 135–137.

Turner, M. E., & Pratkanis, A. R. (1998). Twenty-five years of groupthink theory and research: Lessons from the evaluation of a theory. *Organizational Behavior and Human Decision Processes, 73,* 105–115.

Turner, M. E., Pratkanis, A. R., Probasco, P., & Leve, C. (1992). Threat, cohesion, and group effectiveness: Testing a social identity maintenance perspective on groupthink. *Journal of Personality and Social Psychology, 63,* 781–796.

Turner, R. H., & Killian, L. M. (1972). *Collective behavior* (2nd ed.). Englewood Cliffs, NJ: Prentice Hall.

Tushman, M. L. (1979). Work characteristics and subunit communication structure: A contingency analysis. *Administrative Science Quarterly, 24,* 82–97.

Twenge, J. M. (2001). Changes in women's assertiveness in response to status and roles: A cross-temporal meta-analysis, 1931–1993. *Journal of Personality and Social Psychology, 18,* 133–145.

Tyler, T. R., & Blader, S. L. (2000). *Cooperation in groups: Procedural justice, social identity, and behavioral engagement.* Philadelphia: Psychology Press.

Unger, R. (1990). Conflict management in group psychotherapy. *Small Group Research, 21,* 349–359.

U.S. Department of Labor. (1991). *A report on the Glass Ceiling Initiative.* Washington, DC: U.S. Department of Labor.

U.S. Department of Labor. (1997). *Facts on working women: Women in management.* (http://www.dol.gov/dol/wb/public/wb_pubs/wmgt97.htm)

Van de Ven, A. H., & Delbecq, A. L. (1974). The effectiveness of nominal, Delphi, and interacting group processes. *Academy of Management Journal, 17,* 605–621.

Van Dyne, L., & Saavedra, R. (1996). A naturalistic minority influence experiment: Effects on divergent thinking, conflict, and originality in work-groups. *British Journal of Social Psychology, 35,* 151–167.

Vaughn, S. (2001, July 15). Common ground for differences. *Los Angeles Times,* pp. W1, W3.

Vecchio, R. P. (1987). Situational leadership theory: An examination of a prescriptive theory. *Journal of Applied Psychology, 72,* 444–451.

Veiga, J. F. (1991). The frequency of self-limiting behavior in groups: A measure and an explanation. *Human Relations, 44,* 877–895.

Verdi, A. F., & Wheelan, S. A. (1992). Developmental patterns in same-sex and mixed-sex groups. *Small Group Research, 23,* 356–378.

Volkema, R. J., & Bergmann, T. J. (1997). Use and impact of informal third-party discussions in interpersonal conflicts at work. *Management Communication Quarterly, 11,* 185–216.

Volpe, C. E., Cannon-Bowers, J. A., Salas, E., & Spector, P. E. (1996). The impact of cross training on team functioning: An empirical investigation. *Human Factors, 38,* 87–100.

von Hippel, W., Sekaquaptewa, D., & Vargas, P. (1995). On the role of encoding processes in stereotype maintenance. *Advances in Experimental Social Psychology, 27,* 177–254.

Vroom, V. H. (1991). Leadership Revisited In B. M. Staw (Ed.), *Psychological dimensions of organizational behavior* (pp. 413–423). New York: Macmillan.

Vroom, V. H., & Jago, A. G. (1988). *The new leadership: Managing participation in organizations.* Englewood Cliffs, NJ: Prentice Hall.

Vroom, V. H., & Jago, A. G. (1995). Situation effects and levels of analysis in the study of leader participation. *Leadership Quarterly, 6,* 169–181.

Vroom, V. H., & Yetton, P. (1973). *Leadership and decision making.* Pittsburgh: University of Pittsburgh Press.

Wagner, G. W., Pfeffer, J., & O'Reilly, C. A. (1984). Organizational demography and turnover in top management groups. *Administrative Science Quarterly, 29,* 74–92.

Wagner, J. A., & Gooding, R. Z. (1987). Shared influence and organizational behavior: A meta-analysis of situational variables expected to moderate participation-outcome relationships. *Academy of Management Journal, 30,* 524–541.

Walker, I., & Mann, L. (1987). Unemployment, relative deprivation, and social protest. *Personality and Social Psychology Bulletin, 13,* 275–283.

Walton, R. E., & McKersie, R. B. (1965). *A behavioral theory of labor negotiations: An analysis of a social interaction system.* New York: McGraw-Hill.

Watson, W. E., Kumar, K., & Michaelson, L. K. (1993). Cultural diversity's impact on interaction process and performance: Comparing homogeneous and diverse task groups. *Academy of Management Journal, 36,* 590–602.

Watson, W. E., & Michaelsen, L. K. (1988). Group interaction behaviors that affect group performance on an intellective task. *Group and Organization Studies, 13,* 495–516.

Wayne, S. J., Kacmar, K. M., & Ferris, G. R. (1995). Coworker responses to others' ingratiation attempts. *Journal of Managerial Issues, 7,* 277–290.

Wayne, S. J., Liden, R. C., Graf, I. K., & Ferris, G. R. (1997). The role of upward influence tactics in human resource decisions. *Personnel Psychology, 50,* 979–1007.

Webster, M. (1994). Experimental methods. In M. Foschi & E.J. Lawler (Eds.), *Group processes: Sociological analyses* (pp. 43–69). Chicago: Nelson-Hall.

Webster, M. Jr., & Foschi, M. (1988). *Status generalization: New theory and research.* Stanford, CA: Stanford University Press.

Webster, M. Jr., & Hysom, S. J. (1998). Creating status characteristics. *American Sociological Review, 63,* 351–378.

Weingart, L. R., & Weldon, E. (1991). Processes that mediate the relationship between a group goal and group member performance. *Human Performance, 4,* 33–54.

Weingarten, H. R., & Douvan, E. (1985). Male and female visions of mediation. *Negotiation Journal, 1,* 349–358.

Weirsema, W. F., & Bantel, K. A. (1992). Top management team demography and corporate strategic change. *Academy of Management Journal, 35,* 91–121.

Weisfeld, G. E., & Weisfeld, C. C. (1984). An observational study of social evaluation: An application of the dominance hierarchy model. *Journal of Genetic Psychology, 145,* 89–99.

Weldon, E., & Gargano, G. M. (1988). Cognitive loafing: The effects of accountability and shared responsibility on cognitive effort. *Personality and Social Psychology Bulletin, 14,* 159–171.

Weldon, E., & Weingart, L. R. (1993). Group goals and group performance. *British Journal of Social Psychology, 32,* 307–334.

Welp, M. G. (1998). The treasures and challenges of diversity for white males. In A. Arien (Ed.), *Working together* (pp. 107–116). Pleasanton, CA: New Leaders Press.

Wharton, A. S., & Baron, J. N. (1987). So happy together? The impact of gender segregation on men at work. *American Sociological Review, 52,* 574–587.

Wheelan, S. (1990). *Facilitation training groups.* New York: Praeger.

Wheelan, S. A. (1994). *Group processes: A developmental perspective.* Boston: Allyn & Bacon.

Wheelan, S. A., & Hochberger, J. M. (1996). Validation studies of the Group Development Questionnaire. *Small Group Research, 27,* 143–170.

Wheelan, S. A., & Krasick, C. (1993). The emergence, transmission, and acceptance of themes in a temporary organization. *Group and Organization Management, 18,* 237–260.

Wheelan, S. A., & McKeage, R. (1993). Developmental patterns in small and large groups. *Small Group Research, 24,* 60–83.

Wheeler, L., & Kunitate, M. (1992). Social comparison in everyday life. *Journal of Personality and Social Psychology, 62,* 760–773.

Whetton, D. A., & Cameron, K. S. (1995). *Developing management skills* (3rd ed.). New York: HarperCollins.

White, R. K. (1983). Empathizing with the rulers of the USSR. *Political Psychology, 4,* 121–137.

White, R. K. (1984). *Fearful warriors: A psychological profile of U.S.-Soviet relations.* New York: Free Press.

Whitney, K. (1994). Improving task performance: The role of group goals and group efficacy. *Human Performance, 7,* 55–78.

Whyte, G. (1998). Recasting Janis's groupthink model: The key role of collective efficacy in decision fiascoes. *Organizational Behavior and Human Decision Making Processes, 73,* 185–209.

Whyte, W. F. (1943). *Street corner society.* Chicago: University of Chicago Press.

Williams, K. D., Harkins, S., & Latane, B. (1981). Identifiablity as a deterrent to social loafing: Two cheering experiments. *Journal of Personality and Social Psychology, 40,* 303–311.

Williams, K. D., & Karau, S. J. (1991). Social loafing and social compensation: The effects of expectations of co-worker performance. *Journal of Personality and Social Psychology, 40,* 303–311.

Williams, K. D., Nida, S. A., Baca, L. D., & Latane, B. (1989). Social loafing and swimming: Effects of identifiability of individual and relay performance of intercollegiate swimmers. *Basic and Applied Social Psychology, 10,* 73–81.

Williams, K. D., & Sommer, K. L. (1997). Social ostracism by coworkers: Does rejection lead to loafing or compensation? *Personality and Social Psychology Bulletin, 23,* 693–707.

Williams, K. Y., & O'Reilly, C. A. (1998). Demography and diversity in organizations: A review of 40 years of research. *Research in Organizational Behavior, 20,* 77–140.

Williams, S., & Taomina, R. J. (1993). Unanimous versus majority influences on group polarization in business decision making. *Journal of Social Psychology, 133,* 199–205.

Wilmot, W. W., & Hocker, J. (1998). *Interpersonal conflict* (5th ed.). New York: McGraw-Hill.

Wilson, S. R., Cai, D. A., Campbell, D. M., Donohue, W. A., & Drake, L. E. (1995). Cultural and communication processes in international business negotiations. In A. M. Nicotera (Ed.), *Conflict and organizations: Communicative processes* (pp. 201–238). Albany: State University of New York Press.

Winquist, J. R., & Larson, J. R., Jr. (1998). Information pooling: When it impacts group decision making. *Journal of Personality and Social Psychology, 74,* 371–377.

Wittenbaum, G. M., Stasser, G., & Merry, C. J. (1996). Tacit coordination in anticipation of small group task complexion. *Journal of Experimental Social Psychology, 32,* 129–152.

Wittenbaum, G. M., Vaughan, S. I., & Stasser, G. (1998). Coordination in task-performing groups. In R. S. Tindale, L. Heath, J. Edwards, E. J. Posavac, F. B. Bryant, Y. Suarez-Balcazr, E. Henderson-King, & J. Myers (Eds.), *Theory and research on small groups* (pp. 177–204). New York: Plenum.

Wofford, J. C., & Liska, L. Z. (1993). Path-goal theories of leadership: A meta-analysis. *Journal of Management, 19,* 858–876.

Wood, D., Kumar, V. K., Treadwell, T. W., & Leach, T. W. (1998). *International Journal of Action Methods, 51,* 122–138.

Wood, J. T. (1994). *Gendered lives.* Belmont, CA: Wadsworth.

Wood, W. (1987). Meta-analytic review of sex differences in group performance. *Psychological Bulletin, 102,* 53–71.

Wood, W., & Karten, S. J. (1986). Sex differences in interaction style as a product of perceived sex differences in competence. *Journal of Personality and Social Psychology, 50,* 341–347.

Wood, W., Lundgren, S., Ouellette, J. A., Busceme, S., & Blackstone, T. (1994). Minority influence: A meta-analytic review of social influence processes. *Psychological Bulletin, 115,* 323–345.

Wooten, D. B., & Reed, A. (1998). Informational influence and the ambiguity of product experience: Order effects on the weighting of evidence. *Journal of Consumer Research, 7,* 79–99.

Worchel, S., & Austin, W. G. (Eds.). (1986). *Psychology of intergroup relations* (2nd ed.). Chicago: Nelson-Hall.

Worchel, S., Coutant-Sassic, D., & Grossman, M. (1992). A developmental approach to group dynamics: A model and illustrative research. In S. Worchel, W. Wood, & J. A. Simpson (Eds.), *Group process and productivity* (pp. 181–202). Newbury Park, CA: Sage.

Worchel, S., Hart, D., & Butemeyer, J. (1989, April). *Is social loafing a group phenomenon?* Paper presented at the annual meeting of the Southwestern Psychological Association, Houston.

Yalom, I. D. (1975). *The theory and practice of group psychotherapy* (2nd ed.). New York: Basic Books.

Yalom, I. D. (1995). *The theory and practice of group psychotherapy* (4th ed.). New York: Basic Books.

Yetton, P. W., & Bottger, P. C. (1982). Individual versus group problem solving: An empirical test of a best-member strategy. *Organizational Behavior and Human Performance, 29,* 307–321.

Yoder, J. D. (1994). Looking beyond numbers: The effects of gender status, job prestige, and occupational gender-typing on tokenism processes. *Social Psychology Quarterly, 57,* 150–159.

Yoshioka, M. (2000). Substantive differences in the assertiveness of low-income African American, Hispanic, and Caucasian women. *Journal of Psychology: Interdisciplinary and Applied, 134,* 243–260.

Yukl, G. (1994). *Leadership in organizations* (3rd ed.). Englewood Cliffs, NJ: Prentice Hall.

Yukl, G. (1998). *Leadership in organizations* (4th ed.). Englewood Cliffs, NJ: Prentice Hall.

Yukl, G., & Falbe, C. M. (1990). Influence tactics and objectives in upward, downward, and lateral influence attempts. *Journal of Applied Psychology, 75,* 132–140.

Yukl, G., & Falbe, C. M. (1991). Importance of different power sources in downward and lateral relations. *Journal of Applied Psychology, 76,* 416–423.

Yukl, G., Falbe, C. M., & Youn, J. Y. (1993). Patterns of influence for managers. *Group and Organization Management, 18,* 5–29.

Yukl, G., Wall, S., & Lepsinger, R. (1990). Preliminary report on validation of the management practices survey. In K. E. Clark & M. B. Clark (Eds.), *Measures of leadership* (pp. 223–237). West Orange, NJ: Leadership Library of America.

Yukl, G. A. (1989). *Leadership in organizations* (2nd ed.). Englewood Cliffs, NJ: Prentice Hall.

Yukl, G. A., & Van Fleet, D. D. (1992). Theory and leadership in organizations. In G. A. Yukl & D. D. Van Fleet (Eds.), *Handbook of industrial and organizational psychology* (Vol. 3, pp.147–197). Palo Alto, CA: Consulting Psychologists Press.

Zaccaro, S. J. (1984). Social loafing: The role of task attractiveness. *Personality and Social Psychology Bulletin, 10,* 99–106.

Zaccaro, S. J., Foti, R. J., & Kenny, D. A. (1991). Self-monitoring and trait-based variance in leadership: An investigation of leader flexibility across multiple group situations. *Journal of Applied Psychology, 76,* 308–315.

Zajonc, R. B. (1968). Attitudinal effects of mere exposure. *Journal of Personality and Social Psychology Monograph Supplement, 9,* 1–27.

Zalesny, M. D. (1990). Rater confidence and social influence in performance appraisals. *Journal of Applied Psychology, 75,* 274–289.

Zander, A. (1979). Research on groups. *Annual Review of Psychology, 30,* 417–452.

Zander, A. (1982). *Making groups effective.* San Francisco: Jossey-Bass.

Zander, A. (1994). *Making groups effective* (2nd ed.). San Francisco: Jossey-Bass.

Zander, A. (1996). *Motives and goals in groups.* New Brunswick, NJ: Transaction Publishers.

Zander, A., Forward, J., & Albert, R. (1969). Adaptation of board members to repeated failure and success by their organization. *Organizational Behavior and Human Performance, 4,* 56–76.

Zane, N. W., Sue, S., Hu, L., & Kwon, J. H. (1991). Asian American assertion: A social learning analysis of cultural differences. *Journal of Counseling Psychology, 38,* 63–70.

Zhuralev, A. L. , & Shorokhova, E. V. (1984). The human choice: Individuation, reason and order versus deindividuation, impulse and chaos. In W. J. Arnold & D. Levine (Eds.), *Nebraska symposium on motivation, 17,* 237–307.

Zimbardo, P. G., Banks, W. C., Haney, C., & Jaffe, D. (1973, April 8). The mind is a formidable jailer: A Pirandellian prison. *New York Times Magazine,* pp. 38–60.

Glossary

Abilene paradox Occurs when members are so motivated to get along that they all end up agreeing to something no one wants.

Ability and skill diversity Member differences in abilities and skills.

Acculturation strategies The variety of ways in which individuals and groups can respond to diversity, ranging from the isolation of minority group members to integration.

Achieved status Status that is earned.

Actual productivity A group's potential productivity minus process losses (AP = PP − PL), what they actually accomplish compared to what they could have.

Ad hoc groups An artificial group created solely for the purpose of studying it in a controlled laboratory setting.

Additive multiculturalism (integration) The idea that we should respond to diversity by working to understand and appreciate other groups and integrate diverse perspectives.

Adjourning stage The final stage of the basic model of group development, in which members begin to disengage from social, emotional, and task activities.

Affective stage The third stage of social penetration theory, in which close friendships develop and some intimate details are exchanged, but some barriers remain.

Affiliative constraints When a desire to maintain positive relationships between group members or a reluctance to question powerful members causes members to hold back in decision discussions.

Agenda A written list of specific meeting goals and objectives.

Analytic empathy (realistic empathy) When parties understand what each side cares most about in the conflict and why it matters so much (each sides' true issues), making integration possible.

Arbitration A type of third-party intervention in which the third party's recommendations for settlement are binding.

Ascribed status Status given to individuals by virtue of their having some characteristic that a group has designated as prestigious and valuable.

Assertive behavior Behaviors oriented toward asserting one's own rights, opinions, or boundaries in a way that also respects the rights of others.

Autistic hostility When conflicting parties break off contact, making conflict resolution difficult because there is no opportunity to correct misperceptions.

Autocratic (authoritarian) leaders A highly task-oriented, controlling type of leadership in which leaders use their power to coerce others to follow them and allow them little input.

Autonomy/connection dialectic The relationship tension created by our desire to be independent and our desire to be emotionally connected to another.

Basking in reflected glory How we can be proud and happy for a significant other who performs well on a task that is not important to us.

Behavior theories of leadership Leadership theories that focus on leader behavior and leadership styles.

Bolstering When group members convince themselves that their quick decision is a good one by emphasizing its advantages and overlooking disadvantages and alternatives.

Brainstorming A technique where group members first offer as many ideas as possible without discussion or evaluation, and then discuss the merits of the ideas.

Case studies In-depth profiles of groups.

Centralized communication network A communication structure in which members must go through a central person to communicate with one another and one member is the principal source and target of communication.

Challenge education Games or outdoor activities intended to develop teamwork skills.

Charisma Power that originates in an individual's charm or enthusiasm.

Closed-ended items Questionnaire items that require participants respond to items using the options provided.

Coercive power When a member has power over other members because she or he can deliver punishments to members who do not comply.

Cognitive constraints When a group does not consider all relevant information when making a decision, most commonly because of limited time.

Collective efficacy (group efficacy) Members' beliefs that the team's efforts will lead to success.

Collective effort model Suggests that social loafers slack because they do not think their efforts will increase group performance, increase rewards, or lead to valued outcomes, so they slack.

Collective information-processing model A model emphasizing that individual members possess unique information relevant to the group decision.

Collective memory The combined memory of the group's members, usually superior to the memory of an individual because members remember different things.

Collective mind LeBon's name for his idea that crowds come to act as (one mind) that overrides the minds of individuals.

Collective orientation Having positive attitudes toward working as part of a team.

Collectivistic cultures Cultures that emphasize the importance of the group and community and that value conformity.

Communication The transmission of information and understanding between group members.

Communication structure A group's established communication network, the pattern of information sharing in the group.

Competitive goal structure A conflict context where it is believed that the goals of the two parties are divergent and cannot be reconciled.

Competitive or defensive climate A communication climate in which members distrust one another and communication is competitive.

Concession-convergence model (distributive bargaining) Negotiation model in which each side stakes out a tough position and "baby steps" are made toward agreement.

Confidentiality The researcher's commitment to protect the identities of those studied.

Confirming responses Supportive responses that encourage the sharing of ideas.

Conflict spiraling The escalation of conflict in a progressive pattern of attack and counterattack.

Congruent message When the verbal and nonverbal content of a message are consistent and match.

Construct validity The extent to which a research instrument measures what it is intended to measure.

Constructive conflict A conflict that is primarily cooperative and oriented toward joint problem solving and the maintenance of a working relationship.

Constructive confrontations Calm, well-prepared confrontations that involve clarifying and exploring the issues and the feelings of the participants, and mutual problem solving.

Constructive controversy When parties seek a collaborative agreement in a respectful climate.

Contact hypothesis The assumption that bringing conflicting parties into contact will be enough to reduce conflict.

Context-driven team training Training that is tailor-made for a specific team based on the team's context and task.

Contingency (situational) theories of leadership Leadership theories emphasizing that the situation determines whether a given style of leadership will be effective.

Cooperative education A set of techniques designed to reduce intergroup tensions in educational settings by engineering equal-status contact and superordinate goals.

Cooperative goal structure A context in which conflicting parties believe that they can work together to satisfy both parties' goals.

Cooperative or supportive climate A communication climate in which members feel free to communicate honestly and the communication is directed toward the group's work.

Coordination losses Process losses that occur when group members do not optimally synchronize their efforts.

Corey and Corey's therapy group development model A model describing how trust and cohesion develop in the therapy group so that therapeutic progress can be made.

Correlational methods Nonexperimental methods that tell us whether variables are statistically related but cannot tell us about causality.

Counterdependency and fight stage Stage 2 of the integrative model of group development, in which members conflict as they express their goals and ideas about group structure.

Crew resource management (CRM) Context-driven training in which specific training objectives are identified before training materials are developed.

Cultural distance The extent to which one culture differs from another.

CYA rule ("cover-your-ass rule") When members withhold information or opinions that contradict group leaders to avoid retribution and gain leader approval.

Debriefing Sharing the details and results of the study with research participants at the study's conclusion.

Decay Stage 6 of the developmental model, in which discontent and alienation occur, and the cycle repeats.

Decentralized communication network A communication structure in which information flows between members without going through a central person and communication and access to information are more or less equally distributed.

Decision-making constraints Factors that inhibit effective group decision making, including cognitive, affiliative, and egocentric constraints.

Decision styles Group member differences in approaches to group decision making.

Deep-level diversity Member diversity arising out of attitudinal, belief, and value differences.

Delphi technique A way to collect and synthesize the opinions of a group of experts into a decision using a series of written communications.

Democratic leader A consultative, socioemotional type of leadership in which followers are asked for input and leaders attend to followers' personal needs and wants.

Demographic diversity (social category diversity) Diversity based on attributes such as gender, age, country of origin, or ethnicity.

Dependency and inclusion stage Stage 1 of the integrative model of group development, in which members are dependent on the leader and concerned about being accepted.

Dependent variable (DV) In an experiment, the measured "effect" variable, expected to change depending on the level of the independent variable.

Destructive conflicts Conflicts that damage the group and relationships between members or groups.

Differentiation A part of constructive controversy in which parties illuminate the differences in their positions.

Diffuse-status characteristics Demographically derived status characteristics, such as age, ethnicity, gender, or attractiveness.

Disconfirming responses Unsupportive responses that make members feel disregarded or rejected.

Dissent To challenge group norms.

Diversity How similar or different group members are from one another.

Downward social comparison The comparison of ourselves to others who are worse than we are on a trait, skill, or ability.

Dual-concern model Suggests five conflict resolution styles that vary depending on how concerned the person is with his or her own outcomes as compared with the other party's outcomes.

Dual-process approach to minority influence The idea that majorities and minorities both exert influence on the group, but in different ways.

Dyad A two-person group.

Ecological fallacy The mistaken belief that because two cultures differ, that any two members of those cultures must necessarily differ in that same manner.

Effect size In meta-analysis, a statistic *(d)* that indicates across studies how strong the research finding is.

Effectiveness The ratio of outputs to goals or expectations; whether the group met or exceeded expectations or goals.

Efficiency The ratio of inputs to outputs; how much time and resources it takes a group to produce or achieve something.

Egocentric constraints When members withhold information or opinions because controlling or self-interested members control the discussion.

Emergent leadership The study of who tends to emerge as a leader of a group and how groups choose a leader in an initially leaderless group.

Enemy imagery Stereotypes of the opposing party that suggest they are hostile or evil.

Equity theory Says that people desire equity and decide whether what they receive is fair depending on how it compares to what others receive.

Ethical (positive) charismatics Charismatic leaders who use their power to achieve the collective interests of the group, organization, or society.

Ethical review board A government or university committee that reviews proposed research to determine whether it is in accordance with standard ethical guidelines.

Ethnocentrism The belief that the customs, norms, and values of our ingroup are universally valid and correct.

Ethological approach to status Suggests that the physical strength and size of members influences their status in the group.

Evolutionary norms Norms originating in a member's response to a situation that is adopted as a norm by the group.

Exception-to-the-rule category A schema created to accommodate what a person thinks is a rare case contradicting an otherwise "correct" stereotype.

Expectancy In expectancy-valence theory, a belief about whether increased effort will lead to increased performance.

Expectation states theory Proposes that groups make status assignments based on expectations of each member's ability and potential to contribute to the group.

Experimental confederate A researcher's accomplice who is part of the independent variable manipulation or experimental situation.

Experimental confounds Extraneous factors in a study that confuse our ability to draw clear conclusions about our findings.

Experimental control A key experimental feature that requires that everything in the setting stay the same except for the independent variable.

Experimental method A research method designed to test cause–effect relationships by systematically manipulating hypothesized causal variables while holding all other variables constant.

Expert power When a member is able to influence others because of his or her knowledge or expertise.

Explicit coordination Occurs when members discuss how they will coordinate their actions and make conscious their plans for executing tasks.

Exploratory affective stage The second stage of social penetration theory, in which more information is exchanged, but it is still not very personal.

External validity The extent to which a study's findings can be applied or generalized to other people and settings.

Feedback cycle A cycle in which group members set success criteria, perform, compare the performance with criteria, and set new goals or procedures, before beginning again.

Fiedler's contingency model A contingency theory suggesting that the effectiveness of a leader's style depends on leader–member relations, task structure, and position power.

Field experiment An experiment conducted in a real-world setting.

Field theory Theories suggesting that the behavior of group members is due to an interactive field of influences, including personal, interpersonal, group, and situation.

Final phase The last period in the development of the time-limited task group, in which the group accelerates its production in order to meet the deadline.

Final stage The termination stage of the therapy group; ideally used as another opportunity for personal growth, learning, or adjustment.

Formal communication network A layered communication network officially designated by the group or organization.

Forming stage The first stage in the basic model of group development, in which member participation is hesitant and dependent on the leader and rules.

Forward-backward (F-B) dimension In SYMLOG, whether the behavior of a group member, group, or organization supports the task orientation of the established authority (F) or opposes the established authority (B).

Fraternal deprivation The perception that one's group is unfairly given a low status relative to other groups.

Free rider effects When some members are "free riders" benefiting from others' efforts, usually because they believe that their own efforts are dispensable.

Gender and ethnic job segregation The finding that most jobs are gender typed and that particular ethnic groups are rarely found in some job categories.

Glass ceiling Term used to refer to the invisible barriers hindering the promotion of women and members of other traditionally underrepresented groups into high leadership positions.

Goals The mission, purpose, or objectives that guide the group's actions and allow the group to plan and coordinate members' efforts.

Gossip Communications about other group members that may or may not be factual.

Grapevine The channel through which gossip, rumors, and other unofficial information travels through the group.

GRIT (Graduated and Reciprocated Initiatives in Tension-Reduction) A systematic conflict resolution program in which each side makes increasingly cooperative gestures.

Group Two or more interacting, interdependent people.

Group cohesion A multidimensional concept that includes a sense of we-ness and belongingness, members' liking of the group and one another, and teamwork.

Group communication climate Whether the context in which group communication occurs is cooperative and supportive or defensive and competitive.

Group composition The types of people that comprise the team—their knowledge, skills, abilities, and other traits.

Group coordination The ways in which group members synchronize their actions in order to successfully complete the group task; who does what, when, where, and how.

Group development How groups change over time as members interact, learn about one another, and structure relationships and roles within the group.

Group dynamics The scientific study of group processes with the goal of understanding and improving groups.

Group identification Stage 3 of the developmental approach, in which the dissatisfied subgroup breaks off and forms a new group.

Group performance (group productivity) The quantity or quality of the outcomes produced, or the time required for task completion.

Group polarization The tendency for group discussion to amplify members' initial inclinations so that the average inclination of group members is strengthened.

Group productivity Stage 4 of the developmental approach, in which the new group, having formed a clear identity, turns its attention to accomplishing goals and tasks.

Group socialization Changes in the relationship between the group and each of its members.

Group structure The group's norms and roles, patterns of prestige and authority, and communication network.

Group support systems (GSS) A technique in which group members use computers to interact, often anonymously; intended to increase the number of ideas and reduce normative pressures and groupthink.

Groupness The extent to which an aggregate functions as a group. Smaller groups with a high level of interaction and a past and future are higher in groupness.

Groupthink The defective decision making that arises in a cohesive group when members seek consensus before fully evaluating alternatives.

High-context communication Indirect communication where the meaning of messages is conveyed by how something is said rather than what is said, common in collectivistic cultures.

Incongruent message When the verbal content and the nonverbal content of a message are mixed and suggest different things.

Independent variable (IV) In an experiment, the hypothesized causal variable, systematically varied (manipulated) by the researcher.

Individualistic cultures Cultures that emphasize the importance of the individual, value independence, and view conformity negatively.

Individualism/collectivism The extent to which individuals in a society view themselves as individuals or as part of a group.

Individuation Stage 5 of the developmental model, in which members shift from a focus on the group to a focus on their own goals and needs within the group.

Influence tactics The specific behaviors that individuals use to wield power and influence others.

Informal communication network A group's unofficial communication network.

Information power When a person has power because he or she possesses information that others want.

Informational diversity Member differences in knowledge bases and perspectives.

Informational pressure The pressure to conform because of uncertainty and a need for information.

Informed consent A statement signed by research participants prior to participation in a study; it provides enough information that they can make a knowledgeable decision.

Ingroup bias When members selectively process their own group's actions in order to maintain a positive view of the group.

Initial stage The first stage in the therapy group, in which members are anxious about being rejected and revealing themselves.

In-process planning Ongoing planning that occurs during the group's work; important when tasks are difficult and variable.

Institutional norms Norms that originate in a group's leader or external authorities.

Instrumentality In expectancy-valence theory, a belief that increased performance will be rewarded and recognized.

Integration A part of constructive controversy in which the parties work to combine their positions into a new position.

Integrative model of group development A revised, expanded version of the basic group development model that emphasizes that group development is ongoing and cyclical.

Interaction process analysis (IPA) An observational coding system developed by Bales to reliably measure six task and six socioemotional activities in a group.

Intercultural approach Perspective that emphasizes helping people to understand, accept, and value the cultural differences between groups.

Intercultural competence The ability to interact effectively with people from other cultures.

Intercultural conflict Conflict involving parties from different cultures.

Intercultural exploration A process of sharing cultural assumptions and values that is intended to avert or clarify misunderstandings and misperceptions that arise out of cultural differences.

Intercultural sensitizer (ICS) A programmed training exercise designed to teach that different behaviors have different meanings in different cultures.

Intergroup anxiety The worry and arousal, and consequent avoidance or excessive politeness, that may occur when we interact with people who are not from our group.

Intergroup conflict Conflict between groups.

Internal validity The ability to conclude from the study results that there is or is not a cause–effect relationship between the variables.

Interpersonal conflict Conflict between two group members.

Interpositional training Training designed to promote a team mental model by giving members a working knowledge of teammate duties and tasks, and how they are related.

Interrater reliability The extent to which the ratings of different observers are in agreement; boosted by careful training.

Intragroup conflict Conflict within a group involving more than two members.

Investigation phase The first phase of group socialization, in which the group recruits new members and potential members look for a group that fits their needs.

Isomorphic attribution When we interpret the behavior of others in the same way they intended it.

Leader prototype A mental picture of what a model leader should look and be like; the leader archetype.

Leadership A process that includes influencing the choice of goals and strategies of a group or organization, influencing people to accomplish goals, and promoting a group identity and commitment.

Leadership categorization theory A theory suggesting that we compare potential leaders to our leader prototypes and this determines whether we cast them in leader roles.

Least Preferred Coworker (LPC) Scale Instrument used by Fiedler to classify leaders as task or socioemotionally oriented based on their ratings of a least preferred coworker.

Legitimate power When a member is seen as having the right to tell other members what to do because of his/her position of authority in the group.

Loose culture A culture in which norms are less clear and deviance is tolerated.

Low-context communication Direct and precise communication where value is placed on providing a clear message through words, common in individualistic cultures.

Maintenance phase The third phase of group socialization, in which the person and the group try to reach an agreement that satisfies the goals of both parties.

Marketing argument (cultural rationale) for diversity Suggests that diversity's value lies in its potential to increase profits or create better products or services.

Masculinity/femininity Whether a society's dominant values emphasize assertiveness and materialism (masculine) or other-centeredness and quality of life (feminine).

Mass psychogenic illness The occurrence in a group of people of similar physical symptoms with no apparent physical cause.

Mediation A type of third-party intervention in which advisory recommendations are made but do not have to be heeded by the disputants.

Member heterogeneity Differences among group members.

Member homogeneity Similarity of group members.

Mere exposure effect The more often we are exposed to something, the more we like it; explains why we like familiar things and people.

Message matching The idea that message senders should tailor their message to the target so that the intended message will be understood.

Meta-analyses A quantitative, statistical integration of the research literature done to arrive at an overall estimate of the size of the differences between groups.

Metaconflict A situation in which new issues produced by the conflict overshadow the issues that initially triggered it.

Mindguards Members who protect the group from receiving information that might shake confidence in their decision; a symptom of groupthink.

Minority influence The idea that a minority of group members can influence the majority.

Mirror image The tendency for the two sides in a conflict to perceive each other in a similar, negative way.

Motivational losses Process losses that occur when members reduce their efforts because they do not value the group or goal or do not think their efforts matter.

Mundane realism The extent to which an experiment is similar to real-life situations.

Mutual gains approach (integrative bargaining) Negotiation model in which both sides share what they want and why they want it, with the goal of coming up with a solution that satisfies the major issues of both parties.

Narrative review A method for examining the research literature on a topic by counting the number of studies that support a particular hypothesis.

Negotiation When conflicting parties use an exchange of offers and ideas to come to a settlement.

Nominal group technique (NGT) A technique where group members first brainstorm individually, and are then polled to ensure all ideas are shared.

Nonverbal communication The way we communicate using body language such as gestures, body orientation, touching, personal distance, paralanguage, and facial expressions.

Normative decision model Proposes that how much leaders should consult the group when making a decision depends on decision quality, decision acceptance, and time.

Normative pressure The pressure to conform in order to be socially accepted and avoid rejection.

Norming stage The third stage of the basic model of group development, characterized by group cohesion and the emergence of structure, roles, and "we-feeling."

Norms Group rules or expectations that specify appropriate behavior for group members.

Norms of competition Norms supportive of members' seeking personal goals at the expense of other members.

Norms of cooperation Norms encouraging members to support one another toward the achievement of the group's goals.

Norms Shared expectations about how the members of a group ought to behave.

Novelty/predictability dialectic The relationship tension created by our desire for excitement and our competing desire for the comfort of the familiar.

Observational methods A set of nonexperimental methods in which observers watch groups to gather information.

Open-ended items Questionnaire items that permit participants to answer in whatever way they choose, with no preset options to choose from and no rating scales.

Openness/closedness dialectic The relationship tension created by wanting to reveal ourselves and maintain our privacy.

Organizational supports Systems and resources that organizations and leaders provide to support teamwork.

Orientation stage The first stage of social penetration theory, in which people exchange superficial information about themselves.

Outgroup bias When members of one group selectively process the actions of another group to maintain a negative view of that group.

Paralanguage A form of nonverbal communication that includes voice pitch, rate, quality, and tone as well as nonword communications such as "tsking" and sighing.

Participative decision making (PDM) A leadership continuum reflecting a range of member participation ranging from no participation to joint decision making.

Participant observation An observational method in which the researcher becomes a member of the group being studied and keeps thorough field notes.

Path-goal theory of leadership A contingency theory recommending that leaders vary their style depending on the members and the task, and should clarify how to reach goals.

Pearson r (correlation coefficient) A statistic, ranging from $+1$ to -1, that indicates how strongly two variables are related to one another.

Perceptual distortion The exaggerated misinterpretation and attribution of hostile intentions to an opponent's actions.

Performance expectations Assumptions about the ability of other group members to contribute to the group's goals, often based on status characteristics.

Performance plan Specific description of a time-and-function-linked series of actions designed to lead to a specific goal or outcome; who will do what, when, where, and how.

Performing stage The fourth stage of the basic model of group development, in which the group focuses on task accomplishment.

Period of discontent Stage 1 of the developmental approach, in which some members feel alienated and estranged from the group.

Personal diversity Member differences in attributes such as personality and background.

Personal power Power that arises from a person's individual characteristics; includes expert, referent, persuasive, and charisma power.

Persuasive arguments explanation for group polarization Suggests that group polarization occurs as members hear additional arguments favoring their prediscussion preferences.

Persuasive power Power derived from a person's ability to use rational argument, facts, and persuasion to influence others.

Pluralistic ignorance Occurs when group members mistakenly assume that others know what's going on; a backfiring of informational pressure.

Political behavior Actions taken by group members to gain a power or status advantage over others.

Position power Power that is based in a person's formal position in the group; includes legitimate, reward, coercive, and information power.

Positive-negative (P-N) dimension In SYMLOG, whether the behavior of a group member, group, or organization is friendly (P) or unfriendly (N).

Power The ability of a group member to get other members to do what he or she wants them to do.

Power distance In a culture, the amount of respect and deference less powerful (subordinate) members generally give to more powerful (superior) members.

Precipitating event Stage 2 of the developmental approach, in which a distinctive event has the effect of galvanizing disgruntled members.

Pre-plans Job descriptions, policies, schedules, and standard operating procedures.

Priming effect The more recently a schema has been activated, the more accessible it is to memory, and the more likely it is to be applied in another context.

Process directiveness The way a leader brings out different viewpoints and orchestrates a democratic decision process.

Process gain When group work increases productivity because it causes members to work harder or more efficiently.

Process loss Loss of productivity that results from motivational or coordination losses.

Production norms Norms specifying how hard to work and how much to produce.

Psychological realism The extent to which an experiment triggers relevant psychological and group processes.

Punctuated equilibrium The idea that time-limited task groups alternate between periods of inertia, in which the group acts according to plan, and periods of creativity and change.

Punctuated equilibrium model Gersick's group development model focusing on time-limited task groups with specific deadlines.

Quasi-experiment A correlational method in which real-world groups that differ on a quasi-IV are compared on a dependent variable.

Random assignment A key experimental feature in which research participants have an equal chance of ending up in any of the IV groups.

Reciprocal liking The idea that an important determinant of our liking of others is whether we think they like us.

Referent power When others take up the suggestions of a member out of respect and liking for that member.

Relational dialectics The idea that dyadic relationships constantly change in response to opposing, yet related forces (dialectics).

Reliability An indicator of whether a measure consistently measures what it is intended to measure.

Remembrance phase The final phase of group socialization, in which group membership ends and the person and the group evaluate their experience.

Resocialization phase The fourth phase of group socialization, in which a member again tries to change the group and the group tries to get the member to accept things the way they are.

Reward power When a member has power over other members because he or she controls resources and can administer rewards that other members want.

Ringi Japanese group decision-making techniques that involve everyone in the organization that the decision affects.

Role ambiguity Confusion about what our role is in the group or what is expected of us in our role.

Role conflict When the various demands of our role conflict (intrarole conflict) or when the demands of several roles we occupy conflict with one another (interrole conflict).

Role differentiation The development of distinct roles in the group that occurs as group members take on different assignments.

Role expectations What we expect of members based on their role in the group.

Roles Positions that people occupy within the group, each with different expectations for behavior.

Rumor Unsubstantiated gossip.

Satisficing When a group seizes upon one of the first decision alternatives that meets minimal requirements.

Schemas Cognitive structures that influence how information from the environment is perceived, stored, and remembered.

Self-disclosure The sharing of personal information, perceptions, and reactions with another.

Self-evaluation maintenance theory A variant of social comparison theory that says when close others do better than we do on things that are important to us, we may experience social comparison jealousy.

Self-fulfilling prophecy When our stereotypes lead us to treat stereotyped members differently and this treatment elicits stereotype-conforming behavior from them.

Sequential stage theories of group development Theories suggesting that groups progress through a series of stages in a particular order.

Shared vision When team members are committed to a common purpose and common performance goals.

Similarity attraction paradigm Tendency to be attracted to and to like people who are similar to us in interests, attitudes, values, and demographics.

Situational theory of leadership Hershey and Blanchard's contingency theory recommending one of four styles based on the group's level of development.

Social categorization approach Emphasizes that we categorize members according to preexisting stereotypes, leading to biased perceptions and interactions.

Social comparison explanation for group polarization Suggests that group polarization occurs when members strengthen their prediscussion preferences because they want to be liked and accepted.

Social comparison jealousy Feelings of jealousy that occur when someone close to us outperforms us on an ego-relevant task.

Social comparison theory A theory emphasizing that people evaluate their own abilities and opinions by comparing themselves to others.

Social desirability bias In research, the tendency for people to act in a socially desirable manner or give a socially desirable response instead of a more honest one.

Social dilemma When so many members act selfishly that the group and its members are harmed and productivity is negatively affected.

Social distance The extent to which members of one culture have contact with members of another culture.

Social facilitation How the presence of others increases performance on well-learned tasks.

Social identity That part of a person's self-concept that comes from knowledge of membership in a social group, together with the value and emotional significance of that membership.

Social impact theory A theory stating that conformity depends on strength (how important the group of people is to you), immediacy (how close the group is to you in space and time), and number (how many people are in the group).

Social loafing The tendency for individuals to reduce their effort on group tasks, especially common individual efforts cannot be identified or are not identified.

Social penetration theory A theory of dyadic relationship development suggesting that relationships develop as people gradually engage in reciprocal self-disclosure.

Social power theory A theory that suggests that a group member's power depends on his or her access to different power bases or sources.

Socialization The process by which new group members learn the norms of the group.

Socialization phase The second phase of group socialization, in which the new member tries to change the group while the group attempts to change the person.

Socioemotional behaviors Leadership behaviors focused on reducing tension and enhancing morale; also called employee-oriented and consideration.

Socioemotional roles Roles centered on satisfying the emotional needs of group members by encouraging others, mediating conflicts, and providing warmth and praise.

Sociogram In sociometry, a graphic display of group members' ratings of one another.

Sociomatrix In sociometry, a tabular presentation of group members' ratings of one another.

Sociometric status In sociometry, an average rating of how much a member is liked by other group members.

Sociometry A technique for analyzing the pattern of relationships among group members–in particular, hierarchies, friendship networks, and cliques within the group.

Specific-status characteristics Skill- or experience-related status characteristics.

Stable exchange stage The final, and rare, stage of social penetration theory in which both people share very private feelings and personal possessions.

Stage 4 Of the developmental approach, in which the new group, having formed a clear identity, turns its attention to accomplishing goals and tasks.

Stalemate The point at which it is clear that there is more to gain than lose from collaborating.

Statistical power The ability to detect a difference between groups; when low, we may fail to detect a relationship between the variables even when one exists.

Status A group member's standing in the hierarchy of a group based on the prestige, honor, and deference accorded him or her by other members.

Status characteristics Personal characteristics, such as skills, experience, or demographic factors, that influence performance expectations.

Status characteristics theory A branch of expectation states theory that focuses on how status hierarchies in groups will form consistent with statuses that members possess in society at large.

Status dues system What the group requires of members before they are awarded a higher status.

Status generalization The tendency for group members to use diffuse-status characteristics to assign status in the group, even when the characteristics are irrelevant to the situation.

Status markers Nonverbal and verbal behaviors that signify status, such as strong eye contact and commanding and interrupting others.

Status system The distribution of power and prestige among a group's members, including the "chain of command."

Status violation When low-status members engage in behaviors that are inappropriate given their rank and face resistance from higher-status members.

Stereotype threat How awareness of others' stereotypes of us may create performance anxiety and lead to a self-fulfilling prophecy.

Stereotypes Generalized beliefs about what members of an identifiable group are like that operate as schemas when perceiving members of those groups.

Stonewalling When one party refuses to talk about a conflict.

Storming stage The second stage of the basic model of group development, in which members may disagree about what to do and how, the leadership, and their roles in the group.

Structured (systematic) observational methods Quantitative observational methods in which group behaviors are observed and recorded with an objective coding system.

Subtractive assimilation (subtractive multiculturalism) The idea that people should give up their unique cultural attributes to fit with the majority culture.

Sucker effect When group members who previously compensated for loafing members reduce their efforts because they are tired of being taken advantage of.

Superordinate goal A goal desired by both parties to a conflict.

Surface-level diversity Member diversity arising out of demographic and physical characteristics.

Surveys/questionnaires Paper-and-pencil instruments used to measure various aspects of group functioning, dependent variables in experimental studies, and variables in correlational studies.

System for the Multiple Level Observation of Groups (SYMLOG) A multimethod scheme for studying group behavior developed by Bales and intended to measure member personalities, member relationships, the group's dynamics, and how the group is affected by its organizational context.

Tacit coordination Occurs when members do not specifically discuss how they are going to accomplish the task and operate according to their assumptions.

Task behaviors Leadership behaviors focused on organizing followers toward task accomplishment; also called initiating structure and production-oriented.

Task cues Behaviors that provide information about a member's actual or potential performance on the task and thereby influence performance expectations.

Task roles Roles focused on getting the job done, including providing information, focusing the discussion on tasks, and assigning work.

Taskwork skills The technical competencies of team members.

Team competencies The knowledge, skills, and attitudes (KSAs) necessary for team performance.

Team incentives Monetary or material rewards offered to motivate the team to meet production targets.

Team mental model A shared understanding of the team and its work; the team's transactive memory system.

Team recognition One-time awards given for good team performance, such as cash bonuses, thank-you notes, time off, and expense-paid trips.

Team training Training designed to improve members' taskwork and teamwork skills.

Teams Workgroups composed of people with the right balance of skills who cooperate to do a job within a larger organization.

Teamwork skills Skills related to being able to work as part of a team.

Termination stage Stage 5 of the integrative model of group development, in which the group ends in some form as members leave or tasks are completed.

Theory of idiosyncrasy credits A theory suggesting that to dissent effectively, you must first earn the right by paying conformity dues called idiosyncrasy credits.

Theory of innovation A theory suggesting that a strong, persistent minority can effectively sway the majority and cause true change.

Third-party intervention When an individual or group distinguishable from the conflicting parties interposes itself in an effort to move them toward agreement.

Tight culture A culture in which norms are clear and reliably imposed and deviance is punished through criticism and rejection.

Trait approach to leadership A leadership perspective emphasizing the unique characteristics and personality traits possessed by effective leaders.

Transactional leadership An "ordinary" leadership that is focused on the immediate situation and getting the job done.

Transactive memory system The way groups rely on individual members to be the group's memory in regard to particular subject areas.

Transformational (charismatic) leadership A charismatic and intellectually stimulating leadership that inspires members to create and achieve new visions.

Transition phase A period in the development of time-limited task groups in which old patterns are dropped, the group reengages with outside supervisors, and dramatic progress is made.

Transition stage A stage in the therapy group in which leaders work to create trust and cohesion and overcome defensiveness.

Triangulation When a group member attempts to mediate a conflict and inadvertently maintains or worsens the conflict, or is hurt in the process.

Trust and structure stage Stage 3 of the integrative model where the group lays the foundation for task accomplishment by organizing itself.

Trust building Efforts to rebuild trust after it has been eroded by conflict.

Tuckman's theory of small group development The basic sequential model that postulates five stages: forming, storming, norming, performing, and adjourning.

Two-factor model of leader behavior A behavior theory of leadership emphasizing two dimensions of leader, behaviors, task, and socioemotional.

Ultimate attribution error When each side in a conflict views its own negative actions as justi-fied by the situation, while seeing the other's negative actions as evidence of an evil nature.

Uncertainty avoidance The degree to which individuals in a society feel uncomfortable with situations that are unstructured, unclear, or unpredictable.

Underpayment inequity Occurs when people believe that what they receive is unfair relative to what others receive and act to restore equity by increasing their outputs or decreasing their inputs.

Unethical (negative) charismatics Charismatics who manipulate their followers into obedience to promote their own self-interests.

Unstructured observational methods A type of observational method in which observers provide impressionistic, descriptive accounts of the group.

Upward social comparison The comparison of ourselves to people who are better than we are on a particular trait or ability.

Upward-downward (U-D) dimension In SYMLOG, whether the behavior of a group member, group, or organization demonstrates values of dominance (U), or submission (D).

Valence In expectancy-valence theory, whether the rewards or outcomes that increased performance bring are valued.

Value-in-diversity hypothesis Posits that diversity in groups offers distinct benefits, such as greater creativity and better problem solving.

Verbal communication The way we communicate using words.

Vigilant decision making Decision strategies intended to reduce groupthink, including a thorough information search and evaluation of alternatives, and impartial leadership.

Voluntary norms Norms negotiated by a group, often to resolve conflict and promote smooth functioning.

Worchel's develpmental approach A cyclical group development theory that describes the development of groups that "spin off" from other groups because their needs are not being met.

Work and productivity stage Stage 4 of the integrative model of group development, in which the group turns ideas into products.

Workflow interdependence The extent to which the behavior of one member influences the performance of others and members must cooperate to perform the task.

Working stage A stage in the therapy group in which members are willing to self-disclose and to have direct and meaningful interactions with other members.

Zero-sum conflict A win-lose conflict in which it is believed that anything gained by one side must be lost by the other.

Name Index

Subject Index

Photo Credits